Healthier Societies

Healthier Societies

From Analysis to Action

Edited by

JODY HEYMANN

CLYDE HERTZMAN

MORRIS L. BARER

ROBERT G. EVANS

OXFORD
UNIVERSITY PRESS
2006

OXFORD
UNIVERSITY PRESS

Oxford University Press, Inc., publishes works that further
Oxford University's objective of excellence
in research, scholarship, and education.

Oxford   New York
Auckland   Cape Town   Dar es Salaam   Hong Kong   Karachi
Kuala Lumpur   Madrid   Melbourne   Mexico City   Nairobi
New Delhi   Shanghai   Taipei   Toronto

With offices in
Argentina   Austria   Brazil   Chile   Czech Republic   France   Greece
Guatemala   Hungary   Italy   Japan   Poland   Portugal   Singapore
South Korea   Switzerland   Thailand   Turkey   Ukraine   Vietnam

Copyright © 2006 by Oxford University Press, Inc.

Published by Oxford University Press, Inc.
198 Madison Avenue, New York, New York 10016

www.oup.com

Oxford is a registered trademark of Oxford University Press

All rights reserved. No part of this publication may be reproduced,
stored in a retrieval system, or transmitted, in any form or by any means,
electronic, mechanical, photocopying, recording, or otherwise,
without the prior permission of Oxford University Press.

Library of Congress Cataloging-in-Publication Data
Healthier societies : from analysis to action / Jody Heymann . . . [et al.].
p.   cm.
Includes bibliographical references and index.
ISBN-13 978-0-19-517920-0
ISBN 0-19-517920-X
1. Social medicine. 2. Medical policy—Social aspects. 3. Epidemiology.
4. Social change. 5. Medical geography. I. Heymann, Jody, 1959–
RA418.H3955 2005
362.1—dc22   2005040679

3 5 7 9 8 6 4 2

Printed in the United States of America
on acid-free paper

When our learning exceeds our deeds we are like trees whose branches are many but whose roots are few: the wind comes and uproots them. . . . But when our deeds exceed our learning we are like trees whose branches are few but whose roots are many, so that even if all the winds of the world were to come and blow against them, they would be unable to move them.

—*R'Elazar ben Azariah*

*To Cécile Brault, Tom Robinson, Ralph David Barer, and Geoffrey Robinson,
who influenced the courses of our lives from the earliest stages*

Preface

By the late 1980s, evidence showed that health status among populations through-out the twentieth century had persistently differed according to social and economic status, despite a dramatic change in the major causes of disease and death. Such a finding clearly indicated an important need to further our understanding of the broad and fundamental determinants of health. In 1987, the Population Health Program was launched to take up this challenge by bringing together a multidisciplinary group of researchers with a diversity of perspectives.

The Population Health Program members brought expertise from a broad range of disciplines, including medicine, epidemiology, geography, anthropology, sociology, economics, and policy analysis. This combination resulted not only in a diversity of perspectives brought to the study of determinants of health, but it also caused researchers to look beyond the barriers of their own disciplines and to think in new ways.

Over the course of fifteen years, the program systematically explored socioeconomic status (SES) gradients and their relationship to health outcomes. It is now well established that, on average, people with higher levels of income, education, and social position live longer and are healthier than those with lower incomes and lesser social positions. Moreover, societies with greater variations in income, education, or social position tend to have higher levels of mortality. In the program's final five years, program members furthered studies in this area by examining the SES gradient at the level of the individual life course, as well as at the levels of the neighborhood, community, and society.

In its effort to develop a comprehensive determinants-of-health framework, the program worked to better understand the biological pathways that lead to variations in population health. Program members sought to learn how systematic differences in living circumstances over time can embed themselves in human biology to create susceptibilities to a wide range of diseases.

The program received international recognition for its major contributions in research, particularly its work on synthesizing knowledge from a wide range of disciplines and developing a model of the determinants of health. The program had a substantial impact on health policy at the local, provincial, and national levels.

This book pulls together the work and viewpoints of a wide range of program members and other colleagues who joined us in this unique research program to truly understand how to improve population health—from basic science research to public policy.

—Clyde Hertzman
Director, Program in Population Health
1998–2003

Acknowledgments

The editors and contributors gratefully acknowledge the many years of support given by the Canadian Institute for Advanced Research (CIAR) to the Program in Population Health. Without the support of the CIAR, the ideas presented in this book would not have had a chance to develop and influence thinking in population health around the world.

The network, with its national and international membership, would not have held together nearly as well without the indispensable help of Michele Wiens. In addition to playing countless roles in helping to facilitate the network's collaborations, she played key staff roles in communicating among contributors for this book. Kate Penrose at Harvard University played a similarly invaluable role in staffing this final project and ensuring that this book came to fruition. We're deeply grateful to both for their help.

All good books benefit from a wise and experienced editorial eye, and this book was no exception. Jeffrey House at Oxford University Press brought his experienced eye to this project and gave invaluable suggestions. Carrie Pedersen generously gave of her time to finish the project after Jeffrey House retired from Oxford.

We are deeply indebted to the many colleagues at each of our institutions who have commented over the years on the ideas that have gone into this book and who have debated us, stimulated our thinking, and encouraged us to focus on the best way to create healthier societies.

The seeds for this work were sown early. Cécile Brault, high school teacher and advisor, grounded Jody Heymann in the impact of lived inequalities and in the responsibility we all have to do all we can to address them. Tom Robinson, Clyde Hertzman's seventh-grade teacher, taught him the value of critical appraisal. Morris Barer's father, Ralph David Barer, was truly the first influence on his career track. Geoffrey Robinson, an early colleague of Bob Evans, pioneered the concept of population pediatrics in Vancouver over thirty years ago, steps ahead of the times. This book is dedicated to them and to many more than we can name who influenced the courses of our lives and this work from its earliest stages.

Contents

About the Editors

JODY HEYMANN is the founding director of the Project on Global Working Families, the first project devoted to understanding and improving the relationship between working conditions and family health and well-being throughout the world. She is founding chair of the Initiative on Work, Family, and Democracy. A professor in the Faculties of Medicine and Arts at McGill University, Heymann is founding director of the McGill Institute for Health and Social Policy. Heymann has been awarded a Canada Research Chair in Global Health and Social Policy. Her current and most recent books include *Forgotten Families: Ending the Growing Crisis Confronting Children and Working Parents in the Global Economy* (OUP, 2005); *Unfinished Work* (2005); *Global Inequalities at Work: Work's Impact on the Health of Individuals, Families, and Societies* (OUP, 2003); and *The Widening Gap* (2000).

Heymann has served in an advisory capacity to the World Health Organization (WHO); United Nations Educational, Scientific, and Cultural Organization (UNESCO); the International Labor Organization (ILO); the U.S. Senate Committee on Health, Education, Labor, and Pensions; and the U.S. Centers for Disease Control and Prevention, among other organizations.

CLYDE HERTZMAN is Director of the Human Early Learning Partnership, Professor in the University of British Columbia's Department of Health Care and Epidemiology, and Associate Director of the Centre for Health Services and Policy Research. Nationally, he is a Canada Research Chair in Population Health and Human Development and a Fellow of the Canadian Institute for Advanced Research (CIAR) in the Successful Societies and Experience-based Brain and Biological Development programs. Hertzman has played a central role in creating a framework that links population health to human development, emphasizing the special role of early childhood development as a determinant of health. His research has contributed to international, national, provincial, and community initiatives for healthy child development.

MORRIS L. BARER is the first Scientific Director of the Institute of Health Services and Policy Research, Canadian Institutes of Health Research. He was the founding Director of the Centre for Health Services and Policy Research at the University of British Columbia, where he remains as research faculty. He is also a professor in and director of the Division of Population Health and Health Services Research in the Department of Health Care and Epidemiology at the University of British Columbia. His recent research has focused on the determinants of health care cost increases; pharmaceutical policy in Canada; separating fact from fiction in arguments about access to care, wait lists, the effects of an aging population; health care financing; use of health care services, particularly by seniors; continuity of care; and the roles of research evidence and interests in the evolution of health care policy.

ROBERT G. EVANS is a professor with the Department of Economics at the University of British Columbia. He is a Fellow of the Canadian Institute for Advanced Research and was director of the Institute's Population Health Program from 1987 to 1997. He held a National Health Research Scientist award and has received a Canadian Institutes of Health Research Senior Investigator award. Major publications include "Strained Mercy: The Economics of Canadian Health Care" (1984) and "Why Are Some People Healthy and Others Not? The Determinants of Health of Populations" (1994; as senior editor). Evans's studies of health care systems and policies have led to numerous invitations to provide policy advice to the Canadian federal and provincial governments. He has also been a consultant and lecturer on health care issues to governments and other public agencies in the United States, Europe, Asia, and the South Pacific. Evans has been elected as a Fellow of the Royal Society of Canada and was awarded the Health Services Research Advancement Award.

About the Contributors

PATRICIA BAIRD is a pediatrician and medical geneticist and has been head of the Department of Medical Genetics at the University of British Columbia. She has been a member of many national and international bodies, among them the National Advisory Board on Science and Technology (chaired by the Prime Minister) and the Medical Research Council of Canada. She chaired the Federal Royal Commission on new reproductive technologies. She has served as an advisor to the WHO on genetics in recent years and has published extensively on the policy implications of new genetic and reproductive technologies.

MARNI BROWNELL is a senior researcher with the Manitoba Centre for Health Policy and an assistant professor in the Department of Community Health Sciences at the University of Manitoba. Brownell holds a New Investigator Award with the Canadian Institutes of Health Research and is a core member of the Canadian Institute for Advanced Research New Investigator Network. Her background is in developmental psychology, and her research focuses on the social determinants of child health.

PAUL C. CHAULK is president of the Atlantic Evaluation Group and has ten years of experience covering a broad scope of health research as well as participatory models of program and system evaluation. In particular, he was the project coordinator of the Prince Edward Island System Evaluation Project, which evaluated the 1993 health reforms in that province.

LORI J. CURTIS is a specialist in health economics and econometrics. Curtis was an assistant professor in the Department of Community Health and Epidemiology and the Department of Economics at Dalhousie University when collaborating on this project; she was awarded a Clinical Scholar Award by the Faculty of Medicine. Curtis has recently moved to the Applied Research and Analysis Directorate in Health Canada and is now focusing on health policy research. Research areas have included child and maternal health; the relationship between poverty, health, and health care utilization; gender, labor force participation, and health; and poverty and inequality.

LISE DUBOIS is an associate professor in the Department of Epidemiology and Community Medicine at the University of Ottawa. She is based at the Institute of Population Health at the University of Ottawa, where she holds a Canada Research Chair in Nutrition and Population Health. Her research interest relates to the role of nutrition as a determinant of social health inequalities in different countries. She works mainly on population-based birth cohort data, analyzing the role of nutrition in early years on later social and health inequalities.

JAMES R. DUNN is an assistant professor in the Department of Community Health Sciences at the University of Calgary. He holds a New Investigator Award from the Canadian Institutes of Health Research and a Health Scholar award from the Alberta Heritage Foundation for Medical Research. His background is in the social geography of health, and he has research interests in the relationship between income inequality and population health in North American metropolitan areas and housing as a socioeconomic determinant of health.

ALISON EARLE is a research scientist at the Harvard School of Public Health, where she has taught classes on the translation of public health research into public policy. She currently serves as project director for the Work, Family, and Democracy Initiative, a research effort designed to compare social conditions and public policies influencing the health and well-being of working families globally. Her published research has focused on differences across social classes in the availability of social supports and adequate working conditions, and their impact on children's health and developmental outcomes.

JOHN D. EYLES is a professor at McMaster University and is Director of its Institute of Environment and Health. His main research interests include the appraisal, evaluation, and application of scientific evidence in policy settings; individual, community, and policy responses to environmental events; and the relationships between environmental quality (and degradation) and human health, values, and the environment. Eyles has carried out work for several national and provincial organizations and governments in Canada and has served on several expert panels and advisory committees and boards.

JOHN FRANK is a physician-epidemiologist with special expertise in prevention. In December 2000, Frank was appointed Scientific Director of the Canadian Institutes of Health Research, Institute of Population and Public Health, located at the University of Toronto. Frank's main area of interest is the biopsychosocial determinants of health status at the population level. Frank was the founding Director of Research at the Institute for Work & Health in Toronto and is currently a senior scientist with the institute.

KATHERINE L. FROHLICH is an assistant professor at the Université de Montréal in the Department of Social and Preventive Medicine. Her research interests are the integration of social theory into social epidemiological research and, specifically, how to conceptualize, operationalize, and understand the effects of context on disease outcomes.

GEORGE A. KAPLAN is Professor and Chair of the Department of Epidemiology in the School of Public Health and a Senior Research Scientist at the Institute for Social Research. He is also Director of the Michigan Initiative on Inequalities in Health; the Michigan Interdisciplinary Center on Social Inequalities, Mind and Body; and the Center for Social Epidemiology and Population Health, all at the University of Michigan. Kaplan also directs the newly formed Robert Wood Johnson Foundation Health and Society Scholars Program at the University of Michigan.

ANITA L. KOZYRSKYJ is an associate professor at the Faculty of Pharmacy and Department of Community Health Sciences at the University of Manitoba. Over the past nine years she has been a health services researcher at the Manitoba Centre for Health Policy. Her research has spanned several areas, from population health studies in asthma and other chronic diseases in children to policy research on pharmaceuticals. She is Manitoba Director of the Western Regional Training Centre in Health Services Research. Kozyrskyj holds a Canadian Institutes of Health Research New Investigator Award.

JOHN N. LAVIS is the Canada Research Chair in Knowledge Transfer and Uptake, Associate Professor in the Department of Clinical Epidemiology and Biostatistics, Member of the Centre for Health Economics and Policy Analysis, and Associate Member of the Department of Political Science at McMaster University. His principal research interests include knowledge transfer and uptake in public policy-making environments, the politics of health care systems, and the links between labor market experiences and health.

MARGARET LOCK is Marjorie Bronfman Professor in Social Studies in Medicine in the Department of Social Studies of Medicine and also in the Department of Anthropology at McGill University. She is a Fellow of the Royal Society of Canada and was awarded the Prix Du Québec, domaine Sciences Humaines, the Canada Council for the Arts Molson Prize, and the Canada Council for the Arts Killam Prize. Lock's prize-winning monographs include *Encounters with Aging: Mythologies of Menopause in Japan and North America* (1993) and *Twice Dead: Organ Transplants and the Reinvention of Death.*

GEOFFREY LOMAX is Research Director with the California Environmental Health Tracking Program. He is currently involved in the planning and implementation of a statewide population health surveillance system. He has been conducting environmental and occupational health research since 1985. His doctoral research involved an evaluation of the scientific, ethical, legal, and policy issues related to workplace biomonitoring and genetic testing.

JOHN LYNCH is an associate professor in the Department of Epidemiology, School of Public Health, at the University of Michigan. He has joint appointments at the Center for Human Growth and Development, the Institute for Social Research, and the Center for Research on Ethnicity, Culture, and Health. His main area of research interest is in the life course processes that help generate trends in population health and social inequalities in health.

VERENA MENEC is an associate professor in the Department of Community Health Sciences and the Director of the Centre on Aging at the University of Manitoba. She holds a Tier 2 Canada Research Chair in Healthy Aging. Her main research interests are in the areas of healthy aging and the relationship between health services use and population health, particularly among senior populations.

CAM MUSTARD is a professor in the Department of Public Health Sciences at the University of Toronto and President and Senior Scientist at the Institute for Work and Health. He was Associate Director and Fellow of the Population Health Program of the Canadian Institute for Advanced Research and a recipient of a Canadian Institutes of Health Research Scientist award. Mustard has active research interests in the areas of labor market experiences and health, the distributional equity of publicly funded health and health care programs, and the epidemiology of socioeconomic health inequalities across the human life course.

VINH-KIM NGUYEN, a practicing HIV specialist and medical anthropologist, has been involved in a number of projects to expand access to antiretroviral drugs in West Africa for the past ten years. His research concerns the broader social and political problematic of access to treatment. He is Associate Professor of Family Medicine at McGill University and is also affiliated with the Departments of Anthropology and Social Studies of Medicine.

LARS OSBERG is currently McCulloch Professor of Economics at Dalhousie University. His major fields of research interest have been the extent and causes of poverty and economic inequality, with particular emphasis in recent years on social policy, social cohesion, and the implications of unemployment and structural change in labor markets. Among other professional responsibilities, he has been a president of the Canadian Economics Association and a member of the Executive Council of the International Association for Research in Income and Wealth.

ALECK OSTRY is an assistant professor in the Department of Healthcare and Epidemiology and Center for Health Services and Policy Research at the University of British Columbia. He is a current recipient of a Canadian Institutes of Health Research New Investigator Award as well as a Michael Smith Foundation for Health Research Scholar Award. Ostry teaches courses and conducts research on the social determinants of health. He specializes in research on work and stress.

CHRIS POWER is Professor of Epidemiology and Public Health at the Institute of Child Health in London, UK. She has conducted extensive research on life course epidemiology and social inequalities in health. Currently her research focuses on pathways from childhood circumstances, particularly socioeconomic conditions, through cognitive development, growth and obesity, to adult disease.

NORALOU P. ROOS is a professor in the Department of Community Health Sciences at the University of Manitoba and was founding director of the Manitoba Centre for Health Policy. Roos held a National Career Scientist Award and now holds the Canada Research Chair in Population Health. Roos has been a member of the Prime Minister's National Forum on Health. Her research focuses on using population-wide data on health, education, and social assistance to understand the determinants of health and human development.

NANCY ROSS is Assistant Professor of Geography at McGill University and an associate of the Health Analysis and Measurement Group at Statistics Canada. Ross is a New Investigator with the Canadian Institutes of Health Research, with research interests in the contribution of social environmental conditions to health outcomes. Along with colleagues, she has studied the income inequality and mortality relationship in comparative contexts.

CLAUDIA SANMARTIN is a senior analyst in the Health Analysis and Measurement Group at Statistics Canada. Sanmartin is focusing on issues related to access to health care services in Canada, including waiting times and the effects of income inequality on health. Sanmartin was awardedthe Canadian Institute for Advanced Research doctoral stipend in population health.

ANDREW SHARPE is founder and Executive Director of the Ottawa-based Centre for the Study of Living Standards (CSLS). Established in 1995, CSLS is a national, independent, nonprofit research organization. Its main objectives are to study trends and determinants of productivity, living standards, and economic well-being and to develop policy recommendations to improve the lives of Canadians. Sharpe's earlier positions include Head of Research at the Canadian Labour Market and Productivity Centre and Chief, Business Sector Analysis at the Department of Finance.

GREG L. STODDART is a professor in the Department of Clinical Epidemiology and Biostatistics, a member of the Centre for Health Economics and Policy Analysis, and an associate member of the Department of Economics at McMaster University. He has published widely on both the economics of health care and the economics of health, and he is currently participating in the development of the Program in Policy Decision-Making at McMaster, a new research program that seeks to better understand the public policy decision-making process and the factors that influence it.

TÖRES THEORELL is a professor of psychosocial medicine at the Karolinska Institute and director of the National Institute for Psychosocial Factors and Health in Stockholm, Sweden. He has a background in internal medicine, occupational medicine, and social medicine and has done research in stress physiology and stress epidemiology.

JOACHIM VOGEL is a professor in the Department of Sociology at the University of Umeå, Sweden, as well as senior expert on social indicators, social welfare analysis, and social reporting at Statistics Sweden. He was founder and director for the Swedish annual social welfare surveys located at Statistics Sweden, as well as the official Swedish system of social reporting. His recent research concerns comparative research of welfare regimes and welfare delivery in Europe; social reports on the living conditions of the elderly, youth, and immigrants; and studies of income and material living standards in Europe.

MICHAEL WOLFSON is Assistant Chief Statistician of Analysis and Development at Statistics Canada. This position includes responsibility for analytical activities generally at Statistics Canada, for health statistics, and for specific analytical and modeling programs. In addition to his federal public service responsibilities, Wolfson has been a Fellow of the Canadian Institute for Advanced Research. His recent research interests include income distribution, tax/transfer and pension policy analysis, microsimulation approaches to socioeconomic accounting and to evolutionary economic theory, design of health information systems, and analysis of the determinants of health.

CHRISTINA ZAROWSKY is a physician with a specialization in public health; she is also a medical anthropologist. She leads International Development Research Centre's (IDRC) new Governance, Equity, and Health program initiative, which examines public health and health systems issues from a governance lens. Zarowsky's areas of research include determinants of population health, the politics of humanitarian aid, trauma and social reconstruction among Somali refugees, and the interfaces among community, professional, and government perspectives on health care.

Healthier Societies

Healthier Societies: An Introduction

Jody Heymann and Clyde Hertzman

Failure to Address Social Underpinnings of Health

At an emergency room, an ambulance, with sirens blaring, drives into the bay. Inside is a fifty-year-old man who has had a heart attack at work. As rapidly as possible, emergency medical technicians (EMTs) swing the man out of the back of the van. He has gone into full cardiac arrest, and the emergency medical staff knows that every minute counts in his prognosis. One EMT is pounding on his chest while the other is rapidly rolling the gurney into the emergency room (ER). An ER resident immediately intubates the man. Obtaining an airway but still not finding a pulse, the resident grabs a defibrillator. The nurse readies the crash cart with epinephrine and atropine.

In the meantime, other ER staff members have begun attending to a nine-year-old boy who was raced to the ER by his father because he is clearly having great trouble breathing. Instead of a calm eighteen or twenty times a minute, the boy's respirations are fast, nearly forty per minute. His wheezing is severe enough that the ER staff can hear the whistling sound without a stethoscope. Whenever he tries to get a good breath in, his chest wall retracts far toward his back. Within moments, the boy is receiving oxygen by mask, nebulized beta-agonists, and intravenous steroids.

It is only much later, when the boy is upstairs in the pediatric wing of the hospital and the staff members are doing a postmortem on the man who didn't survive, that more of the details come out. The fifty-year-old man had been a "set-up" for a heart attack: He had been obese, with high blood pressure, and he had never dared to walk in his burned-out neighborhood. The nine-year-old lives in a tenement filled with cockroaches, in a neighborhood congested with smog. His father, who had just lost his job, had been chain smoking on the day of the boy's ER admittance. No one had addressed the social conditions that had placed this fifty-year-old or this nine-year-old at such high risk.

We all want to live in a society where talented ER staff will be available if we or our loved ones need them. We want to have the best care available when we get sick. But we also all know we'd be better off if the illnesses and injuries never happened. We wouldn't hesitate to say that the nine-year-old would have been better off if he had never had an acute exacerbation of his asthma or that the fifty-year-old probably would have lived longer and been better off if the heart attack hadn't occurred. Yet experiences like the boy's and the man's are common. As individuals and as nations, we spend far more time and resources treating illnesses and injuries than we do addressing the conditions that give rise to them. Moreover, in most countries there remains far more political pressure to invest in medical care services for those who are already sick and injured than to invest in the programs and policies that will prevent those illnesses and injuries.

Why the Emphasis on Medical Care?

Although extensive research has demonstrated that social determinants make a difference, at some level, most of us don't truly believe it—not instinctively, not down to our bones. We often do not understand how social conditions can affect biology, and we've been thoroughly enough ingrained with the notion of the *biology* of illness that all explanations starting and finishing with biology seem more plausible than any others.

Another possible reason for our dependence on medical care is that we, as adults, think it's too late to take steps that would help prevent our own health problems. Sure, we all would choose to have our children grow up in a society that invested in the determinants of health and thereby increased our children's likelihood of living many years free of illness and injury. But what about life as an adult? We have already been exposed to many things. Hasn't the die been cast? If our childhood experiences mean that we are already going to have serious health problems, wouldn't it be better for us, as adults, to live in a country that invests almost entirely in medical care?

In addition, we have no idea how to move policy makers. The current political systems know how to make medical care happen. There are departments in federal, state, and provincial governments to address health care. Strong lobbies exist, large amounts of money are already being spent, and the momentum is strong for increasing investment in medical care. In contrast, uncertainty surrounds the prospects for increasing expenditures that would address the social determinants of health.

Healthier Societies: An Overview

This book is designed to address the knowledge gaps behind the barriers to approaching health from a societal perspective. In part I the authors address the following questions: To what extent is health determined by biological factors? To what extent is it determined by social factors? And more fundamentally, how do biological and social factors interact?

In the first chapter, Frank and colleagues deconstruct the simplistic view that genetic research will lead to uniquely effective means of prevention and treatment and demonstrate the extensive role the social environment plays in determining the effect of genetic predispositions on both common and serious diseases. After chapter 1 demonstrates the large role social conditions play even in the expression of genes, chapter 2 dives deeply into the pathways through which social environments affect biology.

In this second chapter, Hertzman and Frank examine what is known about the ways in which social, economic, and psychological environments affect the development of the brain, central nervous system, and other organ systems, as well as how development of neurological and other physiological systems in turn influences the body's immune responses, clotting, and hormonal responses—defense mechanisms that ultimately determine the extent of morbidity and mortality human beings suffer.

Whereas the first two chapters of the book focus on universal findings, chapter 3 contextualizes our understanding of the relationship between the social and biological factors that affect health by demonstrating the enormous degree of local variability in health that occurs even when similar preconditions exist. Lock, Nguyen, and Zarowsky make the case that a wide range of local factors influences the ways in which similar biologic and social conditions contribute to ill health.

An understanding of the ways in which various factors influence health could not be complete if it were just a picture taken at one point in time. The real ways in which social factors and biological factors influence health is through their interaction over time. In chapter 4, Hertzman and Power examine latency models, pathway-dependent relationships, and cumulative effects to highlight the many insights that a life course approach to the social determinants of health can provide.

This first section of the book ends with an examination of the consequences of a preoccupation with medical care as the biological solution to health inequalities. In chapter 5, Roos, Brownell, and Menec demonstrate the extent to which universal medical care systems ensure that those who are poorest, and also burdened with the most disease, receive the most care. At the same time, they make abundantly clear with more than a decade of data that investments in health care alone will neither improve population health as markedly as socioeconomic changes nor adequately reduce inequalities in health.

In part II, the authors examine four case studies that help us see the ways in which social change can dramatically affect adults' health, as well as launch children's lives onto healthy trajectories. This section's authors analyze in detail the cases of nutrition, working conditions, social inequalities, and geographic disparities.

In chapter 6, Dubois provides a historical overview of the relationship between nutrition and population health. She details how the problems of malnutrition have evolved in industrialized countries to a complex mixture of food insecurity, food poverty, ill nutrition, and obesity. Importantly, she provides a nuanced understanding of how nutrition works on a population level, and not merely on the level of individual choice.

In chapter 7, Mustard, Lavis, and Ostry write about the evolving relationship between work and health in industrialized countries. They begin by providing an understanding of the extent to which workplaces have become safer, with respect to physical hazards, and cleaner, with respect to known chemical toxins, yet are having profoundly negative health effects because of the extent to which they are increasingly unstable environments, with employees facing greater threats of termination, job loss, and increasing inequalities—and are plagued more and more with high demands that cannot be met.

Chapter 8 provides a detailed discussion of what is known about the relationship between inequalities and health. Ross and colleagues note that inequality is a particularly important determinant of health in the United States and Great Britain, which have weak employment security, inadequate unemployment protection, and limited social safety nets. In contrast, the level of inequalities in cities and provinces plays a lesser role in determining health in Canada and in Sweden because of the greater safety nets.

This chapter naturally transitions into the discussion in chapter 9 of the role of geography in determining how inequalities affect health and human development. Dunn and colleagues examine the wide range of factors that are associated with geography, from the extent to which housing is heterogeneous, to the availability of child and elder care, to the quality of public transportation.

Yet even when we are convinced that social factors are as important as biological ones in determining health, and even when we believe that their impact is enormous in both adulthood and childhood, the challenge of changing public policies and programs remains. The third section of the book takes a serious look at what would be involved in translating into action research findings like those described in parts I and II. Many books conclude, almost as an afterthought, with a section on what societies should do. Few, however, address the question of how to get it done. This is the goal of the final section.

In chapter 10, Vogel and Theorell build on the discussions in chapters 8 and 9 about how national-level social policies can moderate the impact of inequalities on health. Specifically, they look at a range of social welfare and labor policy models in Europe and analyze how the choices that different countries have made with respect to their public policies have directly affected health.

In chapter 11, Osberg and Sharpe take on the question: How would we measure nations' economic success if we really cared about the impact of economic policies on health? They develop a new measure of economic well-being that includes the factors most salient to health and apply it to a wide range of countries, demonstrating how it performs notably differently from the commonly used measure of gross domestic product (GDP).

Chapter 12 examines a unique public policy experiment that occurred in Canada. Prince Edward Island took the rare step of making a commitment to share resources across public sectors in order to maximize population health. In this chapter, Stoddart and colleagues look at the successes and the challenges that arose when this province sought to improve population health by improving social conditions rather than just by increasing medical care.

Chapter 13 examines three case studies in child policy. Kozyrskyj, Curtis, and Hertzman examine what can be learned from a study of the extent to which national children's policies in Canada, the United States, and Norway were influenced by research on the determinants of child health and well-being.

In concluding, the final chapter seeks to answer, Where do we go from here? In chapter 14, Earle, Heymann, and Lavis provide a conceptual framework for understanding the process of translating research into action. The chapter then analyzes a wide range of historical experiences in which social science research has influenced the public policymaking process in the United States, the United Kingdom, Canada, the Netherlands, and Sweden. The book concludes with recommendations for researchers and policy makers for the best ways to increase their effectiveness at creating healthier societies.

Part I

The Complex Relationship between Social and Biologic Determinants of Health

Chapter 1

Interactive Role of Genes and the Environment

John Frank, Geoffrey Lomax, Patricia Baird, and Margaret Lock

Enthusiasm for discovering genetic correlates of health and disease is currently widespread. This enthusiasm is encouraged by a combination of recent research initiatives, such as the Human Genome Project, and the flurry of media reports announcing that yet another gene–disease association has been identified. Implicit in all these activities, and explicit in many, is the notion that one can attribute health and disease to genetic determinants and that understanding the genome will lead, inexorably, to improvements in population health.[1] The new insights provided by advances in human genetics are exciting because genes hold the codes for molecules that carry out biological processes. Thus, genetic research provides a molecular level of analysis for the study of diseases and their causation. For example, powerful new genetic research techniques allow the researcher to document the molecular changes that occur when a benign cell is transformed into a malignant (cancerous) one. This level of information is proving invaluable in the management of lung and colon cancer (Fong et al. 1999; Dubois 2000).

Information at the molecular genetic level has greatly informed disease diagnosis and management of individuals with inherited conditions due to single genes (i.e., those known as Mendelian conditions). However, these breakthroughs will be counterproductive if they distract attention from other forms of disease causation—especially social structure, physical environmental influences, and lifestyle factors,[2] which are of great importance for the common diseases of industrialized life, all of which are "genetically complex" in that they are the product of many genes interacting with the environment over entire lifetimes (Willet 2002; Ridley 2003; Shostak 2003).

The tendency toward an emphasis on clinical interventions in the new genetics leaves us skeptical that elucidating genetic determinants of disease will imminently lead to improvements in population health. Our skepticism arises from experience suggesting that interventions involving broad-based genetic screening are profoundly difficult to implement and have a limited impact on population health. Further, we are concerned that a disproportionate emphasis on genetic determinants leads us to overlook the importance of population health research—research and policies directed toward the full complement of social, environmental, and lifestyle determinants of health.

Enthusiasm for research linking gene expression to health and disease is understandable. As a branch of risk-factor epidemiology, it lends itself to relatively tightly controlled study, and genetic correlates are more easily grasped than the complex notion of a web of physical, chemical, biological, social, economic, and personal factors interacting over the life course to cause disease. Yet modern epidemiologists have for decades used the metaphor of "webs of causation" in explaining the origins of human health at the population level (MacMahon and Pugh 1970). It is important, therefore, that powerful and intuitively appealing genetic mechanisms be viewed as only part of this web. It is also critical that genetic technologies be applied and used wisely, and their limitations recognized, so that they are not made the object of unrealistic expectations. If the potential of genetic technology is overestimated, it may be applied inappropriately, with resultant harm or, at minimum, with waste of scarce health care resources (Baird 2000).

We argue that knowledge of the actual determinants of human health at the population level—and especially the role of social structure, environment, and lifestyle—should lead to rather modest expectations of a "genetic silver bullet" approach to improving population health status. This argument, in turn, has two main themes:

1. Most common diseases in technologically advanced societies are multifactorial in origin, meaning that they are the product of complex interactions between our genetic endowment and the world around us, acting over the course of a human lifetime.
2. There are profound difficulties in attempting to actually implement broad-based genetic screening and intervention programs at the population level, of the sort that would be required if the new genetic knowledge were to radically alter disease frequency in entire societies.

The Multifactorial Nature of Human Disease

A key observation about rates of disease, as well as indicators of health, is that they are astonishingly variable across populations. Consider the so-called chronic diseases, such as cancer and heart disease, that are the principal causes of death in developed nations. Schottenfeld and Fraumeni (1996) have documented ten- to twentyfold differentials in site-specific cancer incidence rates around the globe, particularly for the most common cancer sites in Westernized populations with high life expectancy: breast, colon, prostate, lung, and bladder. In some cases we know a great deal about why these rates differ; for example, lung cancer's relationship to smoking, at both the population and individual levels of analyses, is common knowledge. However, even with tumors for which we cannot currently explain more than a fraction of cases by known causal exposures in the environment, such as breast and colon cancers, occurrence rates may vary by more than tenfold (Schottenfeld and Fraumeni 1996). This is true even from region to region within those wealthier nations that have sophisticated cancer surveillance registry systems that produce reliable statistics at the level of the subnational region.

What might proponents of genetic disease determination say about such differentials? They would look for varying genetic characteristics across these differently affected populations, for example, in tumor suppressor/promoter gene frequency and/or expression. On the other hand, the public or population health scientist would point to the dozens of published migrant studies in the past few decades as evidence of the clear environmental influence on these disease rates (Marmot et al. 1975; Marmot and Syme 1976; McCredie et al. 1990; Ziegler et al. 1993).

Geographic Variation in Disease Occurrence and Migrant Studies

Researchers who conduct migrant studies take advantage of immigration to compare the disease experience of the immigrant groups with that of both their countries of origin and destination. Many of these studies have shown that, over time, immigrants shed the chronic disease patterns of their countries of origin and take on those of their country of destination. For instance, significant changes in chronic disease rates, including cancer incidence, occur within a generation or two of migration from low-incidence settings to high-incidence settings, and vice versa (Schwab 1998). Genetic differences could not possibly provide the primary explanation for this phenomenon, since genes do not change that quickly in populations. Furthermore, the gene pool of most migrants studied generally changes very little over the first few generations after migration, due to persistent intramarriage within the migrant community after arrival in the new homeland.

High-quality migrant studies demonstrating these patterns abound in the epidemiological literature, but they appear to have been largely overlooked by genetic researchers. A well-executed epidemiological migrant study of disease occurrence is analogous to, but constitutes a distinct improvement upon, the "twins reared apart" study design used by many genetic researchers to help disentangle genetic from environmental influences on health and function (Plomin et al. 1990; Reiss et al. 1991; Cooper 2001). In both study designs, genetics is held constant, while environment is changed. In migratory studies, substantial variation in environmental conditions is guaranteed by the constraint that study subjects have moved from one country to another. In twin studies, all that can be guaranteed is that the twins have not lived together; they may, in fact, live in the same region or in different regions where the disease rates of interest are similar. Thus, well-designed migratory studies may be a more reliable source of information on the influence of environmental factors, "holding genetics constant," than are studies of twins reared apart.

Table 1.1 summarizes some influential migrant studies conducted over recent

Table 1.1. Selected migrant studies of chronic disease

Authors	Study design	Findings	Conclusions
Ziegler et al. 1993	Population-based case–control study of Chinese, Japanese, and Filipinos aged 20–55 migrating to San Francisco–Oakland, Los Angeles, and Oahu	A sixfold gradient in breast cancer risk by migration patterns was observed.	Migrants with 8 or more years in the West had a relative risk of breast cancer 1.8 times the risk of migrants with 2–7 years.
McCredie et al. 1990	Breast cancer rates in migrants to New South Wales (NSW), Australia, from various European countries, compared with native-born women	The relative risk for Italians changed from 0.5 to 1 over a 17-year period. The risk for Welsh changed from 2.75 to 1.5 over the same period.	Rates in groups with previously higher and lower relative risks moved toward risk levels of their new homeland after migration.
McCredie et al. 1990	Colon cancer in migrant males and females to NSW from Italy and Greece, compared with native born	The relative risk for Greeks and Italians changed from 0.2 to approximately 0.8 over a 17-year period. The change was less in Italian women: 0.2 to 0.6.	Immigrant patterns were converging on native patterns.
Marmot et al. 1975; Marmot and Syme 1976	Mortality from coronary heart disease (CHD) among Japanese from Japan, Hawaii, and California	Age-adjusted prevalence rates for definite CHD were: Japan, 5.3; Hawaii, 5.2; and California, 10.8/1,000.	Japanese in California were converging on the native California experience.

Sources: Reprinted, with permission, from Ziegler et al. 1993; McCredie et al. 1990; Marmot et al. 1975; and Marmot and Syme 1976.

decades regarding coronary heart disease (CHD) and the industrialized world's major cancers. These studies demonstrated large increases in the rates of disease within two generations of immigration to high-risk countries from low-risk countries and, occasionally, the reverse pattern in those moving from high- to low-risk settings.

The point of this table is that the most widespread, serious diseases of modern life, all of them conditions more common among older adults, seem to be extraordinarily sensitive to environmental influences. And there is abundant evidence that *environment* in this case includes both physical and chemical exposures, as well as social-psychological experiences. An illustrative example of the role of the environment is explored next in this chapter. The practical public health implication is obvious: Some adverse environmental effects, such as nutrition, acculturation, and "lifestyle" are clearly reversible, since migrants to high-risk areas are protected from adverse consequences of such environmental exposures only one generation before migration and a few thousand miles away.

Finnish Height Study

It is often thought that the extent of genetic determination of a trait—its heritability—is clear-cut, quantifiable, and fixed. But this is not the case, in that heritability differs from environment to environment. Heritability can be expressed in a statistical index (ranging from a value of 0 to a value of 1) reflecting the proportion of the variation in the characteristic or condition that is genetically transmitted among individuals in a defined population. It can be derived from a variety of study designs, including studies of monozygotic (identical) and dizygotic (fraternal) twins. An elegant Finnish study of height clearly demonstrated that complex gene–environment interactions make the heritability of even a "simple" human trait, such as height, highly context sensitive.

The Finnish researchers used an established national twin registry with 33,534 pairs of adult twins, born before 1958 and both still alive in 1974 (Silventoinen et al. 2000). Using data from two mailed questionnaires on height and factors determining zygosity (e.g., appearance, gender), 3,466 identical and 7,450 fraternal pairs of twins' data were analyzed. The results showed a clear time trend in the heritability of height across the following four birth cohorts: those born before 1928; between 1929 and 1938; between 1939 and 1946; and between 1947 and 1957. The heritability of height steadily increased during this period of gradually improving living conditions in Finland, from 0.76 to 0.81 in men and from 0.66 to 0.82 in women. This finding fits with global data showing that in developing countries with widespread malnutrition and infectious diseases associated with suboptimal child growth, heritability of height is generally lower—for example, 0.56 in one West African study (Solomon, Thompson, and Rissanen 1983). Thus, the degree of genetic determination of this basic human trait is not a constant but will vary in different environments.

Genetic determination is greatest when environmental factors adversely affecting height are least prevalent, and it is least when these factors are most widespread. This contextual "relativity" of causation in human biology has long been described by epidemiologists (Rothman 1986; Pearce 1996, 1999). It is due to the fact that we can observe the influence of only those causal factors that *vary* in given settings. The role of genetics in determining height (and many other human attributes and conditions) is not fixed but is subject to alteration in the face of different environmental circumstances, such that our genetic height "potential" cannot always be realized in our actual living conditions. The net genetic determination of a trait, observed in a study of a specific population, such as Finns over the past century, is inevitably "filtered" through that population's environmental exposures.

The Thrifty Gene

The idea that the observed genetic contribution to a specific trait in a population is always filtered through environmental exposures is important. As we suggested in the example of cancer, differential rates of disease within and between populations tend to be attributed, upon superficial examination, to genetic factors. The problem is that this simplistic view of the meaning of disease variation may distract attention from the complex processes actually at play.

Consider the observation of a clustering of non–insulin-dependent diabetes mellitus (NIDDM) in certain South Pacific ethnic groups. This clustering has been attributed to the existence of a "thrifty" genotype[3] that enabled the carrier to use food more efficiently during times of famine but that has become less of an asset now than in the feast-or-famine days of hunting–gathering and seafaring cultures (Neel 1999). The underlying hypothesis is that the thrifty genotype became a risk factor for NIDDM only when the food supply became stable and more than adequate. But, as more and more people have been exposed to the late-twentieth-century Western lifestyle, it has become clear that obesity and NIDDM are the response of diverse populations, regardless of whether a specific thrifty gene is present (McDermott 1998; Wareham et al. 2002; Pearce et al. 2004). A high intake of energy-dense refined foods (animal fats and sugar), combined with low exercise levels and a lack of micronutrients from fresh fruits and vegetables—the typical dietary pattern of individuals in lower social classes living a Western lifestyle—appears to be the high-risk scenario for NIDDM. The nutritional influences of the environment act to filter the expression of the genetic predisposition to NIDDM. However, an imbalanced focus on genetic determinants of the condition in affected ethnic groups diverts attention from more appropriate dietary interventions that can actually preempt or reverse NIDDM. The genes matter, but they were always there. What has changed—and rapidly so—is the environment.

Coronary Heart Disease

This brings us to the central reason why profound preventive impact will not readily result from genetic technology for coronary heart disease (CHD), most cancers, and chronic diseases in general: These diseases are all profoundly *multi-factorial*. For example, CHD, which is still the major killer in the developed world and the top cause (after childbirth) of hospital admissions in most developed countries, has more than twenty known independent risk factors of biological significance,[4] only a few of which are primarily genetically determined.

Figure 1.1 summarizes, without intending to be exhaustive, the levels of causation currently known or thought likely to independently affect the occurrence of CHD, categorized according to their position in the causal pathway. More "up-stream" (or exogenous) risk factors, such as social position and environment, are distinguished from more intermediary risk factors, such as blood pressure and cholesterol levels. The latter are biological characteristics that are under homeostatic control in the human body—that is, they are regulated by internal feedback systems that are influenced, in turn, by a complex range of factors from the external environment and the internal milieu. These mechanisms are, in turn, controlled

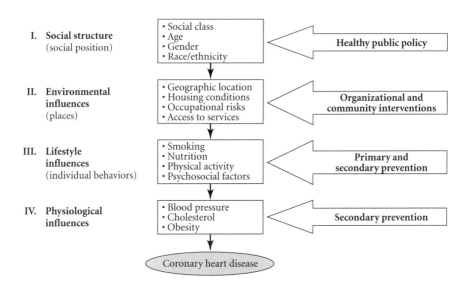

Figure 1.1. Levels of causation of coronary heart disease and corresponding types of health intervention

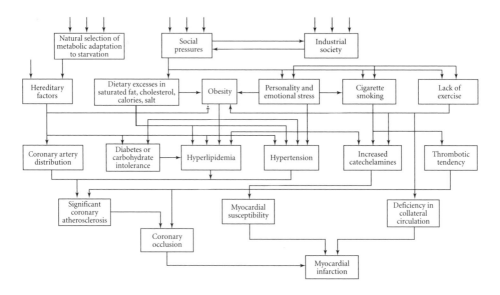

Figure 1.2. The web of causation for myocardial infarction: A current view

partly by our genetic endowment and partly by cumulative environmental influences throughout life.

The interrelationships between these many established levels of influence—all of them putative causes of CHD—are so complex and so poorly understood that we are aware of no recent publication that has attempted a comprehensive causal path diagram depicting them. However, it is instructive to examine, in figure 1.2, such a figure published more than a decade ago by Friedman (1987) in *Primer of Epidemiology*. Complex though the figure is, many recently discovered risk factors, such as perinatal characteristics, antioxidant intake, and recent antibiotic use, are absent from this schema (Danesh et al. 1997; Jha et al. 1995; Mattila et al. 1998). However, one can readily see that the full "causal web" for CHD, even as currently understood, probably involves interactions among these and dozens of other co-factors acting over the entire life course. Again, only a small subset is primarily genetic in their determination.

The Contribution of Geoffrey Rose

Fortunately, a conceptual framework has been advanced that places these causal processes in a broader context. The British cardiovascular epidemiologist Geoffrey Rose, in his landmark 1985 paper "Sick Individuals and Sick Populations," proposed the framework (see chapter 4 for another discussion of Rose's work). Rose pointed out that risk factors for chronic diseases such as CHD can be thought of as either conferring risk because they shift *entire* human populations' distributions of exposure or because they shift an *individual's* position within a particular societal distribution of exposure. For example, serum low-density lipoprotein (LDL) cholesterol can be thought of as conferring more CHD risk on some individuals in Western countries than others, according to whose measured levels are higher or lower. However, the entire bell curve distribution in Western countries has been so enormously shifted upward that even relatively "low" individual LDL cholesterol levels in these populations confer considerable CHD risk, compared with the markedly lower distributions of LDL cholesterol in most developing countries. Rose pointed out that research seeking to identify only the determinants of an *individual's* level of this CHD risk factor, as compared with the levels of others in the same society, will fail to uncover the fundamental causes of the population-level shift in CHD. Only through comparison with samples of individuals from preindustrial populations, whose cholesterol levels are not shifted upward en masse, can the true nature and underlying causal factors of the modern epidemic of CHD in richer nations be understood.

Most common diseases today show a very strong inverse gradient by social class (Evans et al. 1994). As noted earlier, the common fatal diseases of our society are due to interactions between genotype and environmental factors. Yet genotypes do not differ strongly by class[5]; rather, marked class differences in disease incidence are due to different exposures to environmental "triggers." Genes affect *who* may get sick within a class if exposed, but environmental factors, such as those previously listed for CHD, determine the *relative frequency* of sickness across social classes. Rose went on to make many useful points for those who would seek to change dietary, exercise, and other human habits at the individual level of intervention. He warned that only modest impacts on population-level disease burden can ever be expected from approaches targeted at particular individuals who are outliers on the societal distribution curve for the risk factors. The best we can do, clinically, is therapeutically truncate the high end of the risk curve by risk factor modification. To substantially reduce a population's level of chronic disease, one needs to seek the causes of incidence that shift entire risk factor distributions at the population level, not simply the causes of cases at the individual level.

For our discussion here, however, there is another implication of Rose's pioneering conceptual framework. It turns out—as Rose noted—that for many chronic-disease risk factors (including serum lipids, blood pressure, and perhaps serum levels of key toxic or protective nutrients such as homocysteine or folic acid), the determinants of entire populations' distributions of risk are largely environmental, whereas the factors affecting an individual's level of risk, within any population, are much more likely to have a genetic component. An example has been provided in data from controlled trials of lipid-lowering diets for high-cholesterol individuals (Denke 1994; Denke and Grundy 1994). These trials have shown that only 30% to 50% of treated individuals have a substantial serum lipid response to dietary management—one that primary care doctors would consider successful as first-line treatment of elevated LDL cholesterol (Ramsay and Yeo 1991). Other individuals are not very responsive to diet, and genetic factors are thought to be important in this difference.

Many people with elevated lipids are genetically sensitive to diet, and our culture has evolved so as to expose virtually all of us to unhealthy diets. Sijbrands and colleagues (2001) examined mortality over two centuries in a large pedigree with familial hypercholesterolemia, a condition that leads to high serum levels of LDL cholesterol arising from mutations in the LDL receptor gene. Mortality in the pedigree was lower than in the surrounding general population in the nineteenth century, but it rose after 1915 to reach a peak about 1950. Sijbrands and colleagues suggested that increased LDL concentrations may have protected people from infectious diseases more common in earlier centuries but that the absence of environmental risk factors, such as widespread cigarette smoking, a high-fat diet, and sedentary physical activity patterns in the nineteenth century may have been equally important. In other words, the decline in the former class of threats and the rise in the latter over the past two centuries transformed a genetically low-risk state into a high-risk one. Today, the many citizens of affluent societies with high cholesterol have that condition due to environmental conditions *peculiar to their specific historical and cultural context,* interacting with their individual metabolic/ genetic constitution (Kaprio 2000).

The point is that gene–environment interactions codetermine the most common chronic and lethal diseases. The way in which genes and environment interact to cause the major diseases of our time is such that patients with overwhelmingly "genetic" conditions or overwhelmingly "environmental" conditions are relatively few. Rather, occupying the top positions in the rank orderings of major public health problems are conditions where both genes and environment interact, such as heart disease, stroke, cancer, and diabetes. Even the effect of smoking, which is a clear environmental hazard for individuals who smoke and for those around them, differs in interaction with genetic constitution. It has been known for decades that not all smokers suffer equally from the health consequences of their habit. Indeed, basic scientific research has demonstrated several genetically mediated mechanisms by which some smokers develop lung cancer, chronic obstructive lung disease, and other adverse health consequences of the habit, whereas others do not (Haugen et al. 2000; Hemminki et al. 2001; Larrson 1978). (Rose himself [1985] pointed out that lung cancer would be regarded as a largely genetic disease if we happened to live in a society wherein every person smoked.) So even a clear environmental risk factor like smoking has genetically codetermined health effects. Even though the elimination of smoking would be very beneficial to the population overall, some individuals would not benefit as much as others because of being less likely to suffer detrimental consequences from tobacco smoke exposure in the first place, presumably on a genetic basis (Haugen et al. 2000).

The environmental codetermination of most chronic disease means that increased genetic knowledge, enabling more powerful genetic interventions, will not be sufficient to broadly improve population health. Such interventions are not likely to have a major impact unless we start to die or become disabled from very different causes than we do today. Purely genetic manipulations undoubtedly will confer specific health benefits on those at very high risk for largely genetic reasons—for example, single-allele conditions such as Huntington's chorea, some familial hypercholesterolemias, or hemochromatosis.[6] The fact is, the vast majority of single-allele conditions are quite rare (<0.1% prevalence) (Baird et al. 1988). To understand the conditions that affect most people in their later years, and eventually lead to death, will require a combined genetic and environmental approach. The multiplicity of causal pathways to the common chronic disease end points of adulthood and the complexity of interacting factors over the life course make it unlikely that there will be a widely applicable "genetic silver bullet" for these diseases. Indeed, emerging evidence indicates that such diseases have their roots in pre- and perinatal life, and in early childhood, due to complex gene–environment interactions "embedding" themselves in human physiology and leading to frank disease decades later (Barker and Medical Research Council 1992; Barker 2001; McCormack et al. 2003; also, see chapters 2 and 4 in this volume).

Problems in Moving from Science to Society: Some Examples of Difficulties in Genetic Program Implementation at the Population Level

A typical layperson's response to news of any genetic advance, particularly the discovery of a new gene associated with a specific disease, is that we can soon expect breakthroughs that will reduce the disease's impact on society. Implicit in this expectation is the belief that widespread screening for, and/or genetic manipulation of, the defective gene will bring net health benefits. However, a few examples reveal that (to paraphrase the ancient Greek poet Homer, and other writers) "there are many slips 'twixt cup and lip" in the practical use of genetic technologies to improve health across entire populations. This is especially true among persons currently well, who are only at risk of future illness. For these people, genetic screening may be ineffective and actually cause substantial harm.

Breast Cancer Genes

There can be little doubt that the discovery of the BRCA1 and -2 genes in recent years has led to many requests for breast cancer risk screening by women and their physicians. This trend has constituted a substantial additional workload for the health care system, in terms of assessing women's risk, counseling them appropriately, and testing those who can genuinely benefit. Does this constitute a cost-effective use of resources to reduce the incidence of breast cancer? Existing reviews and recent studies (Ford, Easton, and Peto 1995; Langston et al. 1996; Tambor et al. 1997; Lock 1998; Collins 1996; Elwood 1999a, 1999b; Evans et al. 2001; Haga, Khoury, and Burke 2003; Khoury et al. 2004; Lerman et al. 1997; Lynch et al. 1997; Malone et al. 1998) have suggested the following reasons to doubt that this new clinical genetic activity will markedly reduce the future incidence of breast cancer:

- Early estimates of the proportion of all breast cancers occurring in carriers of these two genes were substantially inflated. That proportion is now believed to be less than 5%, although it is slightly higher for cancer patients less than thirty-five years of age. This overestimation occurred because genetic investigators based their estimates, uncritically, on studies of high-risk families (Bleutler et al. 2000; Begg 2002). They did not employ proper epidemiological techniques to reduce the potential for bias in generalizing the experience of very atypical (high-risk) families to the broader population, so that other unidentified genetic and environmental risk factors in these families crept in and artificially inflated their risk estimates. Thus, even if it were possible to completely remove the effects of these two genes, there would be little impact on breast cancer rates in the population.

- Similarly, early notions of the frequency of these genes in the general population were exaggerated. It is now clear, for example, that BRCA1 occurs in only 0.12% to 0.2% (12 to 20 per 10,000) of women in North America. Thus, even if it were possible to offer lifelong tamoxifen or raloxifene to all carriers and have them comply with such chemoprophylaxis, population-based screening efforts to identify women with these genes would be extraordinarily inefficient—2,500 individuals would require testing to prevent one case of cancer (Vineis et al. 2001).

- Furthermore, even if screening the whole population of women were seen as desirable from a societal perspective, there are disincentives to being screened, from the patient's perspective. For example, it has been found that even among proven, multicase BRCA1-carrier families, only 43% of women invited for testing participated fully and wanted their test results. Of the remainder, fear of loss of health insurance was a major reason given for refusal of testing or for having testing but not wanting results personally.

- Even simple screening decisions themselves may have adverse psychosocial consequences for persons merely offered screening. Among the women in the carrier families, six-month follow-up revealed a decline in depression among those tested and found to be noncarriers, no change in those testing positive, and an increase in depression among the substantial subset that had declined testing.

- Women in families that have been affected by breast cancer tend to greatly overestimate their own risk of the disease, and their misapprehensions are not reduced by intensive counseling from a trained genetic educator. Analogous effects on the broader population of low-risk women, if screening is offered to them, are a matter of speculation at present.

The point of these findings is *not* that BRCA1 and -2, or similar gene testing, has no place in the rational and compassionate management of breast cancer risk among high-risk families. Rather, the public health concern is the balance of risks, benefits, and costs of widespread, unrestricted use of these tests, beyond their selective use in women with clear-cut positive family histories of breast cancer (Holtzman and Marteau 2000; Burke et al. 2002; Grann and Jacobson 2002). The spread of testing is of special concern because commercially oriented testing labs seeking to expand their market will inevitably exploit low-risk women's anxieties about breast cancer (Lock 1998). Therefore, there is reason to be concerned that the demand for such breast cancer gene testing in the general population will greatly exceed the medically justifiable indications for test use (Elwood 1999a, 1999b; Helmes, Bowen, and Bengal 1999). This is worrisome, in that the risks and costs of such testing among low-risk women would predictably exceed any potential health benefits (Khoury et al. 2003). In short, there is precious little promise of net health benefits and, in fact, much potential for both harm and waste of health care resources as a result of overly enthusiastic use of such technology. Fortunately, in this case the cautionary perspectives of evidence-based medicine and public health coincide. But it is not clear that this meeting of perspectives will be enough to restrain the market for screening (Baird 2002).

Fragile X Syndrome

In 1995 the American College of Human Genetics issued testing guidelines to detect the gene for fragile X syndrome.[7] The guidelines included recommendations that all males and females with any physical or behavioral characteristics of the syndrome, individuals with a family history of the disease, and those asymptomatic individuals deemed to be at risk for this disease should be tested (American College of Medical Genetics 1995). The incidence of fragile X syndrome is estimated to be about one per 1,500 males and one per 2,500 females (Warren and Nelson 1994). It is associated with mental impairment and mild learning difficulties or hyperactivity, though the latter is often estimated to be in the normal range (Brown et al. 1993). In common with a good number of other so-called genetic diseases, the involved genes exhibit incomplete penetrance—that is, not all individuals with the genotype will manifest the disease, for unknown reasons. It is estimated that about 20% of males and 70% of females with the mutation express no symptoms, making the designation "at risk" extremely problematic. Moreover, the severity of symptoms varies enormously and cannot be predicted. Benefits from therapeutic and educational interventions have not been shown (Caskey 1994).

In 1993 a testing program for fragile X syndrome was put in place in the Colorado public school system as part of an effort to develop an inexpensive test that could be used as a model for a national program (Hubbard and Wald 1993). The project, funded by the private biotechnology company Oncor, was carried out by a university–industry consortium and was explicitly designed to save later public expenditure on children with mental deficits. Before the program was set up, a report was published by the Colorado Health Sciences Center and the University Business Advancement Center that argued that screening could enhance economic efficiency. The estimated cost to families and the estimated public expenditure for care of fragile-X patients were carefully calculated, and the conclusion was that "the savings to the state would be tremendous" from implementation of a screening program (Lauria and Webb 1992).

The research team developed a checklist of "abnormal" behavioral and physical characteristics associated with the disease, including hyperactivity, learning problems, double-jointed fingers, and prominent ears. They tested selected children but not in a clinical setting. After two years, the program failed to turn up the anticipated number of cases, was deemed uneconomical, and was suspended (Hubbard and Wald 1993). Yet the impact on the lives of those children who did test positive was significant—including their becoming targets of discrimination by health insurance companies. Ironically, even though the predictive quality of the test was uncertain, many parents not only cooperated but also actively encouraged its use. At the time, a report by the Office of Technology Assessment noted that the finding of a "genetic underpinning" to various behavioral and psychiatric problems had given "enormous relief to many families" (Flynn 1993). This cautionary tale demonstrates that population-based genetic screening programs can readily develop a momentum of their own, driven by political, economic, and cultural forces, without regard for the actual risks and benefits to participants.

Preimplantation Diagnosis

There are many fields of medicine, covering the whole life cycle, in which genetic identification may be applied, even starting before embryo implantation in the uterus, for example. If in vitro fertilization is carried out, the early embryo can be genetically tested before it implants. A cell may be taken from the cluster of cells making up the zygote, and either genetic probes may be used to identify particular genes or the chromosomes may be examined. Only those embryos without an identified "undesirable" genotype may then be transferred to the woman's uterus.

The number of instances appropriate for offering preimplantation diagnosis (PID) is extremely small because most common diseases are not determined by single-gene or chromosome abnormalities. Further, it is appropriate to offer PID only when a couple has already been identified as being at increased risk for having a child with a particular serious single-gene or chromosomal disorder, because it is necessary to know what condition to test for. This identification will usually be made because of the previous birth of an affected child. But such couples already have the option of prenatal genetic diagnosis for those disorders for which PID might be used, and prenatal diagnosis is far less costly, is more accurate, and has fewer health risks for the woman. These considerations further reduce the proportion of pregnancies for which it is appropriate to offer PID—it is relevant only for people unwilling to have prenatal diagnosis because of, for example, religious or personal reasons.

Despite the preceding points, private clinics providing this technology can be expected to market and promote it, since the more services they provide, the more successful they are as businesses. In 1997, a private fertility clinic in Toronto offered to screen embryos for risk of genetic disease before implantation for a fee of $6,500 to $9,800 per cycle of treatment. It offered PID to the public for twenty-seven genetic diseases—some of which, such as breast cancer, show no close correspondence between a single gene (allele) and the disease (Mitchell 1997). The clinician involved said, "This is the beginning of the end of genetic disease," and added that the roster of diseases the clinic would identify could grow dramatically over time and that this development should have "the same impact antibiotics did to bacterial disease" (Mitchell 1997). Through such hyperbolic promotion, private clinics market the technology as "quality control for parents." Less invasive, less costly approaches are available for those couples at high risk who wish to avoid having a child that is affected by a particular serious genetic disease. Simply letting the market determine the use of genetic testing at this stage of life, however, is likely to lead to misleading promotion and inappropriate use.

Prenatal Diagnostic Testing

Expansion of prenatal diagnostic testing, mentioned earlier, can be unwise if the use is beyond serious single-gene–determined disorders, as it has been applied to date, to conditions in which the role of genes is less clear. There are rapidly rising numbers of genes that have been, and continue to be, identified through the Human Genome Project. Increasingly, genes said to be associated with particular traits or seen as conferring an increased risk of a disease can now be identified, and a growing range of genes (presently several hundred) related to various traits and susceptibilities can be detected (Vogel and Motulsky 1997; Weaver 1999). In view of the incentives for doctors and laboratories to provide ever more testing services, prenatal testing for a range of such genotypes could become widely disseminated unless it is regulated to ensure that the costs, risks, and benefits have been rigorously established.

Genetic-risk information for diseases with complex causal pathways, such as most cancers and CHD, usually comes in the form of probabilities. As noted previously, semiquantitative phrases such as "associated with," "increased risk," and "related to" are used in this context. It is clear, from the environmental risk perception literature, that probability statements have limited meaning for most people, even when such statements are not being manipulated for marketing purposes (Gwyn et al. 2003). Thus, the public may not readily understand that having a particular gene does not inexorably lead to having its "related" disease, depending on intervening lifelong exposures. Letting prenatal genetic testing develop ad hoc is a recipe for letting anxiety and marketing trump sober analysis. Most people would like to have healthy children, and marketing of prenatal diagnostic testing could play into that natural aspiration exploitatively and misleadingly. Feeling they "should do all they can to have a healthy child," people are understandably susceptible to such marketing. If it is to bring health benefits to a population, prenatal testing should be offered only in programs with clear protocols, demonstrated benefit, demonstrable expertise, and resources for counseling and follow-up.

On a Brighter Note: Promising Genetic Interventions

Having considered the precautions for populationwide genetic interventions, we return now to the genuinely promising potential for understanding and managing multifactorial diseases that result from the interaction of genes and the environment, and are of great public health importance. There are several such conditions for which we are on the verge of quantum leaps in our understanding of prevention, and new genetic technologies are playing a critical role in expanding this knowledge (Zimmern 1999a, 1999b; Kaprio 2000; Thier et al. 2003). In the cases we explore next, genetic insights serve a dialectical purpose—that is, knowledge of the relevant genes and their functions allows us to characterize, with much greater precision, the environments in which they create increased risk. Thus, genetic insight leads, paradoxically, to the opportunity for environmental remedy.

Asthma

Asthma is a disease characterized by an abnormal immunological response to environmental stimuli. There are more than 17 million Americans with asthma—including almost 5 million children—and their numbers are increasing. (Indeed, the very fact that major increases in the frequency of asthma have occurred in recent decades is proof that a considerable portion of its determination cannot be purely genetic.) It is estimated that asthma-related costs in the United States exceeded $16.1 billion in the year 2004 (National Heart, Lung, and Blood Institute 2004). Several specific gene–environment interactions have been implicated as risk factors for asthma (Holgate et al. 1995; Holgate 1999; von Mutius 2001; McKeever et al. 2002). For example, an association has been reported between human leukocyte antigen (HLA) genes and susceptibility to toluene-diisocyanate–induced occupational asthma (Mapp et al. 2000). This knowledge clearly has public health relevance because it enables us to further elucidate the web of causation that, in this example, should inform environmental changes—namely, substitution of hazardous chemicals and improvements in exposure control measures. As more and more genes are defined and their functions in relation to the expression of allergic disease are established, a major task will be to assess the relative importance of each gene and integrate the complex series of genetic and environmental factors into a coherent understanding (Barnes and Marsh 1998). Primary exposure prevention will generally be the most efficacious method for promoting a healthy population, and with that approach, genetic information in aid of individually targeted environmental preventive measures will be secondary.

Nutrition and Tuberculosis

Tuberculosis has been projected to be the largest single infectious cause of death, globally, between 1990 and 2020 (Murray and Lopez 1997a). Susceptibility to disease after infection is influenced by environmental and genetic factors. Epidemiological risk generally results from dietary deficiency and tuberculosis exposure (Bellamy 2000). Vitamin D deficiency generally results from inadequate dietary intake, but the vitamin's protective effects may also be influenced by genetic variation in the vitamin D receptor gene. Preliminary research has suggested that tuberculosis risk increases tenfold in patients with a genetic variation that influences the serum concentration of vitamin D metabolites (Wilkinson et al. 2000). However, these patients represent a small portion of all tuberculosis cases, and the gene variation is relevant only under conditions in which the individual is likely to be exposed to the tuberculosis pathogen. Such conditions are increasingly rare in the established market economies, where genetic technologies are accessible, but these conditions are highly prevalent in less-developed regions, where tuberculosis is still rampant (Murray and Lopez 1997b). Clearly, the nutritional health of the population in general is paramount in reducing tuberculosis. Genetic information, in this case, serves to inform specific dietary supplementation in limited populations, such as health care workers in communities with large immigrant populations, but the impact of this intervention on the overall burden of disease will be modest at best.

　These examples demonstrate that current advances in our understanding of gene–environment interactions will almost certainly improve our capacity to prevent and treat subsets of some common multifactorial diseases. Targeting specific environmental and lifestyle changes to reduce risk and developing individually tailored therapies (pharmacogenomic tools) for sick individuals are easily foreseeable. However, widespread genetic testing must meet stringent criteria for both proof of safety and preventive effectiveness, as well as for the protection of the rights and privacy of those tested. It must also be judged against the opportunity cost of forgoing measures such as pollution controls, tobacco use reduction, or agricultural- and food-marketing policies that would improve the environment generally and would benefit the health of the population.

Conclusion

The determinants of most common diseases are complex, with environmental and genetic/biological factors interacting over the life course, embedded in a social context. Focusing exclusively on the genetic strand of this intricate web of causation—although profitable for some—will not address many other important disease determinants. An overemphasis on genetic approaches is particularly likely to lead to a passive neglect of environmental codeterminants of health and is unlikely to be the best way to better the population's health status. There are forces in our society (e.g., biotechnology-pharmaceutical industries, testing-service providers and labs, and those wishing to deny socioeconomic factors' role in health determination) pushing for a purely genetic approach to ill health, and this means we are at risk of using genetic technology in an inappropriate and unbalanced way. However, there is promise that, if we can achieve an appropriate and balanced use of new genetic technologies, we will improve our understanding of how genes and environment interact to cause many common diseases. Such a goal would be in the spirit of Rose's maxim to "seek causes of incidence" in populations rather than simply the "causes of cases" among individuals.

Notes

1. For example, at a recent Organization for Economic Cooperation and Development workshop, one speaker claimed that approximately 70% of cancers and cardiovascular diseases are due to inherited susceptibility (Vineis et al. 2001).

2. Note that these levels of causation are frequently aggregated as environmental influences. Here, environment refers to the influence of places. The distinction between social, environmental, and lifestyle is useful because each requires a distinct type of health intervention (McKinlay and Marceau 1999).

3. "Genotype" is the gene determining the identity of an individual, which may or may not be expressed in actual form and function of the body, which is referred to as "phenotype."

4. In this case, the term biological significance means that there is a moderate "strength of association" (Hill 1965) between the risk factor and an incident CHD outcome (as measured by the relative risk of disease occurrence with the risk factor present, compared with that risk without the risk factor present). This means that the relative risk of disease is, say, two or more for dichotomous risk factors such as gender. (Or this can be calculated from the interquartile "dose" of continuous risk factor. This is the amount of exposure equivalent

to the difference between an exposure distribution's twenty-fifth and seventy-fifth percentiles in a given study population, for a risk factor measured on continuous scale, such as blood pressure or serum cholesterol.) The term is used to distinguish risk factors with strong enough disease associations to constitute "substantial" prima facie evidence of causation from those with mere statistical significance, but dubious biological or clinical significance, in a given study.

5. It is difficult for social classes to become strongly associated with genotypes unless there is stable and complete marital isolation of each class for thousands of years—which has not been possible, at least not in Western industrialized countries. Alternatively, if marital selection were strongly associated with heritable traits—for example, only blue-eyed individuals were thought suitable mates for blue-eyed suitors—one could envisage those traits becoming highly associated with certain population groups. But social class, although often the subject of formal marriage taboos in many societies, has rarely proved such an impassable barrier for human affection in the long run.

6. New population-based evidence has suggested that the commonest gene for this last disorder actually causes clinical symptoms in only 1 out of 150 homozygotes, suggesting that previous estimates of the gene's "penetrance" (i.e., predictive validity for disease) were far too high, due to overgeneralization from high-risk families studied (Bleutler et al. 2002).

7. The fragile X syndrome is the most common form of heritable moderate mental retardation and the second most common among all causes of mental retardation, after Down's syndrome in males. It is due to multiple excessive (more than 200) repeats of a single DNA base-pair triplet, CGG, located in the 5' untranslated region of the first exon of a gene called "FMR1" on the X chromosome, leading to loss of gene function (Nussbaum et al. 2001).

References

American College of Medical Genetics. Working Group of the Genetic Screening Subcommittee of the Clinical Practice Committee. 1994. Fragile X syndrome: Diagnostic and carrier testing. *American Journal of Medical Genetics* 53:380–381.

Baird, P. A. 2000. Genetic technologies and achieving health for populations. *International Journal of Health Services* 30:407–424.

———. 2002. Identification of genetic susceptibility to common diseases: The case for regulation. *Perspectives in Biological Medicine* 45:516–528.

Baird, P. A, T. W. Anderson, H. B. Newcombe, and R. B. Lowry. 1988. Genetic disorders in children and young adults: A population study. *American Journal of Human Genetics* 42: 677–693.

Barker, D. J. P. 2001. *Fetal Origins of Cardiovascular and Lung Disease*. New York: M. Dekker.

Barker, D. J. P., and Medical Research Council (Great Britain), Environmental Epidemiology Unit. 1992. Fetal and infant origins of adult disease: Papers. *British Medical Journal*.

Barnes, K. C., and D. G. Marsh. 1998. The genetics and complexity of allergy and asthma. *Immunology Today* 19:325–332.

Begg, C. B. 2002. On the use of familial aggregation in population-based case probands for calculating penetrance. *Journal of the National Cancer Institute* 94:1221–1226.

Bellamy, R. 2000. Evidence of gene–environment interaction in development of tuberculosis. *Lancet* 355:588–589.

Bleutler, E., V. J. Felitti, J. A. Koziol, N. J. Ho, and T. Gelbart. 2000. Penetrance of 845G→ A (C282Y) HFE hereditary haemochromatosis mutation in the USA. *Lancet* 359:211–218.

Brown, W. T., G. E. Houck Jr., A. Jeziorowska, F. Levinson, X. Ding, C. Dobkin, N. Zhong, J. Henderson, S. S. Brooks, and E. C. Jenkins. 1993. Rapid fragile-X carrier screening and prenatal diagnosis using a nonradioactive PCR test. *Journal of the American Medical Association* 270:1569–1575.

Burke, W., D. Atkins, M. Gwinn, A. Guttmacher, J. Haddow, J. Lau, G. Palomaki, N. Press, C. S. Richards, L. Wideroff, and G. L. Wiesner. 2002. Genetic test evaluation: Information needs of clinicians, policy makers, and the public. *American Journal of Epidemiology* 156: 311–318.

Caskey, C. T. 1994. Fragile-X syndrome—improving understanding and diagnosis. *Journal of the American Medical Association* 271:552–553.

Collins, F. S. 1996. BRCA 1—lots of mutations, lots of dilemmas. *New England Journal of Medicine* 334:186–188.

Cooper, B. 2001. Nature, nurture and mental disorder: Old concepts in the new millennium. [Review] *British Journal of Psychiatry* (suppl. 40):91–101.

Danesh, J., R. Collins, and R. Peto. 1997. Chronic infections and coronary heart disease: Is there a link? *Lancet* 350:430–436.

Denke, M. A. 1994. Individual responsiveness to a cholesterol-lowering diet in postmenopausal women with moderate hypercholesterolemia. *Archives of Internal Medicine* 154: 1977–1982.

Denke, M. A., and S. M. Grundy. 1994. Individual responses to a cholesterol-lowering diet in 50 men with moderate hypercholesterolemia. *Archives of Internal Medicine* 154:317–325.

Dubois, R. N. 2000. Review article: Cyclooxygenase—a target for colon cancer prevention. *Alimentary Pharmacology and Therapeutics* 14 (suppl. 1):64–67.

Elwood, M. J. 1999a. Public health aspects of breast cancer gene testing in Canada, part 1: Risk and interventions. *Chronic Diseases in Canada* 20:3–13.

———. 1999b. Public health aspects of breast cancer gene testing in Canada, part 2: Selection for and effects of testing. *Chronic Diseases in Canada* 20:14–20.

Evans, J. P, C. Skrzynia, and W. Burke. 2001. The complexities of predictive genetic testing. *British Medical Journal* 322:1052–1056.

Evans, R. G., M. L. Barer, and T. R. Marmor. 1994. *Why Are Some People Healthy and Others Not? The Determinants of Health of Populations*. New York: Aldine de Gruyter.

Flynn, L. L. 1993. *Understanding the Role of Genetic Factors in Mental Illness*. Washington, DC: Office of Technology Assessment.

Fong, K. M., Y. Sekido, and J. D. Minna. 1999. Molecular pathogenesis of lung cancer. *Journal of Thoracic and Cardiovascular Surgery* 118:1136–1152.

Ford, D., D. F. Easton, and J. Peto. 1995. Estimates of the gene frequency of BRCA1 and its contribution to breast and ovarian cancer incidence. *American Journal of Human Genetics* 57:1457–1462.

Friedman, G. D. 1987. *Primer of Epidemiology*. New York: McGraw-Hill.

Grann, V. R., and J. S. Jacobson. 2002. Population screening for cancer-related germline gene mutations. *Lancet Oncology* 3:341–348.

Gwyn, K., S. W. Vernon, and P. M. Conoley. 2003. Intention to pursue genetic testing for breast cancer among women due for screening mammography. *Cancer Epidemiology, Biomarkers, and Prevention* 12:96–102.

Haga, S. B., M. J. Khoury, and W. Burke. 2003. Genomic profiling to promote a health lifestyle: Not ready for prime time. *Nature Genetics* 34:347–350.

Haugen, A., D. Ryberg, S. Mollerup, S. Zienolddiny, V. Skaug, and D. H. Svendsrud. 2000. Gene–environment interactions in human lung cancer. *Toxicology Letters* 112:233–237.

Helmes, A. W., D. J. Bowen, and J. Bengal. 1999. *Genetic Testing for Breast Cancer: An Issue of Money*. Report on the Second National Conference on Genetics and Public Health, Genetics and Disease Prevention: Integrating Genetics into Public Health Policy, Research, and Practice. Baltimore: Karger.

Hemminki, K., I. Lonnstedt, P. Vaittinen, and P. Lichtenstien. 2001. Estimation of genetic and environmental components in colorectal and lung cancer and melanoma. *Genetic Epidemiology* 20:107–116.

Hill, A. B. 1965. The environment and disease: Association or causation? *Proceedings of the Royal Society of Medicine* 58:295–300.

Holgate, S. T. 1999. Genetic and environmental interaction in allergy and asthma. *Journal of Allergy and Clinical Immunology* 104:1139–1146.

Holgate, S. T., M. K. Church, P. H. Howarth, E. N. Morton, A. J. Frew, and R. Djukanovic. 1995. Genetic and environmental influences on airway inflammation in asthma. *International Archives of Allergy and Immunology* 107:29–33.

Holtzman, N. A., and T. M. Marteau. 2000. Will genetics revolutionize medicine? *New England Journal of Medicine* 343:141–144.

Hubbard, R., and E. Wald. 1993. *Exploding the Gene Myth: How Genetic Information Is Produced and Manipulated by Scientists, Physicians, Employers, Insurance Companies, Educators, and Law Enforcers*. Boston: Beacon Press.

Jha, P., M. Flather, E. Lonn, M. Farkouh, and S. Yusuf. 1995. Antioxidant vitamins and cardiovascular disease—a critical review of epidemiologic and clinical trial data. *Annals of Internal Medicine* 123:860–872.

Kaprio, J. 2000. Science, medicine, and the future—genetic epidemiology. *British Medical Journal* 320:1257–1259.

Khoury, M. J., L. L. McCabe, and E. R. McCabe. 2003. Population screening in the age of genomic medicine. *New England Journal of Medicine* 348:50–58.

Khoury, M. J., Q. Yong, M. Gwinn, J. Little, and W. D. Flanders. 2004. An epidemiologic assessment of genomic profiling for measuring susceptibility to common diseases and targeting interventions. *Genetics in Medicine* 6:38–47.

Langston, A. A., K. E. Malone, J. D. Thompson, J. R. Daling, and E. A. Ostrander. 1996. BRCA1 mutations in a population-based sample of young women with breast cancer. *New England Journal of Medicine* 334:137–142.

Larrson, C. 1978. Natural history and life expectancy in severe α1-antitrypsin deficiency, Pi Z. *Acta Medica Scandinavica* 204:345–351.

Lauria, D. P., and W. J. Webb. 1992. The economic impact of the Fragile X syndrome on the state of Colorado. In Hagerman, R. F. and P. McDenzie, eds. *International Fragile X Conference Proceedings*: Dillon, CO: National Fragile X Foundation and Spectra Publishing.

Lerman, C., B. Biesecker, J. L. Benkendorf, J. Kerner, A. Gomez-Caminero, C. Hughes, and M. M. Reed. 1997. Controlled trial of pretest education approaches to enhance informed decision-making for BRCA1 gene testing. *Journal of the National Cancer Institute* 89:148–157.

Lock, M. 1998. Breast cancer: Reading the omens. *Anthropology Today* 14 (4):7–17.

Lynch, H. T., S. J. Lemon, C. Durham, S. T. Tinley, C. Connolly, J. F. Lynch, J. Surdam, E. Orinion, S. Slominski-Caster, P. Watson, C. Lerman, P. Tonin, G. Lenoir, O. Serova, and S. Narod. 1997. A descriptive study of BRCA1 testing and reactions to disclosure of test results. *Cancer* 79:2219–2228.

MacMahon, B., and T. F. Pugh. 1970. *Epidemiology: Principles and Methods*. Boston: Little Brown.

Malone, K. E., J. R. Daling, J. D. Thompson, C. A. O'Brien, L. V. Franciso, and E. A. Ostrander. 1998. BRCA1 mutations and breast cancer in the general population: Analyses in women before age 35 years and in women before age 45 years with first-degree family history. *Journal of the American Medical Association* 279:922–929.

Mapp, C. E., B. Beghe, A. Balboni, G. Zamorani, M. Padoan, L. Jovine, O. R. Bari Cordi, and L. M. Fabbri. 2000. Association between HLA genes and susceptibility to toluene diisocyanate-induced asthma. *Clinical and Experimental Allergy* 30:651–656.

Marmot, M. G., and S. L. Syme. 1976. Acculturation and coronary heart disease in Japanese-Americans. *American Journal of Epidemiology* 104:225–247.

Marmot, M. G., S. L. Syme, A. Kagan, H. Kato, J. B. Cohen, and J. Belsky. 1975. Epidemiologic studies of coronary heart disease and stroke in Japanese men living in Japan, Hawaii and California: Prevalence of coronary and hypertensive heart disease and associated risk factors. *American Journal of Epidemiology* 102:514–525.

Mattila, K. J., V. V. Valtonen, M. S. Nieminen, and S. Asi Kainen. 1998. Role of infection as a risk factor for atherosclerosis, myocardial infarction, and stroke. *Clinical Infectious Diseases* 26:719–734.

McCormack, V. A., I. dos Santos Silva, B. L. De Stavola, R. Mohsen, D. A. Leon, and H. O. Lithell. 2003. Fetal growth and subsequent risk of breast cancer: Results from long-term follow-up of Swedish cohort. *British Medical Journal* 326:332–348.

McCredie, M., M. S. Coates, and J. M. Ford. 1990. Cancer incidence to migrants to New South Wales from England, Wales, Scotland and Ireland. *British Journal of Cancer* 62: 992–995.

McDermott, R. 1998. Ethics, epidemiology and the thrifty gene: Biological determinism as a health hazard. *Social Science and Medicine* 47:1189–1195.

McKeever, T. M., S. A. Lewis, C. Smith, J. Collins, H. Heatlie, M. Frischer, and R. Hubbard. 2002. Early exposure to infections and antibiotics and incidence of allergic disease: A birth cohort study with the West Midlands General Practice Database. *Journal of Allergy and Clinical Immunology* 109:43–50.

McKinlay, J. B., and L. D. Marceau. 1999. A tale of 3 tails. *American Journal of Public Health* 89:295–298.

Mitchell, A. 1997. A clinic to sift out bad genes. *Globe and Mail* (Toronto), September 24, p. A1.

Murray, C. J. L., and A. D. Lopez. 1997a. Alternative projections of mortality and disability by cause 1990–2020: Global Burden of Disease Study. *Lancet* 349:1498–1504.

———. 1997b. Global mortality, disability, and the contribution of risk factors: Global Burden of Disease Study. *Lancet* 349:1436–1442.

National Heart, Lung, and Blood Institute. 2004. *Morbidity and Mortality: 2004 Chart Book on Cardiovascular, Lung, and Blood Diseases.* Accessed April 14, 2005, at http://www .nhlbi.nih.gov/resources/docs/04_chtbk.pdf.

Neel, J. V. 1999. Diabetes mellitus: A "thrifty" genotype rendered detrimental by "progress"? *Bulletin of the World Health Organization* 77:694–703.

Nussbaum, R. L., R. R. McInnes, and H. F. Willard. 2001. *Thompson & Thompson Genetics in Medicine.* Philadelphia: Saunders.

Pearce, N. 1996. Traditional epidemiology, modern epidemiology, and public health. *American Journal of Public Health* 86:678–683.

———. 1999. Epidemiology as a population science. *International Journal of Epidemiology* 28:S1015–S1018.

Pearce, N, S. Foliaki, A. Sporle, and C. Cunningham. 2004. Genetics, race, ethnicity, and health. *British Medical Journal* 328:1070–1072.

Plomin, R., P. Lichtenstein, N. L. Pedersen, G. E. McClearn, and J. R. Nesselroade. 1990. Genetic influence on life events during the last half of the life span. *Psychology and Aging* 5:25–30.

Ramsay, L. E., and W. W. Yeo. 1991. Hypertension and coronary artery disease—an unsolved problem. *Journal of Cardiovascular Pharmacology* 18:S31–S34.

Reiss, D., R. Plomin, and E. M. Hetherington. 1991. Genetics and psychiatry: An unheralded window on the environment. *American Journal of Psychiatry* 148:283–291.

Ridley, M. 2003. *Nature via Nurture: Genes, Experience, & What Makes Us Human.* Toronto: HarperCollins Canada.

Rose, G. 1985. Sick individuals and sick populations. *International Journal of Epidemiology* 14:32–38.

Rothman, K. J. 1986. *Modern Epidemiology.* Boston: Little Brown.

Schottenfeld, D., and J. F. Fraumeni. 1996. *Cancer Epidemiology and Prevention.* New York: Oxford University Press.

Schwab, M. 1998. *Genes and Environment in Cancer.* New York: Springer.

Shostak, S. 2003. Locating gene–environment interaction: At the intersections of genetics and public health. [Review] *Social Science and Medicine* 56:2327–2342.

Sijbrands, E. J. G., R. G. J. Westendorp, J. C. Defesche, P. H. E. M. de Meier, A. H. M. Smelt, J. J. P. Kastelein, and J. Kaprio. 2001. Mortality over two centuries in large pedigree with familial hypercholesterolemia: Family tree mortality study. *British Medical Journal* 322: 1019–1023.

Silventoinen, K., J. Kaprio, E. Lahelma, and M. Koskenvuo. 2000. Relative effect of genetic and environmental factors on body height: Differences across birth cohorts among Finnish men and women. *American Journal of Public Health* 90:627–630.

Solomon, P. J., E. A. Thompson, and A. Rissanen. 1983. The inheritance of height in a Finnish population. *Annals of Human Biology* 10:247–256.

Tambor, E. S., B. K. Rimer, and T. S. Strigo. 1997. Genetic testing for breast cancer susceptibility: Awareness and interest among women in the general population. *American Journal of Medical Genetics* 68:43–49.

Thier, R., T. Bruning, P. H. Roos, H. P. Rihs, K. Golka, Y. Ko, and H. M. Bolt. 2003. Markers of genetic susceptibility in human environmental hygiene and toxicology: The role of selected CYP, NAT and GST genes. *International Journal of Hygiene and Environmental Health.* 206:149–171.

Vineis, P., P. Schulte, and A. J. McMichael. 2001. Misconceptions about the use of genetic tests in populations. *Lancet* 357:709–712.

Vogel, F., and A. G. Motulsky. 1997. *Human Genetics: Problems and Approaches* (3rd ed.). New York: Springer.

von Mutius, E. 2001. The increase in asthma can be ascribed to cleanliness. *American Journal of Respiratory and Critical Care Medicine* 164:1106–1109.

Wareham, N. J., P. W. Franks, and A. H. Harding. 2002. Establishing the role of gene–environment interactions in the etiology of type 2 diabetes. [Review] *Endocrinology and Metabolism Clinics of North America* 31:553–566.

Warren, S. T., and D. L. Nelson. 1994. Advances in molecular analysis of fragile X syndrome. *Journal of the American Medical Association* 271:536–542.

Weaver, D. D. 1999. *Catalog of Prenatally Diagnosed Conditions* (3rd ed.). Baltimore: Johns Hopkins University Press.

Wilkinson, R. J., M. Llewelyn, Z. Toossi, P. Patel, G. Pasvol, A. Lalvani, D. Wright, M. Latif, and R. N. Davidson. 2000. Influence of vitamin D deficiency and vitamin D receptor polymorphisms on tuberculosis among Gujarati Asians in west London: A case-control study. *Lancet* 355:618–621.

Willet, W. C. 2002. Balancing life-style and genomics research for disease prevention. *Science* 296:695–698.

Ziegler, R. G., R. N. Hoover, and M. C. Pike. 1993. Migration patterns and breast cancer risk in Asian-American women. *Journal of the National Cancer Institute* 85:1819–1827.

Zimmern, R. L. 1999a. Genetic testing: A conceptual exploration. *Journal of Medical Ethics* 25:151–156.

———. 1999b. The human genome project: A false dawn? *British Medical Journal* 319:1282–1284.

Chapter 2

Biological Pathways Linking the Social Environment, Development, and Health

Clyde Hertzman and John Frank

In this chapter we have three purposes. First, we present an overview of current knowledge regarding the biological pathways by which socioeconomic, psychosocial, and developmental experiences "embed" themselves in human biology *over the life course*. The interest here is in understanding not only how systematic differences in health status emerge among groups of people whose life experiences differ from one another but also how the variations are translated into differential risks of conditions such as coronary heart disease, mental illness, and Alzheimer's disease. Second, we offer a conceptual framework for comprehensively integrating and accommodating the rapidly growing body of evidence on the biological pathways that contribute to this process, which we have come to call *biological embedding*. Finally, we identify key research opportunities and challenges in furthering our understandings in the field.

How the Environment Gets under the Skin

What follows here is a discussion of selected observations that require a coherent understanding of biological embedding in order to be properly explained. They cross the life course—early, middle, and late—giving examples wherein human experiences in different socioeconomic, psychosocial, and developmental environments, as well as human biological regulatory and defense systems, are closely connected. A formal discussion of biological embedding follows these examples, rather than preceding them, so that the reader will understand the nature of the phenomena that a concept of biological embedding must explain.

Early Life

The prenatal environment can affect health later in the life course. There is consistent evidence that infants who are born at term but are small for gestational age may be at increased risk for adult-onset diabetes, high blood pressure, and heart disease several decades later (Barker 1990; Bateson et al. 2004). At the same time, it has long been understood that low-birth-weight or small-for-gestational-age babies are at increased developmental risk (Shenkin et al. 1932; Richards et al. 2001; Sorensen et al. 1997; Matte et al. 2001). However, our recent research has suggested that the gestational effect is fundamentally modified by early socioeconomic circumstances (Jefferis et al. 2002). Taking math achievement in grade school as an example, we have shown that high-socioeconomic-status (SES) children, on average, start school with above-average skills, and their advantage grows from age seven to sixteen. Low birth weight reduces, but does not eliminate, the advantage of growing up in a high-SES family. Conversely, low-SES children start school, on average, with below-average math skills, and this disadvantage increases from age seven to sixteen. Low birth weight among children growing up in a low-SES family exacerbates this disadvantage. We have shown that, when these effects are combined, low-birth-weight children from privileged backgrounds still have a developmental advantage over normal-birth-weight children from underprivileged backgrounds. Thus, socioeconomic disadvantage and gestational factors have both declared their developmental impacts by early in the life course, and both go on to confer a risk of diabetes, high blood pressure, and heart disease later in life. Understanding the processes by which this happens raises questions of biological embedding.

Work over the past half century has demonstrated how the newborns' immediate postnatal social environment has profound, long-lasting influences on subsequent health and development. A prime example is infant attachment to a parental figure (usually the mother) in both higher primates and humans. The parental figure's failure to provide the full set of necessary visual, tactile, and auditory—and, perhaps, olfactory—inputs during a "critical early window" of infant development leads to profound developmental delay. Indeed, in cases of severe neglect, this deprivation can result in adult stunting or even death, despite the availability of theoretically adequate physical nourishment, warmth, and other material necessities. Furthermore, there is much less effect of this form of psychosocial deprivation when it occurs at later ages, as if the infant is "prewired" to require this input at precisely a certain developmental stage. This finding mirrors a very large body of animal and human research on critical windows of other sorts, recently reviewed elsewhere (Cynader et al. 1999; chapter 4 in this volume).

A legitimate concern here is the potential for overgeneralization of the critical window hypothesis. The concern is that notions of critical periods could be converted to policies of "social immunization," wherein young children's needs receive special attention, whereas "doomed" older children who have not had appropriate early experiences are abandoned in child development policy and programs (Hertzman 1994). In reality, developmental windows open throughout the full course of childhood, as well as into adulthood. The brain continues to sculpt itself, albeit at a declining rate, such that the brain does not reach its "adult" state until the end of the second or beginning of the third decade. For instance, key executive functions, regarding how an individual responds to social and emotional stimuli, develop in the prefrontal cortex from approximately age three to nine. At the same time, there is evidence that neural connections to the prefrontal cortex, from centers in the midbrain that sense environmental threats, develop earlier. Thus, it may turn out that, although the physiological sense of threat is developed at a very young age, the repertoire of responses to a sense of threat may develop later and may be subject to effective intervention at later ages. Quantifying this issue—the degree to which later intervention can compensate for early disadvantage—is crucial. At present, however, our knowledge in this area is rudimentary.

Insights suggesting subtle interactions between children's social environments and their "personality traits" have come from the work of Boyce, among others. Liang and Boyce (1993) showed that children with "reactive" cardiovascular systems (i.e., those who show large fluctuations in heart rate and blood pressure in response to stressors) appeared to experience higher accident rates than less-reactive children in child-care centers with frequent stressful events, as noted by trained observers; but the same type of children experienced lower accident rates than their peers in less-stressful centers. Subsequent work (Boyce et al. 1995) showed the same pattern of individual–environment interaction for respiratory infections and CD19+ cell counts (a short-lag-time marker of up-regulated cellular immune function that may be followed by immune suppression). Findings in rhesus macaques by Suomi and colleagues (Bennett et al. 2002) suggested that these "personality traits" are not in fact fixed, genetically or in utero, but rather can be modified by parental rearing practices.

Other childhood experiences have also been shown to profoundly influence subsequent development and health status (Keating and Hertzman 1999). Indeed, North American culture has completely internalized—some might say excessively—the adage "As the twig is bent, so grows the tree." Later we discuss some very specific mechanisms, as exemplified in the hypothalamic-pituitary-adrenal (HPA) axis "life story," by which health outcomes over the entire life course may be set in motion via early life embedding of experience in physiological system functioning—especially in the psychoneuroendocrine (PNE) and psychoneuroimmune (PNI) response repertoires.

Midlife

The most important issue in midlife is the extent to which adults' place in society, their living conditions, and the individual adult's understanding of these circumstances have biological roots and biological consequences. There may in fact be a systematically changing sequence of predominant biological pathways in our response to the stresses of daily living as we age. Early in life (and *early* is only a relative term here), one would tend to expect a sympatho-adrenal-medullary (SAM)–mediated response to threatening, challenging circumstances. In other words, when confronted with a challenge, a person's physiological response would be to support acts of coping by causing the "adrenaline to flow." But over time, the experiences of people in lower socioeconomic circumstances will tend to convert their physiological responses to "learned helplessness." That is, because their life experiences will have led them to expect that they cannot, or do not have the resources to, solve the problems of daily living, they would come to respond (consciously or unconsciously) as though the stressors that challenge them are likely to defeat them. Lundberg's hypothesis is that learned helplessness has a physiological dimension—namely, a gradual switchover may occur from a SAM-type "mobilize-the-energy" physiological reaction, typically involving heart rate and blood pressure responses, to an HPA-type "defeat" reaction, involving increased secretion of cortisol. Although this is only a hypothesis, it is recognized here as a model thoroughly consistent with the emergence of socioeconomic gradients in health status across the life course.

The research literature abounds with evidence of biological pathways that could help explain gradients. There are many studies of adults' health outcomes being influenced by psychosocial stressors, through a variety of specific PNE/PNI mechanisms. Cohen and colleagues (1997), for instance, showed that clinical manifestations of upper respiratory infection were strongly related to the frequency and quality of social contacts among healthy subjects exposed to a standard dose of cold virus. The investigators also measured laboratory parameters of immunocompetence, which correlated with disease outcomes. Apparently extensive, supportive social connections protect people from infections' clinical consequences—although doubters will wonder whether part of the mechanism may be the larger cumulative exposure to, and thus prior immunological experience with, a range of germs, among those with a larger social circle. Many studies have correlated a variety of depressed immune responses with bereavement and other acute emotional stressors, such as student exams (Kiecolt-Glaser 1999; Kiecolt-Glaser et al. 2002a; Kiecolt-Glaser et al. 2002b; Kiecolt-Glaser and Glaser 2002).

Kristensen's (1998) work, comparing fifty-year-old "healthy" men from Sweden and Lithuania, is central to the question of biological embedding. In Eastern Europe over the past twenty years there has been a mounting health crisis, exacerbated by the political, social, and economic dislocations at the end of the Soviet era. Whereas heart disease mortality rates for middle-aged men were similar in Sweden and Lithuania in the mid-1960s, by the mid-1990s they were fourfold higher in Lithuania than in Sweden. An early report on the East–West "life expectancy gap" suggested that the difference between Eastern Europe and the West could be thought of as analogous to SES differences (Hertzman et al. 1996). In other words, the experience of life for people in Eastern Europe in recent decades was, in some respects, like that of low-SES groups in the West. Kristensen's work was designed to test that idea. She studied fifty-year-old men from one Lithuanian city and one Swedish city and examined their cortisol response pathways, using a challenge protocol. This involved three stress tests: psychosocial, mental-intellectual, and straightforwardly physical (inserting the subjects' hands into cold water). What she found was that the pattern of salivary cortisol before, during, and after these standardized stressors was such that the Lithuanian men had a higher baseline cortisol level and then a blunted response to the stressor (what she described as a "burnout" pattern). The Swedish men had lower baseline levels, a sharp response to the stressor, regardless of which one, and then a quicker return to baseline levels; ultimately, the Swedes' cortisol levels came down further.

Kristensen found that the Lithuanian pattern tended to be associated with low self-esteem, a lower sense of coherence (i.e., a sense of conjunction between of one's lived experience and one's sense of what life should bring) (Antonovsky 1993), and increased reported job strain (according to the Karasek model [Karasek and Theorell 1990]). In general, the Lithuanians showed decreased decision latitude in their jobs, increased "vital exhaustion," and increased depression, according to self-reports. This "psychosocial risk factor complex" association with coronary heart disease risk was quite specific. Other biological variables known to predict coronary heart disease risk that were examined—such as serum cholesterol and blood pressure levels—could not, in themselves, explain the two populations' very different heart disease rates. The Swedish men's cortisol levels were reminiscent of Sapolsky's findings in socially dominant baboons (described shortly), whereas the Lithuanian men tended to have the cortisol response pattern of socially subordinate baboons—at least during periods of stable living conditions (Sapolsky 1995). In Lundberg's (1996) terms, these are the physiological differences of greater or lesser degrees of learned helplessness. Kristensen's work supports the hypothesis that systematic differences in living conditions among societies can influence the HPA axis such that by adulthood the range of HPA axis functioning will be different in different societies.

Late Life

Here, the leading hypothesis is that the principal host defense systems (the HPA, SAM, and PNI systems) age at differential rates, depending on the quality of the environments where their hosts have grown up, lived, and worked, as well as on the relative success or failure of individual–environment interactions across the life course. This hypothesis may help to explain, in broad terms, why socioeconomic differences emerge, at a given age, in the rates of diseases whose incidence tends to rise with age. If the HPA, SAM, and PNI systems age at differential rates across the socioeconomic spectrum, then it is not that hard to imagine how gradients that cut across a wide range of disease processes could emerge. All individuals in society are on a similar trajectory of increasing risk of a range of diseases with increasing age, but life circumstances (and the biological responses to them) determine how rapidly individuals move along that trajectory.

Take, for instance, the immune system. Its aging has been likened to a spring, and physiological stresses that challenge the immune system lead to aging like forces on the spring. If a spring is "sprung" too often over time, it will start to lose its "elasticity" and, thus, its ability to return to the original shape after being stretched. If the immune system is too frequently and severely challenged over time, the analogy goes, this process may prematurely age the system, leading to "dysregulation" in either of two ways. First, the normal immune response involves two basic immune subsystems (known as TH1 and TH2) that respond to challenge in a balanced way. Dysregulation could mean an increasingly imbalanced response to physiological stresses over time. Second, it could mean vulnerability to a generalized under-or overstimulation of the immune system. Immune dysregulation, in turn, has been associated with vulnerability to coronary heart disease, allergic conditions (asthma, hives), and autoimmune conditions. It also has been viewed as creating windows of opportunity for pathogenic organisms and infection (Glaser and Kiecolt-Glaser 1998; Glaser et al. 1999; Glaser et al. 2001).[1]

The spring model resembles the concept of "allostatic load" that has been developed by life course researchers whose principal focus is on aging (McEwen and Wingfield 2003) rather than the early years. Allostatic load, in essence, proposes that the "set point" for physiological homeostasis is different in different individuals, such that daily perturbations of homeostasis (i.e., springing of the spring) will affect aging differently in those with different set points. The physiological set point in this model can be equated with the degree to which the spring's shape at rest reflects loss of elasticity. If the physiological set point is influenced by earlier life experiences, then the concept of biological embedding, inferred from observations early in life, could be merged with allostatic load, based on aging, to encompass the entire life course. That is, biological embedding would help explain how an individual's allostatic load came to be "set" where it is in midlife, and allostatic load would, in turn, help explain systematic differences in health status during late life.

Kiecolt-Glaser and colleagues (1995) studied isolated elderly spouse-caregivers of Alzheimer's patients by giving them a standardized, small puncture wound (of the sort routinely used for skin biopsies) and observing closely to see how long it took for the wound to heal. They found dramatically reduced rates of wound healing compared with those among age-matched controls not providing care to others. These researchers suggested that there was a connection between a strong chronic-stress–induced cortisol response in caregivers and tissue levels of interleukin 8 (IL-8) and IL-1. These substances are cytokines, which are secreted by a range of body cells during inflammatory responses in order to assist wound healing. These regulatory substances also feed back from the immune system to the brain. When not inhibited by chronic stress, they are critical in bringing into a wound the cells that set up the body's complex series of healing responses. The second phenomenon these investigators examined was humoral (antibody) response to routine annual influenza immunization. Once again, they found dramatically reduced rates of developing a competent humoral response among Alzheimer's caregivers compared with those of age-matched controls. They found that, even five to six years after the spouse had died, the sluggish immune response was still present, suggesting clear embedding with prolonged effects.

Biological Embedding

Biological embedding is an overarching hypothesis that seeks to explain how systematic differences in human experience can systematically affect the healthfulness of life across the life course (Hertzman and Wiens 1996). The detailed hypothesis can be stated as follows. Systematic differences in the qualities of emotional, social, intellectual, and physical circumstances are found in different socioeconomic, psychosocial, and developmental environments. From the time of conception through the first several years of life and at a diminishing pace thereafter, these differences will affect the development of the brain and the central nervous system, and will, in turn, have systematic effects on cognitive, social, emotional, and behavioral development. The central nervous system, which plays a key role in interpreting the environment, interacts closely with a variety of host defense systems, such as the immune, hormone, and clotting systems. The same factors that influence development will also influence the conditioning of these pathways.

Thus, systematic differences in socioeconomic, psychosocial, and developmental environments across the life course will ultimately influence five factors:

- the "objective" degree of stressfulness of the circumstances of daily life
- the degree to which given circumstances are experienced as stressful
- the cognitive, social, and emotional coping skills people bring with them into adulthood
- the physiological pattern of host response to the stresses of daily living
- the individual's biological responses to the circumstances and experiences of daily life

Systematic differences across these five factors day by day, week by week, and year by year over the life course will lead to systematic differences in the function of organ systems and create systematic differentials in morbidity and mortality that will cut across a wide variety of disease processes.

The preceding description is a statement about human biology, yet the primary insights that motivated it did not come from research in human biology. They came, instead, from the field of population health—in particular, from several insights into the ubiquitous and persistent socioeconomic gradient in human health, as follows:

First, the gradient is found, to a greater or lesser degree, for most major causes of morbidity and mortality. It has shown the potential to replicate itself for new, emerging conditions such as heart disease (during the mid-twentieth century) and HIV (at the end of the twentieth century), soon after they have become endemic in society. Thus, explaining the gradient requires recognizing a general pattern of resilience and vulnerability that operates *in addition to* factors that increase the risk for specific diseases only. It is exceedingly difficult to conceive of panpathological vulnerability or resilience (i.e., generalized resilience or vulnerability to whatever the major diseases of the day might be) without focusing on the developmental biology of the host resistance and stress response, which, in turn, requires a life course perspective.

Second, the widespread socioeconomic gradient in health status found in adult life is paralleled by socioeconomic gradients in cognitive and behavioral development in early life (Keating and Hertzman 1999). In Canada and the United States, these developmental gradients are already well established by kindergarten age and are related to differential access, by socioeconomic status, to "developmental priming mechanisms" for healthy child development in the first years of life: opportunities for secure attachment; encouragement of exploration; mentoring in basic skills; celebration of developmental advances; guided rehearsal and extension of new skills; protection from inappropriate disapproval, teasing, or punishment; and a rich and responsive language environment (Ramey and Ramey 1998). The reasons for differential access are many. Some, like secure attachment, can be profoundly affected by factors such as work-life/home-life time conflicts that are more difficult to control for those with little workplace flexibility. Others, such as the richness and responsiveness of the language environment, can be related to parental education, consciousness of the importance of early intellectual stimulation, or access to quality child-care arrangements.

Third, evidence from longitudinal studies has shown that early child development and the socioeconomic and psychosocial environments of childhood are linked to adult health status through latent, pathway, and cumulative effects (see chapter 4). Biological embedding comprises all those biological developmental mechanisms by which early life exposures and experiences are translated into influences on health and functioning through the balance of the life course (Hertzman and Wiens 1996; Keating and Hertzman 1999).

Finally, there is new research, scattered throughout this chapter, showing that those who have experienced different circumstances across the life course react to common experiences of daily living—especially to *stressful* experiences—in physiologically different ways that, in turn, are associated with differences in subsequent health.

Notwithstanding these insights, there are substantial epistemological problems with fully understanding biological embedding. The intellectual task is easy enough to state: to understand how socioeconomic, psychosocial, and developmental environments influence biological processes that, in turn, engender systematic differences in health status and function over the life course. This inquiry starts by focusing on differences in the qualities of early childhood environments and then follows the subsequent effects on human biological parameters across the life course. Put differently, the task is identifying the spectrum of specific biological mechanisms by which health is determined, through embedding of the environment in human functioning, with varying lag times (or latencies), as well as pathway and cumulative effects, from childhood to old age (chapter 4 in this volume; Hertzman et al. 1994).

In practice, however, the task is daunting. It means merging two fundamentally different perspectives: one that focuses on large-sample, long-term epidemiological studies of entire populations in varying environments and another that involves short-term, intensive follow-up of relatively small samples of individuals, studied in fine biological detail. It means convincing those who have made a lifelong commitment to understanding social causation that they cannot ignore insights from human biology. It also means convincing investigators who work with small samples of people in the laboratory to think in population terms. Finally, it means motivating researchers who spend their careers doing highly focused studies of developmental processes to think in broader, simpler terms, as well as convincing those who work with delicate bioassays and biological processes that unfold over the very short term to think also in life course terms. We return to this challenge later, in some detail, when we suggest a future research agenda to help bridge these diverse but essential disciplinary perspectives in this quintessentially transdisciplinary field.

Current Theses about Biological Embedding

For decades, biological and behavioral investigators have been conducting research focused on particular organ systems' functioning, host defense mechanisms, and behavioral responses at different points in the life course. These efforts have made it possible for those interested in biological embedding to extract specific research findings from a wide range of disciplines and then recast them to help explain how systematic differences in health and well-being across a variety of disease processes can emerge as the life course unfolds. Before considering some of the most illuminating of these research findings, however, we need to briefly review for the general reader some basic principles and biological systems that underlie the embedding concept.

- Children spend the many years required for full human brain development in socioeconomic, psychosocial, and developmental environments of radically differing qualities, leading to systematic differences in brain structure and function.
- Differential brain structure and function associated with differing socioeconomic, psychosocial, and developmental environments are closely associated with systematic differences in the function of at least three important physiological control systems: the HPA axis (which controls cortisol secretion), the SAM axis (which controls epinephrine and norepinephrine secretion), and the PNI axis (which involves central nervous system influences on immune system function and blood clotting factors).
- The SAM, HPA, and PNI axes all have a "life" within individuals in society that, in turn, has an empirically demonstrable role in producing systematic (e.g., SES) gradients in health over the life course.

This thesis contends that early life experience profoundly shapes the ways these axes develop; that these body-regulatory and defense systems, in turn, experience the environment and respond to it in radically different ways in different individuals, over the short and long terms; that these responses affect the individual's lifelong health; and finally, that systematic differences in these responses across SES groups in a society affect health differentially. The interest here is in the interplay—moment to moment, hour to hour, day to day—between the environments where people live, work, and grow up, on the one hand, and the development and responses of the SAM, HPA, and PNI axes, on the other, which lead to systematically differing health expectancy over a lifetime. In particular, there is a special capacity of these axes to influence far-reaching latent, pathway, and cumulative effects of early life experiences, later in life (Hertzman and Wiens 1996; Power and Hertzman 1997). As a well-developed example of this, we tell in some detail, as follows, the "life story" of the HPA axis, as it is beginning to be understood, throughout the full span of mammalian developmental stages.

Case Study of the "Life Story of the HPA Axis" in Society

The first place to look for evidence of biological embedding is in what might be called the life story of the HPA axis, as it unfolds in individuals differentially positioned in society. This axis is key because of its role in our perception of, and response to, stressful circumstances. HPA stimulation leads to the secretion of the hormone cortisol, which, in turn, has widespread metabolic effects on various human organ systems. These effects are adaptive in the acute stress-response phase, focusing the body's energy on the immediate task at hand and reducing metabolic processes that do not contribute to the immediate response. But, over the long term, cortisol can damage these same organ systems as a result of high exposure (McEwen 1998).

Animal studies provide a preliminary model of the role the HPA axis may play in general vulnerability and resistance to disease. Three lines of evidence are particularly pertinent here. First, Meaney (Sapolsky 1992) has shown that, in rats, apparently minimal intervention (i.e., handling) in early life can permanently condition the way the HPA axis responds to stressful conditions over the remainder of the life course. This conditioning effect can be detected only during a limited and specific period in early life, which suggests that it depends on appropriate stimulation during a highly circumscribed window of opportunity in brain development (i.e., a critical period). Most important, once the HPA axis has been conditioned, the effects appear to be lifelong. In the study conducted by Meaney, rat-pup handling reduced total lifetime exposure of corticosterone—the rat equivalent of cortisol in humans—to the brain. Chronic overexposure to corticosterone, in turn, endangered selected neurons in the brain's hippocampus, such that the rate of loss of hippocampal neurons was reduced in the handled rats over their life span. Because of cognitive functions' sensitivity to relatively small degrees of hippocampal damage, the handled rats, by twenty-four months of age (elderly by rat standards), had been spared some of the cognitive deterioration typical of aging.

To fully test this hypothesis, the researchers tested these rats on learning and memory tasks throughout their lives. At age six months—full maturity for a rat—both the handled and nonhandled rats, when thrown into a vat of murky water, were able to find their way out after a short period of swimming. By twelve months of age, a clear difference, in favor of the handled rats, started to emerge in the time it took these rats to get out of the murky water. By age twenty-four months—old age for a rat—the difference in time to exit was threefold. Rats not handled as pups showed a progressive deterioration in their memory, cognitive processing, and learning performance with age; in contrast, much less deterioration occurred in aged rats handled in infancy (Meaney 2001; Sapolsky 1992).

There is a fascinating subtext here. The apparently simple handling of the baby rats meant in practice that they were removed for half an hour per day from their cages, from week 3 to week 9 of their lives—a protocol that involved putting them on a sheet and gently agitating them. At the time, the researchers thought this was the main intervention. However, the de facto intervention turned out to be something different. When the researchers returned the baby rats to their cages, the mothers, who had been without them, then engaged in extra licking, grooming, and other affectionate and stimulating behavior that was not offered to the unhandled baby rats. Subsequent biochemical studies have shown that, after the intervention, the handled rats showed a more adaptive, or functional, cortisol response pattern to stress: a low basal cortisol level, an abrupt response to acutely stressful circumstances, and an abrupt decline to baseline thereafter. Among the nonhandled rats there was a much broader range of responses, typified by higher baseline levels and a more blunted response to stressful circumstances. Thus, the cumulative lifetime exposure to the rat hormonal equivalent of cortisol was higher for the nonhandled rats than for the handled rats, leading to a sort of hippocampal neuronal damage documented by Sapolsky (1992) after chronic stressor exposure. Again, it is striking that when the researchers tried the handling protocol later in life, rather than during the critical window between three and nine weeks of age, it did not work. They did not see the prolonged change in the cortisol response pattern or the differential aging of learning and memory functions. This elegant study presents a model of a discrete stimulus occurring at a critical point in early development and affecting a basic biological function relevant to host stress re- sponse, defense, and organ-system aging—a latent effect that then had lifelong consequences for health, well-being, and competence.

A second series of experiments adds important depth to the story of early ex- perience and life course consequences as just described. By comparing the devel- opment of rat pups that were frequently, versus infrequently, licked and suckled by their mothers, Meaney and colleagues (2001) were able to elucidate a mecha- nism by which systematic differences in the function of the HPA axis emerge. They showed that licking and suckling initiate a biochemical cascade that leads to alter- ations in the expression of genes influencing the development not only of response patterns in the HPA axis but also of higher-order executive functions in the brain (Weaver et al. 2004; Szyf 2003). In colloquial terms, Meaney speaks about a "life is going to suck" pattern, wherein the less-licked-and-suckled rats end up with a more highly reactive HPA axis (good for fight-or-flight, but bad for sustaining learning and memory functions over time) and a reduction of neuron-to-neuron synapses in the cerebral cortex. It is a model wherein high-quality early nurturance leads, *through genetic mediation*, to a more tranquil HPA axis and a greater capacity for sophisticated learning.

Perhaps most important, these investigators have shown that the benefits of lick- ing and suckling can be transmitted from one generation to the next. This series of experiments began with distinct subgroups of rats that had histories of either high or low licking and suckling. However, when female rat pups from the low-licking and -suckling group were "cross-fostered" with high-licking and -suckling mothers, they experienced the same benefits as the natural offspring. Most important, they adopted the high-licking and -suckling behavior when they became mothers. In other words, a pattern of intergenerational learning was taking place that trans- mitted the more adaptive nurturing pattern to those who had been "predisposed" to the nonadaptive pattern. Taken as a whole, Meaney and colleagues' research gives a complete working model of biological embedding over the life course with respect to a key host defense system.

Lightman has further suggested (Lightman, personal communication 1999) that a hypothalamic "long-term memory" exists for stressful experiences. He described an experiment in which the researchers injected young rats with a substance that created a flu-like condition, whereas control subjects received no injection. At a much later rat age, they injected both experimental and control animals with water only. The controls did not react, but the experimental animals reacted in a pronounced way, as though the active substance were in the second injection. Lightman suggested that the hypothalamus, having processed the traumatic experience of injection early in life, had maintained the memory of that experience. Much later on in the life course, if something comes along that "reminds" the hypothalamus of that early experience, this event can stimulate a cortisol stress response identical to that seen in reaction to the rat pup's exposure to the actual event.

Suomi (1999) has demonstrated the complex relationship among nature, nurture, social mobility, and the life of the HPA in rhesus monkeys. He has shown that approximately 15% of rhesus monkeys are born predisposed to be highly reactive to stressors, in terms of both behavioral and endocrine/metabolic responses. The behaviors are not adaptive, in that they involve avoidance of novel stimuli, as well as anxious and depressive reactions to maternal separation in early life, which is a normal feature of rhesus monkeys' rearing practices. On the endocrine/metabolic level, the HPA axis is overstimulated in these high-strung individuals, with exaggerated cortisol responses to the routine stresses of daily living. Under normal rhesus monkey rearing conditions, high-strung youngsters often provoke frustrated reactions in their mothers that, in turn, increase the stressfulness of their early experiences. In adulthood, highly reactive males are usually low status, and highly reactive females are at increased risk of neglecting their offspring. However, Suomi has shown that arranging to have highly reactive rhesus monkeys raised by exemplary parents (i.e., ones with strong rearing skills) can transform all these tendencies: reactive behavior is transformed into vigilance on behalf of the troop; the HPA axis is stabilized; adult males tend toward high status; and adult females adopt the parenting styles of their foster parents, becoming much better mothers (Suomi 1999).

Interplay of the HPA Axis with Environments and Experiences Spanning the Life Course

Suomi's and Meaney's experiments illustrate the biological embedding of early experience on the HPA axis, its subsequent role in the life course, and the prospects for intergenerational transmission of embedded experience. These models, however, leave out the interplay of the HPA axis with the environments and experiences of the balance of the life course—analogous to human socioeconomic and psychosocial conditions. For this, we turn to Sapolsky's studies of free-ranging baboon populations of the Serengeti (Sapolsky 1995; Abbott et al. 2003).

From his intimate knowledge of the prior life circumstances of each baboon under study, Sapolsky defined four factors that lead to variation in basal cortisol levels in the wild. In terms of the life story of the HPA axis, lower basal cortisol levels can be thought of as the healthier state, in terms of a sense of well-being. These four factors are as follows:

1. *Rank*: When all other factors are held constant, an individual's higher social rank in the baboon community is correlated with lower basal cortisol level.

2. *Social stability and its enforcement*: When baboon societies are stable, those in dominant positions have lower basal cortisol levels than they do during periods of social instability. When stability is imposed by high levels of violence and coercion, the nondominant baboons have higher basal cortisol levels than when stability is maintained with low levels of violence and coercion.

3. *The experience of rank, stability, and enforcement*: When social instability occurs (as with drought or famine), some nondominant baboons will actually experience decreases in basal cortisol. This is because their relationships with those above them in the hierarchy are traditionally stressful, but stressful interactions may be easier to avoid when the more dominant baboons are preoccupied by each other, such as during fights for supremacy in turbulent times. Other low-ranked baboons, however, will do worse, as they become victims of displaced aggression perpetrated by the losers in the struggle for social dominance.

4. *Personality and coping styles*: Individual characteristics matter, too. Increased well-being results from the ability to distinguish seriously threatening situations from ruses and bluffs, to distinguish winning from losing a fight, to relieve stress by displacing aggression, and to develop friendships and strategic alliances. These coping skills are not entirely fixed at birth: They can be modified by the circumstances of upbringing and by mentorship in early adult life. Here, the potential connection to the findings of Suomi and Meaney is compelling.

Does the HPA axis truly have the same sort of life story in human society that it seems to among animals? Evidence on this point has been much slower to accumulate. However, there are at least seven lines of inquiry that converge with the evidence just presented. Two of these, the work of Lundberg and Kristensen, were described in an earlier section. An additional five follow:

• Gunnar and Nelson (1994) have shown that the quality of early maternal–child attachment (discussed earlier) affects both the HPA axis function and behavior, such that poorly attached toddlers have both more reactive HPA axes and less adaptive behavioral responses in social conflict situations. Early in infancy there are differences in cortisol reactivity that are associated, on the one hand, with differences in the level of attachment and, on the other, with infant behaviors that reflexively affect the infant's social environment. There is an important interaction between the individual's behavior and the qualities of his or her immediate environment. Attachment, for example, is under considerable social control, but the environment's failure to properly signal and set up the reactions of positive attachment in the child's HPA axis and brain means that the child will be at risk of missing significant social cues. This, in turn, can make the child less easy for caregivers and peers to relate to, which, in turn, can lead to deterioration of the child's immediate social environment, making it more stressful. This vicious circle, in turn, can have significant consequences for the child's social, emotional, and cognitive development.

- An extreme example of the situation just described is the plight of Romanian orphans studied by Gunnar and colleagues (2001). After some years of relative neglect since infancy in poorly administered, neglectful orphanages, these children have tended to become high-cortisol reactors and to suffer various behavioral disturbances—ranging from "psychosocial dwarfism," among children who never received minimal infant love and attention, to minor, and apparently often reversible, developmental delay in those only orphaned later and for a brief period.

- There are systematic social class differences in basal cortisol levels among both primary and secondary school children (Lupien et al. 2001). Early morning, prepeak salivary cortisol levels vary widely among children from different social classes. Lupien and colleagues found that in the elementary school population the early morning cortisol levels were higher in children from families with low parental income, education, and employment status, and higher levels of parental depression (Lupien et al. 2001). This was especially so among the children who "did not think that much was possible in their lives," an attitude that was more common among lower- than higher-SES children.

- The work of Kirschbaum and colleagues (Kudielka et al. 1998; Kudielka et al. 1999; Ockenfels et al. 1995; Pruessner et al. 1997; Pruessner et al. 1999) demonstrates that the biology of response to a single stress is very different from the response to the same stress repeated many times over days and weeks. These researchers measured the salivary cortisol response in an acute stressor test versus repeats of the same stressor over days and weeks. There were two very different adaptations to the recurrent stressor—one more functional than the other. The key factor discriminating between the two sorts of subjects was self-esteem. For men tested with their spouse present, they would tend to shift from a maladaptive type of cortisol response to a more adaptive response. Spousal support mattered (perhaps somehow it influences self-esteem). There were also correlations with hostility and a sense of "not trusting people in general." (Similarly, Kawachi and colleagues [1997] found a general lack of trust to be a common survey response in U.S. states with higher overall mortality rates.)

• Berkman and colleagues have been studying cortisol patterns in conjunction
  with psychosocial and socioeconomic factors in elderly populations (Berkman,
  personal communication 1999). Overall, there was cognitive decline in their
  subjects, despite the fact that all of them began the study as well persons with
  a relatively high level of functioning. But not everyone declined at the same
  rate. The researchers observed a steady reduction in the rate of cognitive decline with advancing age as they went from the study subjects with the lowest
  income level to the highest one. In other words, high-income elderly subjects
  had a lower rate of cognitive decline with age than low-income elderly subjects.
  Berkman and colleagues also have pointed out that at low income levels, being
  socially well integrated provided the elderly subjects with a buffering or protective effect in relation to the rate of cognitive decline; however, at higher
  income levels, the buffering effect disappeared. Most important here, these
  differences were closely associated with variations in cortisol secretion (Berkman, personal communication 1999). This is a significant, though complex
  model, bringing together socioeconomic, psychosocial, and biological pathways
  considerations in later life.

The Complex Relationship between Physiological and Social Factors Affecting Health

Taken together, the studies of different species suggest that the life story of the
HPA axis in socially positioned individuals parallels the socioeconomic determinants of health in human societies. Hierarchy and social stability are, fundamentally, characteristics of whole societies, although they may be inscribed either within
society as a whole (social stability) or in the individual (place in the hierarchy).
There is a parallel between the pattern of lower average basal cortisol in baboon
communities with low levels of violence and coercion; and research findings in
human populations that social equity, trust, and strong collective social security
mechanisms (Wilkinson 1992, 1997; Kaplan et al. 1996), plus shallow social class
gradients in health (Vagero and Lundberg 1989), are correlates of increased longevity. The experiences of hierarchy in times of prosperity and stability, as well as
in the opposite sorts of times—as manifested in the day-to-day experiences of
good times, as in a positive workplace and home life, and of bad times, due to
lack of control at work, layoffs, or long-term unemployment—are closely related
to "civil society" functions, which reside in an intermediate zone between the
individual and the state. Personality and coping styles are embedded in the individual, but they interact profoundly with the social environment over the life
course. The importance of the latter point has been reinforced by the work of both
Meaney and Suomi.

The preceding discussion has not been intended to suggest that the HPA axis is the only biological pathway from socioeconomic position to the systematic gradients in health status that emerge across the life course. Other pathways operating through perceptual mechanisms, such as the SAM axis, play an important role. Moreover, life circumstances may help create gradients through mechanisms that have no perceptual or cognitive/conscious element at all. For example, lack of food, clothing, and shelter; toxic chemical exposures in the environment; and repeated adverse physical exposures (e.g., demanding physical labor) can all have profound biological impacts without reference to perception. We suspect that, as societies become increasingly wealthy, the mechanisms that operate through perception, memory, and learned response become increasingly important in explaining how health inequalities emerge, and the nonperceptual mechanisms become increasingly less important. This issue, at present, is at the forefront of population health research.

Future Research Opportunities and Challenges

Transdisciplinary synthesis is very much the current challenge in this field (Sakata and Crews 2004). We need to find ways to integrate the tantalizing biological insights previously described into a more comprehensive, long-term scenario that will explain how biological pathways, such as those we have discussed, embed the health effects of various socioeconomic, psychosocial, and developmental environments in human biology. In addition, we need to determine how much any given "embedding pathway" contributes, and in what manner, to systematic differences in health status over the life course.

Above all, there is not yet an overarching conceptual framework through which researchers can integrate this research, and thus summarize and communicate it simply and clearly. Most of the existing PNE/PNI reviews, for example, have been written from a distinctly specialized disciplinary perspective—often biological laboratory based, psychological, and/or clinical—with inadequate attention to both the precipitating "upstream" social factors per se and the resulting "downstream" health effects, particularly when considered over the entire life course. In an effort to remedy this situation, we suggest that the sort of schematic depicted in figure 2.1 may be useful. It clearly suggests the need to design better longitudinal studies of upstream social environmental exposures/determinants and downstream health outcomes (the usual approach of social epidemiology), as well as a need to include in these studies specific biological measurements of intermediary pathways that link exposures and outcomes.

Figure 2.1 offers a conceptual model that posits six complementary research activities as essential elements that must be integrated in this intensely transdisciplinary field:

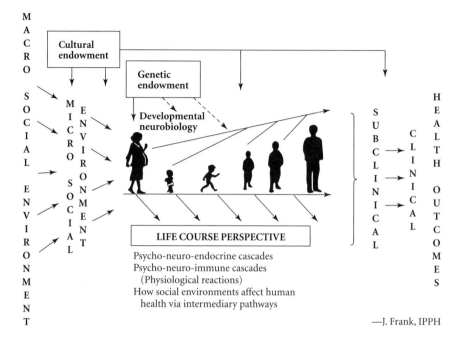

Figure 2.1. **Biological embedding in population health**

- Measurement of the key *social factor "exposures"* that influence human health—not all of which are attributes of individuals; some, such as the income or wealth of entire groups or populations, can be defined and measured only at the aggregate level (Wilkinson 1997; Diez-Roux 1998).
- Identification of the relevant *biological endowments* present in early life (presumably genetic and intrauterine in origin) that interact with such environmental exposures to codetermine human health (see chapter 1 of this volume).
- Measurement of the critical intervening, intermediate *psychological constructs/ reactions* that initiate the embedding process, of which some leading candidates are perceived control over work and life, feelings of being socially supported and loved, and self-esteem/mastery.
- Measurement of the actual *biopathways*—HPA, SAM, and PNI—that further "insert under the skin" the socioeconomic, psychosocial, and developmental factors described earlier (whether or not these reactions to the environment are detectable by questionnaires or exist as conscious constructs for the individual).

There is much technical work to be done here. For example, various researchers have extensively studied chronically dysregulated HPA, but they have viewed very differently the best ways of measuring the degree of dysregulation and, as a result, of identifying strong associations with individuals' elevated future risk of disease. International scientific consensus is urgently needed on the best means for assessing dysregulated HPA axis function in large epidemiological studies—for example, taking salivary cortisol samples at multiple times during the day to assess diurnal biorhythm versus using a standardized stressor-test response over some hours.

- *Epidemiological validation*, preferably nested inside large prospective cohort studies, of the association between perturbed biopathway markers and subsequent disease risk. For example, given the high cost of exhaustive biological marker measurements on large cohorts typically needed for studies of the etiology of chronic disease, there are design and analytic strategies (e.g., nested case-control and case-cohort designs) that can greatly improve study efficiency and reduce costs.
- *Biostatistically robust modeling of the interrelationships between all of the preceding factors*, explicitly from a longitudinal, life course perspective. For example, repeat-measures methods are available that can flexibly but robustly adjust for autocorrelations between exposure or biological pathway measures in the same subjects over time (Zeger and Liang 1986).

We recognize the difficulty of designing—and obtaining funding for—the sort of novel and potentially expensive interdisciplinary study that can prospectively validate these exact embedding relationships against both prior environmental exposures and subsequent health outcomes. Indeed, most epidemiologists are not yet familiar with statistical analytic methods for "three compartment" designs such as that suggested in figure 2.1, wherein intermediary variables' links to both upstream exposures and downstream outcomes must be modeled. Importation (from sociology, psychology, and econometrics) into the field of structural equations modeling is just beginning and may yet yield important insights. Certainly, we doubt the capacity of simple one-step risk regression, the analytic workhorse of epidemiologists for more than thirty years now, to meet this challenge.

We suggest that the key to facilitating this new transdisciplinary research is to increase the mixing of professionals from the relevant disciplines—including the basic biologists—during their periods of advanced training. This approach is perhaps best accomplished in postdoctoral work, when individual egos and professional identities are adequately developed to cope with the potentially threatening experiences involved, but before professionals' ossification in the ways of the respective disciplines is too far advanced. Of course, such integrated training programs will succeed only to the extent that meaningful collaboration with mentoring senior scientists is actually occurring. For such collaboration to become more commonplace, the creation of more explicitly mission-driven research centers, spanning traditional university departments, will probably be necessary.

To conclude, there is immense promise in the integration of the diverse scientific perspectives we have described. We believe that quantum leaps in our understanding of biological embedding can occur by fostering creative cross-fertilization and that these insights will be very useful to those in charge of both public health and social policies and programs, who seek to reduce inequalities in health.

Note

1. It is important to distinguish here between a model of the immune system's aging and an explanation for the causes of specific immune-related disorders that may be affected by aging. For example, there is evidence that increases in childhood asthma may be related to *reduced* stimulation of the immune system, rather than overstimulation. Although this may be important for explaining the current rise in childhood asthma in an era of declining air pollution, it does not detract from a separate line of understanding as to how immune dysregulation may unfold over the life course.

References

Abbott, D. H., E. B. Keverne, F. B. Bercovitch, C. A. Shively, S. P. Mendoza, W. Saltzman, C. T. Snowdon, T. E. Ziegler, M. Banjevic, T. Garland, Jr., and R. M. Sapolsky. 2003. Are subordinates always stressed? A comparative analysis of rank differences in cortisol levels among primates. *Hormones and Behavior* 43:67–82.

Antonovsky, A. 1993. The structure and properties of the sense of coherence scale. *Social Science and Medicine* 36:725–733.

Barker, D. J. P. 1990. Fetal nutrition and cardiovascular disease in later life. *British Medical Bulletin* 51:96–108.

Bateson, P., D. Barker, T. Clutton-Brock, D. Deb, B. D'Udine, R. A. Foley, P. Gluckman, K. Godfrey, T. Kirkwood, M. M. Lahr, J. McNamara, N. B. Metcalfe, P. Monaghan, H. G. Spencer, and S. E. Sultan. 2004. Developmental plasticity and human health. *Nature* 430:419–421.

Bennett, A. J., K. P. Lesch, A. Heils, J. C. Long, J. G. Lorenz, S. E. Shoaf, M. Champoux, S. J. Suomi, M. V. Linnoila, and J. D. Higley. 2002. Early experience and serotonin transporter gene variation interact to influence primate CNS function. *Molecular Psychiatry* 7:118–122.

Boyce, W. T., M. Chesney, A. Alkon, J. M. T. Schann, S. Adams, B. Chesterman, F. Cohen, P. Kaiser, S. Folkman, and D. Wara. 1995. Psychobiologic reactivity to stress and childhood respiratory illness: Results of two prospective studies. *Psychosomatic Medicine* 57: 411–422.

Cohen, S., W. J. Doyle, D. P. Skoner, B. S. Rabin, and J. M. Gwaltney. 1997. Social ties and susceptibility to the common cold. *Journal of the American Medical Association* 277:1940–1944.

Diez-Roux, A. V. 1998. On genes, individuals, society, and epidemiology. *American Journal of Epidemiology* 148:1027–1032.

Glaser, R., and J. K. Kiecolt-Glaser. 1998. Stress-associated immune modulation: Relevance to viral infections and chronic fatigue syndrome. *American Journal of Medicine* 105:35S–42S.

Glaser, R., J. K. Kiecolt-Glaser, P. T. Marucha, R. C. MacCallum, B. F. Laskowski, and W. B. Malarkey. 1999. Stress-related changes in proinflammatory cytokine production in wounds. *Archives of General Psychiatry* 56:450–456.

Glaser, R., R. C. MacCallum, B. F. Laskowski, W. B. Malarkey, J. F. Sheridan, and J. K. Kiecolt-Glaser. 2001. Evidence for a shift in the Th-1 to Th-2 cytokine response associated with chronic stress and aging. *Journals of Gerontology Series A—Biological Sciences and Medical Sciences* 56:M477–M482.

Gunnar, M. R., and C. A. Nelson. 1994. Event-related potentials in year-old infants: Relations with emotionality and cortisol. *Child Development* 65:80–94.

Gunnar, M. R., S. J. Morison, K. Chisholm, and M. Schuder. 2001. Salivary cortisol levels in children adopted from Romanian orphanages. *Development and Psychopathology* 13: 611–628.

Hertzman, C. 1994. The lifelong impact of childhood experiences: A population health perspective. *Daedalus* 123:167–180.

Hertzman, C., and M. Wiens. 1996. Child development and long-term outcomes: A population health perspective and summary of successful interventions. *Social Sciences and Medicine* 43:1083–1095.

Hertzman, C., J. Frank, and R. G. Evans. 1994. Heterogeneities in health status, and the determinants of population health. In *Why Are Some People Healthy and Others Not?*, ed. R. G. Evans, M. L. Barer, and T. R. Marmor, 67–92. New York: Aldine de Gruyter.

Hertzman, C., S. Kelly, and M. Bobak, eds. 1996. *East-West Life Expectancy Gap in Europe: Environmental and Non-Environmental Determinants.* Dordrecht, The Netherlands: Kluwer Academic Publishers.

Jefferis, B., C. Power, and C. Hertzman. 2002. Birth weight, childhood socioeconomic environment and cognitive development in the 1958 birth cohort. *British Medical Journal* 325:1–6.

Kaplan, G. A., E. R. Pamuk, J. W. Lynch, R. D. Cohen, and J. L. Balfour. 1996. Inequality in income and mortality in the United States: Analysis of mortality and potential pathways. *British Medical Journal* 312:999–1003.

Karasek, R., and T. Theorell. 1990. *Healthy Work, Stress, Productivity, and the Reconstruction of Working Life.* New York: Basic Books.

Kawachi, I., B. P. Kennedy, K. Lochner, and D. Prothrow-Stith. 1997. Social capital, income inequality, and mortality. *American Journal of Public Health* 87:1491–1498.

Keating, D., and C. Hertzman, eds. 1999. *Developmental Health: The Wealth of Nations. Social, Biological, and Educational Dynamics.* New York: Guilford.

Kiecolt-Glaser, J. K. 1999. Norman Cousins Memorial Lecture 1998. Stress, personal relationships, and immune function: health implications. *Brain, Behavior, and Immunity* 13: 61–72.

Kiecolt-Glaser, J. K., and R. Glaser. 2002. Depression and immune function. Central pathways to morbidity and mortality. *Journal of Psychosomatic Research* 53:873–876.

Kiecolt-Glaser, J. K., L. McGuire, T. F. Robles, and R. Glaser. 2002a. Emotions, morbidity, and mortality: New perspectives from psychoneuroimmunology. *Annual Review of Psychology* 53:83–107.

———. 2002b. Psychoneuroimmunology and psychosomatic medicine: Back to the future. *Psychosomatic Medicine* 64:15–28.

Kristensen, M. 1998. The LiVicordia study: Possible causes for the differences in coronary heart disease mortality between Lithuania and Sweden. Linkoping University medical dissertations no. 547, Linkoping University, Linkoping, Sweden.

Kudielka, B. M., J. Hellhammer, D. H. Hellhammer, O. T. Wolf, K. M. Pirke, E. Varadi, J. Pilz, and C. Kirschbaum. 1998. Sex differences in endocrine and psychological responses to psychosocial stress in healthy elderly subjects and the impact of a two-week dehydroepiandrosterone treatment. *Journal of Clinical Endocrinology and Metabolism* 83:1756–1761.

Kudielka, B. M., A. K. Schmidt-Reinwald, D. H. Hellhammer, and C. Kirschbaum. 1999. Psychological and endocrine response to psychosocial stress and dexamethasone/corticotropin-releasing hormone in healthy postmenopausal women and young controls: The impact of age and a two-week estradiol treatment. *Neuroendocrinology* 70:422–430.

Liang, S. W., and W. T. Boyce. 1993. The psychobiology of childhood stress. *Current Opinion in Pediatrics* 5:545–551.

Lundberg, U. 1996. Influence of paid and unpaid work on psychophysiological stress responses of men and women. *Journal of Occupational Health* 1:117–130.

Lupien, S. J., S. King, M. J. Meaney, and B. S. McEwen. 2001. Can poverty get under your skin? Basal cortisol levels and cognitive function in children from low and high socioeconomic status. *Development and Psychopathology* 13:653–676.

Marmot, M., and M. Wadsworth, eds. 1997. Fetal and early childhood environment: Long-term health implications. *British Medical Bulletin* 53:210–221.

Matte, T. D., M. Bresnahan, M. D. Begg, and E. Susser. 2001. Influence of variation in birth weight within normal range and within sibships on IQ at age 7 years: Cohort study. *British Medical Journal* 323:310–314.

McEwen, B. 1998. Protective and damaging effects of stress mediators. *The New England Journal of Medicine* 338:171–179.

McEwen, B. S., and J. C. Wingfield. 2003. The concept of allostasis in biology and biomedicine. *Hormones and Behavior* 43:2–15.

Meaney, M. J. 2001. Maternal care, gene expression, and the transmission of individual differences in stress reactivity across generations. *Annual Review of Neuroscience* 24:1161–1192.

Ockenfels, M. C., L. Porter, J. Smyth, C. Kirschbaum, D. H. Hellhammer, and A. A. Stone. 1995. Effect of chronic stress associated with unemployment on salivary cortisol: overall cortisol levels, diurnal rhythm, and acute stress reactivity. [Review] *Psychosomatic Medicine* 57:460–467.

Power, C., and C. Hertzman. 1997. Social and biological pathways linking early life and adult disease. *British Medical Bulletin* 53:210–221.

Pruessner, J. C., J. Gaab, D. H. Hellhammer, D. Lintz, N. Schommer, and C. Kirschbaum. 1997. Increasing correlations between personality traits and cortisol stress responses obtained by data aggregation. *Psychoneuroendocrinology* 22:615–625.

Pruessner, J. C., D. H. Hellhammer, and C. Kirschbaum. 1999. Burnout, perceived stress, and cortisol responses to awakening. *Psychosomatic Medicine* 61:197–204.

Ramey, C. T., and S. L. Ramey. 1998. Prevention of intellectual disabilities: Early interventions to improve cognitive development. *Preventive Medicine* 27:224–232.

Richards, M., R. Hardy, D. Kuh, and M. E. Wadsworth. 2001. Birth weight and cognitive function in the British 1946 birth cohort: Longitudinal population-based study. *British Medical Journal* 322:199–203.

Sakata, J. T., and D. Crews. 2004. Developmental sculpting of social phenotype and plasticity. *Neuroscience and Biobehavioral Reviews* 28:95–112.

Sapolsky, R. M. 1992. *Stress, the Aging Brain, and the Mechanisms of Neuron Death*. Cambridge, MA: MIT Press.

———. 1995. Social subordinance as a marker of hypercortisolism: Some unexpected subtleties. *Annals of the New York Academy of Sciences* 771:626–639.

Shenkin, S. D., J. M. Starr, A. Pattie, M. A. Rush, L. J. Whalley, and I. J. Deary. 1932. Birth weight and cognitive function at age 11 years: The Scottish Mental Survey. *Archives of Diseases of Childhood* 85:189–196.

Sorensen, H. T., S. Sabroe, J. Olsen, K. J. Rothman, M. W. Gillman, and P. Fischer. 1997.

Birth weight and cognitive function in young adult life: Historical cohort study. *British Medical Journal* 315:401–403.

Suomi, S. J. 1999. Developmental trajectories, early experiences, and community consequences: Lessons from studies with rhesus monkeys. In *Developmental Health and the Wealth of Nations,* ed. D. P. Keating and C. Hertzman. New York: Guilford.

Szyf, M. 2003. *DNA Methylation Enzymology, Encyclopedia of the Human Genome.* New York: Macmillan Publishers, Nature Publishing Group.

Vagero, D., and O. Lundberg. 1989. Health inequalities in Britain and Sweden. *Lancet* 2:35–36.

Weaver, I. C. G., N. Cervoni, F. A. Champagne, A. C. D. Alessio, S. Sharma, J. R. Seckl, S. Dymov, M. Szyf, and M. J. Meaney. 2004. Epigenetic programming by maternal behavior. *Nature Neuroscience* 7:847–854.

Wilkinson, R. G. 1992. Income distribution and life expectancy. *British Medical Journal* 304: 165–168.

———. 1997. Health inequalities: Relative or absolute material standards? *British Medical Journal* 314:591–595.

Zeger, S. L., and K. Y. Liang. 1986. Longitudinal data analysis for discrete and continuous outcomes. *Biometrics* 42:121–130.

Chapter 3

Global and Local Perspectives on Population Health

Margaret Lock, Vinh-Kim Nguyen, and
Christina Zarowsky

A great deal of research on the impact of social conditions on health has focused on popularizing the notion of "determinants of health." In contrast, this chapter is grounded in the assumption that neither biological variables nor social and cultural phenomena should be understood as *determinants* of health and disease. In taking this position, we are attempting to move away from universal cause-and-effect models to focus instead on both biological and social variables as contributors to disease causation, rather than as determining factors. We argue that, when trying to answer the question of why some populations are healthier than others, the problem is one of establishing what constellation of biological and social processes are most significant in specific settings, and of elucidating how these processes interact with one another in actual practice to precipitate specific outcomes.

Abject poverty and highly virulent pathogens result, almost without exception, in disease and death. But, aside from such extreme examples, both social and biological factors that produce ill health can be either constrained or exacerbated by the specific contexts in which they occur. They are therefore contributory and not universal determinants of the health outcome. However, we are not simply claiming that variables should be understood as necessary but insufficient with respect to disease causation. Rather, we are arguing for a more radical reformulation of ideas about the many factors so often thought of as determinants in population health research. Two approaches are particularly useful for rethinking determinisms. First, investigators supporting such a reformulation have not treated biology as a "black box"—that is, in effect, as a universal base over which social and cultural variations are layered. This approach is consistent with a wide range of evidence cited by population health researchers and is reflected in chapters 1 and 2. Second, investigators taking this approach have avoided bias and misrepresentation by recognizing that central concepts—represented by such terms as *social cohesion, social determinants of health, stress, family, class, race,* and *ethnicity*— must reflect the meanings, if any, attributed to them by specific populations and groups of people under study. This approach contrasts with that taken by many other researchers who, though well aware that such terms signify only working concepts, nevertheless proceed as though the terms are unproblematic because they permit easy systematization of data. That underlying assumption raises difficulties when such categories are "essentialized" and applied as though factual. It is very doubtful, for example, whether it is appropriate to use the concept of class when doing research in Japan or, for that matter, many other countries where ideas about hierarchies are structured entirely differently than was true in nineteenth-century Britain. Indeed, even the more encompassing terms *society, culture, population,* and even *biology* are not timeless categories but rather nineteenth-century inventions that we have come to assume are ubiquitous.

For example, most of the world's people do not use the term *family* to refer to a nuclear household or even to a one-generation, vertically extended household. Similarly, the significance of morbid events is usually registered in terms of their impact on locally meaningful social units (e.g., the household), rather than on individuals. Stress is a thoroughly modern concept. Although in numerous languages it is possible to describe sensations that closely approximate what we think we mean by the term *stress*, theories of etiology and the psychophysiological and social manifestations of stress like states are highly varied and are imbued with a wealth of different meanings in different linguistic settings (e.g., see Kleinman 1986; Lock 1990). Even those categories that appear unproblematic call for caution in their application cross-culturally. For example, although the importance of learning is no doubt recognized everywhere, the idea of receiving a formal education is not. In fact, pursuing a formal education can be perceived as a threat to the social order in many settings because participating children are not available for work; do not learn the skills needed for daily life; and, as the result of their exposure to foreign ideas may, it is believed, spearhead local unrest as they mature. Similarly "income" and "occupation" (but not "work," of course) are modern concepts that have had no place, until recently, outside capitalist economies. As a result, considerable caution must be exercised before assuming that concepts are commensurable.

We are also arguing for greater recognition of biological diversity than generally existed through the second half of the twentieth century. This shift would involve recognition that genetic variation among human populations is extensive; that lifestyle and nutrition affect individuals' and communities' physical health; and that dynamically evolving environments—particularly, rapid transformations in pathogens and toxins of various kinds—produce rapid changes in individual bodies.

In sum, appreciation of the contingency of local contexts—social, cultural, linguistic, and biological—is indispensable when accounting for health and disease in human populations. In the following discussion we build our argument by presenting three case studies about very different problems: female aging and menopause, the AIDS epidemic in West Africa, and the refugee experience of Somalis in Ethiopia. Before introducing the first two case studies, in which the relationship of biology, culture, and politics is focal, some further elaboration of our position is in order.

Interpenetration of the Biological and the Social

Research in medical anthropology has documented the role of culture as a prism through which symptoms and signs of bodily distress are categorized, interpreted, and acted upon. Studies of local and sometimes regional systems of knowledge for managing misfortune have shown how differing cultural logics influence not only how disease classification varies historically and among cultures but also how the natural history of diseases in individuals and populations may be affected (Brown 1987; Kleinman 1986; Kleinman and Good 1985; Lock 1980). On the basis of these findings it is legitimate to ask, even though pathology has always existed, whether or not specific diseases predate the cultural frameworks for their recognition and management. The strongest evidence for this approach emphasizing the interpenetration of biology and culture is found in connection with psychiatric illnesses and life-course transitions that have recently been medicalized as though their etiology is entirely biological. Moreover, there is substantial evidence that "somatic" disease entities—including low blood pressure, diabetes, Alzheimer's disease (AD), and various immune system disorders—are not universal entities but entities that vary in their incidence, distribution, and physical manifestations. By no means can all of this variation be attributed to environmental factors. Alzheimer's disease, for example, was "discovered" early in the twentieth century, then lost, then rediscovered, and is currently being reconceptualized yet again as a result of neuroimaging and genetic findings. The relationship between autopsy findings, long thought to be conclusive evidence of AD pathology, and specific behavioral changes in mental functioning seen in patients is currently undergoing revision. The reality of plaques and tangles in the brain of most demented patients is not in question, but their significance is.

In addition to the provisional nature of disease categories, recent research has shown that biological variation within and among human populations is considerably more complex than has heretofore been acknowledged, making any assumption about the universality of diseases and morbid events highly problematic. Two of the well-known examples of biological variation are the forms and severity of sickle-cell anemia and the distribution of the lactase deficiency enzyme associated with milk metabolism.

Changes in local environments, linked to the expression of biological diversity, are brought about as the result of local economies, politics, and shared cultural values. Frequently, political and environmental stressors—notably warfare, epidemics, or famines—instigate major change in which technological innovations are also implicated. Over thousands of years the impact of these social changes can be great enough to effect selection pressure on human populations, thereby altering the frequency of genes that confer susceptibility or resistance to environmental threats (Durham 1991). Typically, these social changes engender a host of cultural transformations that impinge more immediately but indirectly on human biology, either by restructuring local pathogen ecologies, changing nutritional options, or forcing exposure to unfamiliar environments. Recent work has suggested that local environments, starting with early attachment, can actually change the manner in which a common set of genes is expressed (see chapter 2). The time frames for emergence of the resulting genetic diversity may vary greatly, however. As a result, the biological makeup of each one of us living today—our individual genomes and the specific proteins associated with them—in effect represents a microcosm of the historical transformations that our ancestors have undergone. Failure to recognize biological diversity and its interrelationship with ongoing transformations in social, political, and technological complexes is a major obstacle to advancing research in population health, particularly in a global perspective.

Local Biologies, Biological Diversity, and the Experience of Menopause

It is widely recognized today that as aging populations become increasingly common throughout the world, research into the possible effects of menopause on the health of women as they age is very significant. Medical knowledge about menopause has been created in large part out of the symptom reporting and experiences of small samples of women in clinical situations, almost all of them living in Europe or North America. These women have visited doctors because of their physical and emotional distress, and many of them have had hysterectomies. These patients are not representative of women in general, and until very recently virtually no research had been done into the subjective experiences of samples taken from the population at large (to be discussed shortly). Medical knowledge about menopause is being produced and circulated, therefore, without reference to the lived experience of most women and is therefore biased, in particular with respect to the frequency and type of symptom reporting.

Survey research carried out with more than 1,300 women in Canada, nearly 8,000 in the United States, and more than 1,200 in Japan—all aged forty-five to fifty-five and drawn from the populations at large—showed that the menopausal transition was not a difficult time for the majority (Avis and McKinlay 1991; Kaufert et al. 1992; Lock 1993). Moreover, Japanese women going through *kônenki* (the term usually glossed as menopause) reported very few of the supposedly classical symptoms of menopause—namely, hot flashes and night sweats. Through extensive open-ended interviews with more than 100 women and other confirmatory exercises, Lock concluded that this finding had little to do with a lack of willingness to cooperate with the researcher, women's shyness about reporting symptoms, or the lack of a clear and unambiguous signifier in Japanese that refers exclusively to hot flashes in female middle age. Those relatively few Japanese women in the study (12.3%) who had experienced one or more hot flashes in the two weeks prior to answering the questionnaire were able to talk about them unambiguously. In Canada and the United States 31% and 35%, respectively, of surveyed women reported hot flashes in the previous two weeks, and the severity and frequency were greater than in Japan. Fewer than 25% of peri- and postmenopausal Japanese women reported that they had at some time experienced a hot flash, whereas approximately 75% of both Canadian and American women reported having had hot flashes. Similarly, reporting of night sweats was much lower in Japan. The difference between Japan and North America was quantitative, not qualitative, and it was statistically significant (Lock 1993).

Local Biologies, Embodiment, and Biological Diversity

The term *local biologies* was created to account for these differences in symptom reporting. *Local biologies* is not used to convey the idea that the categories of the biological sciences are historically and culturally constructed, nor does the concept refer to measurable biological difference across human populations, although this contributes to the argument. Rather, *local biologies* refers to the way in which physical sensations, well-being, health, illness, and so on are experienced differently, depending on evolutionary, historical, life-span, social, and individual factors that vary from place to place. In other words, *local biologies* refers to the way in which biosocial interactions produce local regularities in human physiology.

But in addition, subjective experience is influenced by how the body is represented, both by oneself and by others, drawing on cultural, medical, and political influences. These representations vary in time and space, and they are indispensable in shaping embodied experience and, above all, making it available to language and public expression. Over the past hundred years understanding about the body and its representation has increasingly been influenced by the biological sciences. This biologically oriented knowledge is now dominant in the West and is available and drawn on around the globe. Biomedical knowledge does not usurp local knowledge entirely, however; more often than not, biomedical knowledge is incorporated selectively among different communities, often with major modifications.

Here, we introduce the concept of "embodiment," which complements the term *biological embedding* as described by Hertzman and Frank in chapter 2. *Biological embedding* refers to the process by which systematic differences in lived experience can lead, over the life course, to systematic differences in biological responses to common experiences. Hertzman and Frank's emphasis is on how differing life experiences can alter biological potentials that are, in principal, held in common. In contrast, embodiment is the lived experience of the interaction of local biologies and culture and is, by definition, internalized and individualized. Each of us is unique in terms of both genetics and lived experience, and to this extent embodiment is personal. On the other hand, most embodied experiences are shared by us all—pain, the biological changes of aging (although this is inevitably modified by sex), fever, and so on. But even these most basic of biological events are variable, as many studies have shown. One reason for this variability is the uniqueness of individuals. Another is that some kinds of embodied experiences (e.g., living in the arctic or at a high altitude; having survived a major traumatic event such as the Holocaust or the genocide in Cambodia or Rwanda; being chronically malnourished) are relatively common across groups of people or populations who share particular environments, histories, language, behaviors, biological attributes, and values.

Biological attributes, described with reference to the concept of biological populations, are not contiguous with historical and cultural space or with self-defined ethnic groups but very often overlap considerably. Given migration since prehistoric times and the current accelerated globalization, biological populations are widely dispersed. Even so, until late in the twentieth century, most people other than those living near major historical trade routes tended to stay within a short distance of where they had been born, resulting in high levels of overlap between biological populations and human social groupings.

No simple one-to-one relationship exists between local biologies and societies, nation-states, ethnicity, or communities. Even so, lived experience shaped to some extent by partially shared local biologies may contribute to the creation of a shared discourse about health, distress, illness, and life-course transitions that appears natural and inevitable to those who are implicated. Taking local biologies seriously means that subjective reporting of symptoms and distress is less in danger of being exoticized and dismissed as "all in the mind." Patients are less likely to be labeled as hypochondriacal, noncompliant, or lacking in willpower. When local categories of knowledge do not correspond to dominant biomedical categories, the local ones can be marginalized, possibly resulting in iatrogenesis. But, in addition, paying systematic attention to subjective reporting across populations can highlight theoretical bias in research methods.

Implications of Variations in Menopausal Symptom Reporting

The very different form that menopause-related symptom reporting takes in Japan and North America is not fully accounted for even by the fact that *kônenki* in Japan is not understood in the same way as is menopause in the West or that experiences of these life-course transitions are shaped by differing cultural attitudes toward aging, autonomy, and technological intervention into bodily states (Lock 1993). The average Japanese tends to be more in tune with bodily changes than is the average North American, and the Japanese language allows speakers to make many distinctions about bodily states that English or French does not permit. It would be entirely out of place for Japanese women not to pay attention to hot flashes if they experienced those, particularly if flashes took the form that they do for some North American women, that of causing a great deal of sweating and sleep loss. It is probably safe to assume that the Japanese women who took part in the study tended, if anything, to overreport possible symptoms because of an eagerness to facilitate the research. The statistically significant difference in symptom reporting is best explained both by culturally informed values and by local biologies.

There is some evidence that a diet high in phytoestrogens, or naturally occurring estrogenic plant compounds (and in Lock's research, specifically, a diet high in soybean consumption), may in part account for the difference; but it could also be due to genetics, other dietary differences, the environment, and possibly other biological factors, together with cultural variables. One other finding of interest in this research was that Japanese doctors, when asked to list the symptoms of *kô-nenki*, rarely named hot flashes (although today they do, due to the worldwide medicalization of menopause). These physicians had alternative ways to account for changes associated with *kônenki*, including a theory about destabilization of the autonomic system (an idea that was introduced to Japan from Germany at the beginning of the twentieth century). Japanese doctors, unlike many of their European and North American counterparts, did not describe middle-aged women as suffering from a deficiency disease, and many were reluctant to prescribe hormone replacement therapy (HRT) to patients (although this has changed somewhat in recent times). Instead, a good number of Japanese gynecologists recommended herbal therapy.

Studies carried out in India, Indonesia, Taiwan, Hong Kong, Singapore, China, Korea, the Philippines, Thailand, and Malaysia, as well as among Africans living in Israel, have all revealed low reporting of hot flashes and night sweats, although incidence among these studies varied considerably (for a summary of this work, see Lock and Kaufert 2001; Lock 2002). In response, some medical researchers have suggested that the women who participated in these studies in effect biased the research findings. These researchers have argued that because individual responses to menopause are influenced by culture, inattention to hot flashes is essentially learned behavior. However, one could equally well hypothesize that little attention is given to hot flashes in many cultures because so few women experience them at all or so mildly that they hardly notice them.

If one accepts an argument for an inseparable relationship between biology and culture, it seems more appropriate to start out with this latter hypothesis rather than the one assuming, in effect, that the rate of symptom reporting in Europe and North America is the norm and that any deviation from this norm is due to a deficiency in culture. Aside from anything else, it is remarkably difficult to ignore the reality of hot flashes. Such an argument does not dispose of the insight that language and culture influence how symptoms are experienced; clearly, selective attention is paid to bodily symptoms, and this varies among individuals and is influenced by culture. But it is a mistake to set out by assuming that low reporting of symptoms is due to a cultural blindness to these symptoms.

Beyene (1989), in her work among rural Mayans living in the Yucatán, Mexico, where women have numerous pregnancies and extended cycles of amenorrhea associated with prolonged lactation and malnutrition, found no reporting at all of hot flashes or cold sweats. Moreover, it has been shown that Mayans have endocrine changes at menopause similar to those reported for women in the United States. We know that plasma, urinary, and vaginal levels of estrogens are not correlated directly with hot flashes. Changes in sweat rates, capillary blood flow, and deregulation of core body temperature provide valuable information in the laboratory about physiological changes associated with hot flashes, but these changes also do not coincide very well with the subjective reporting of hot flashes by individual women. The physiological mechanism of the hot flash, although better understood than formerly, has by no means been explained fully, and it too may well reflect local biologies and exhibit variation. Whatever is being measured in a laboratory situation clearly does not fully account for the experiences of individual women; but a "physiological determinism" tends to override subjectivity, and women are all too often accused of misreading their own bodies.

In summary, local biologies interact with cultural variables to produce experiences with and accounts of this stage of the female life course that differ from one geographical location to another. The dominant North American account, in which women's bodies are viewed through the lens of pathology, does not mesh well at all with the reality of women's experience (Avis and McKinlay 1991), and the fact that only approximately 15% of women for whom HRT is recommended take it for longer than a year or two highlights this discrepancy (Hill et al. 1999; Santoro et al. 1999). In the case of Japan, as *kônenki* has been gradually medicalized, the mesh between Japanese women's lived experience and the medical model has become even more incongruent. Globally, HRT has been recommended primarily to fend off diseases of aging, in particular, heart disease, osteoporosis, and Alzheimer's disease. The recent announcement by the U.S. National Institutes of Health (NIH) that they had decided three years ahead of schedule to halt the eight-year, randomized, controlled trial designed to demonstrate the long-term benefits of HRT came as a bombshell to many (NIH 2002). In terms of the population of post-menopausal women as a whole, researchers had determined that the risks exceeded the benefits of taking this medication for more than a few years at the time of menopause. This announcement, however, capped many years of dispute about HRT's effectiveness (Santoro et al. 1999). Moreover, universal recommendations for HRT have always been highly problematic in view of the fact that the incidence of heart disease, Alzheimer's disease, osteoporosis, and breast cancer varies significantly from one geographical location to another, making it highly likely that local biologies are implicated.

The next case study also elaborates on how biology interacts with social and cultural variables. Its focus is not, however, on subjectivity and symptom reporting but on the way in which inequality and globalization, mediated through local contexts of biology and culture, affect the trajectory the HIV epidemic takes among specific communities of people.

The Origins of HIV Epidemics and Local Biologies

Infectious diseases caused by "old" pathogens that have recently "reemerged" in new forms (Farmer 1999; Lena and Luciw 2001) and by "new" pathogens about which we know relatively little (see Garrett 1994) pose a major threat to population health globally in the twenty-first century. One prime example is the HIV/AIDS epidemic, since more than 35 million cases and 10 million deaths have been reported to date and since the epidemic is spreading largely unchecked in most parts of the world. Although it may be tempting to view HIV/AIDS as exceptional—as a disease that is overwhelmingly social because of its sexually transmitted spread—the renewed outbreaks of many kinds of infectious diseases (for example, tuberculosis, antibiotic-resistant bacteria, variant Creutzfeld-Jacob diseases [vCJD], West Nile virus, SARS [sudden acute respiratory syndrome], and avian flu) suggest that understanding HIV/AIDS as an exception is not appropriate. The emergence of these new—and non–sexually transmitted—infections is intimately linked to both globalization and local social practices, and they pose a threat to population health worldwide. Whereas social practices, initially in agriculture and animal husbandry, have always been the medium through which humans and their pathogens have coevolved, it now appears that humans are the principal force driving evolution in our global ecosystem (Palumbi 2001).

As a result, the study of how epidemics emerge must be a priority for population health research. Certain types of pathogens, such as RNA viruses, usually first emerge as significant pathogens for evolutionary reasons (Burke 1998), and advances in parallel computing and molecular epidemiology have considerably enriched our understanding of these processes. For some time, commentators have argued that it is important to understand how social forces permit epidemics to emerge, but how these social forces interact with biological phenomena remains poorly understood (Farmer 1999). In the following case study we focus on the HIV/AIDS epidemic in West Africa and contend that a shift in conceptual approach is necessary to furthering our understanding of the population health implications of emerging epidemics.

Origins of the HIV Epidemic: Three Theories

Consideration of three currently competing theories about the origins of the HIV epidemic can now be viewed with the benefit of considerable historical hindsight, and it highlights the interrelation of biological and social factors in the emergence of epidemics. Controversy over the origins of the AIDS epidemic was reignited with the publication of Hooper's *River* (1999). Using extensive fieldwork and archival research, Hooper argued that HIV's ancestor virus (SIVcpz) crossed the species barrier in the late 1950s through wide-scale inoculation of Africans with an experimental oral polio vaccine (OPV) allegedly derived from chimpanzee kidney cells. This hypothesis—the basis for what has become known as the OPV theory—has been countered with molecular evidence that diversification of simian immunodeficiency virus (SIV) strains had begun almost thirty years earlier. Therefore, most researchers view Hooper's hypothesis as implausible, since the polio vaccine trials would have had to separately transmit nine different strains of HIV to explain its current genetic diversity. In addition, it appears highly unlikely that SIV could have survived the processes used to prepare the vaccine, even if contaminated chimpanzee cells had been used.

A second theory, often referred to as the natural transfer theory, argues that SIV crossed the species barrier through "normal" contact between humans and apes, which intensified in the 1930s as a result of changes brought about by colonialism. As SIVcpz is tens of thousands of years old, this theory requires either that (1) novel practices increased exposure to simian viruses, perhaps through intensified butchering of bushmeat and/or (2) behavioral or biological changes in the human population allowed for isolated transmission events to trigger an epidemic.

Wide-scale disruption of indigenous African populations, with resulting famines, is thought to have led to an increased reliance on bushmeat for sustenance, thus providing a greater opportunity for SIV transmission to humans. In addition, the construction of the Congo–Ocean railroad by the French has been implicated, together with business-related practices in what was then known as Belgian and French Equatorial Africa (encompassing what is now Côte d'Ivoire, Senegal, and the Democratic Republic of Congo) (Headrick 1994; Chitnis et al. 2000). In these colonies, companies were granted concessions to exploit the dense rain forest for the production of rubber. The companies relied on native labor, and workers lived in appalling conditions, with the result that mortality was extraordinarily high. Forced-labor practices persisted into the interwar period, even though the concessionary regime ended earlier in the Belgian Congo. Devastating trypanosomiasis epidemics, as well as epidemics of sexually transmitted infections introduced by Europeans, spread like wildfire in work camps and wreaked havoc. Under these conditions the precipitation of a new, zoonotic epidemic (e.g., one involving animal-to-human communication of a disease) has been considered far from implausible. SIVsm, the simian immunodeficiency virus found in sooty mangabey monkeys who are native to the tropical forests of West Africa, is the putative ancestor of HIV-2, a sister virus to HIV-1, whose biological behavior resembles that of its namesake. However, research done in Sierra Leone, Liberia, and Côte d'Ivoire has documented an extremely low rate of transmission of SIVsm to humans (Chen 1997). As a result, investigators have considered as low the likelihood that a "natural transfer" of SIVcpz triggered an epidemic in humans.

The third origin story suggests that biomedical practices may have triggered the epidemic. Quantitative data on the industrial production of needles and their cost have shown that needle use skyrocketed in the immediate postcolonial period (the 1960s) before the unit cost of needles decreased enough to discourage reuse (single-use needles did not become widely available until the mid-1970s). These practices, argue this theory's proponents, could have passed SIV from an infected human to multiple others, amplifying the effect of rare cross-species infection events and selecting for more virulent strains (Marx et al. 2001).

All three of these theories—the OPV theory, the natural transfer theory, and the reused-needles theory—indict the social and biomedical technologies imported by colonial powers. Ultimately, whichever theory one favors, the origin of the epidemic coincided with social changes that initially accompanied colonization of Africa's interior—notably, forced labor, massive migration, and corresponding changes in sexual networks. However, these social changes cannot be considered independently of other widespread changes that occurred simultaneously and acted directly to bring about a worsening of the population's health. Famines, accompanied by epidemics of various diseases, resulted in an increased use of biomedicines and other biomedical technologies, including the equipment to administer injections.

Introduction of HIV into a population in some, and perhaps most, cases results in no epidemic at all, as has been shown by the retrospective uncovering of isolated cases of deaths attributable to AIDS in Africa, the United States, and Europe. Comparative epidemiology has shown that the course of the epidemic varies in different situations. The following case study demonstrates how correlating the spread of the epidemic in space and time with contemporaneous biosocial changes gives insights into how specific biosocial changes condition the emergence and development of the different forms that epidemics take.

Comparative Epidemiology of HIV in West Africa

Abidjan, the economic capital of Côte d'Ivoire, is the epicenter of the epidemic in West Africa. Through the 1980s, infection rates skyrocketed, and by 1989 AIDS had been demonstrated to be the leading cause of death among young men (De Cock et al. 1990). The current national seroprevalence rate of adults is estimated at 10.76%. However, rates in Abidjan are thought to be higher, and estimates range from 15% to 20%; of pregnant women attending prenatal clinics in the city, 13% are HIV-positive. This situation contrasts markedly with that in Senegal, farther west along the coast. That country has recently been touted as a success story for AIDS control, because an epidemic has never taken place. Adult seroprevalence is estimated at 1.77%; the rate among individuals who attend prenatal clinics in the Dakar metropolitan area is less than 1%. An intermediate case is in Burkina Faso, Côte d'Ivoire's northern neighbor, where epidemiological figures are sketchier due to its poor health care infrastructure and capacity for epidemiological monitoring. However, current estimates peg the adult seroprevalence rate for that country at 6%, which is also the rate for women attending antenatal clinics in major urban areas (United Nations Program on HIV/AIDS [UNAIDS] 2004).

How can one explain these differences in the epidemic's evolution? The Abidjan epidemic has been attributed to steep social inequality during the years of the so-called Ivoirian miracle, when the city was the hub of exchange in West Africa, a time when it was easy to make money, and the streets were lined with glamorous call-girls (Gould 1993). The role of prostitutes has, in fact, been repeatedly invoked as contributing to the epidemic. However, this explanation is unpalatable to some researchers both because it singles out prostitutes as vectors of the epidemic and because it is far too simplistic. Steep socioeconomic gradients (and prostitutes) existed elsewhere at the time—notably, in nearby Nigeria, where the epidemic, by all indications, did not achieve the same magnitude, at least until very recently. Epidemiologists have pointed to the role that migration, in addition to social inequality and sexual behavior, has played in the epidemic's spread in Côte d'Ivoire. Each of these contributory factors must be placed in historical perspective to get a fuller picture of why Abidjan emerged as the West African epicenter of the HIV epidemic.

Abidjan was established as a transportation hub for the new French colony of the Ivory Coast in 1903. The colonial plantation economy and the development of an infrastructure to service it constituted a magnet for enormous migratory flows during the colonial period as demand for labor skyrocketed. The city developed rapidly as a trading zone where the plantation economy's products were exchanged for imported goods. Its fastest rate of growth was in the period immediately after independence. Even prior to this time Abidjan had long been a multiethnic city of new migrants with little in common but the shared experience of migration and the colonial power's language and imposed cultural mores. After independence in 1961, social change was accelerated by urbanization and nurtured by the postcolonial state's vision of a modern, capitalist society. Not surprisingly, these social changes were reflected in interpersonal relationships, as the new citizens of Côte d'Ivoire increasingly identified themselves as modern city dwellers. Beginning in the mid-1950s, the state introduced an economic and social modernization program. Through urban planning and educational policies, an attempt was made to create a society in which individuals—apart from their ethnic identity—were made responsible for their own lives, work choices, and behavior. This policy came hard on the heels of earlier practices of enforced dependency and ethnic identification that had been enacted by the colonial state.[1]

The sexual freedom of Abidjan rapidly became legendary throughout West Africa, but this was less a reflection of an increased quantity of sexual activity than of the fact that sexuality became one of the ways in which individuals expressed their individuality. New amorous relationships, both hetero- and homosexual, were fodder for the popular press from the 1970s on—a form of sexual modernity that does not seem to have happened with the same intensity in other West African urban centers. The rapid emergence of these changes in Abidjan was associated with both its cosmopolitan nature and the booming economy that made it a magnet for so many migrants.

The collapse of the global market in primary commodities, including Côte d'Ivoire's main exports of coffee and cocoa,[2] led in 1979 to a profound economic crisis that lasted fourteen years. Incomplete building projects littered the city, highways ended suddenly, and gleaming hospitals stood empty, their equipment stolen and auctioned off. Entry into secondary school was severely curtailed, and these *goulots d'étranglement* (bottlenecks) created a generation of "deschooled" youth. The Ivoirian miracle had been transformed into a mirage and, with state downsizing and economic shrinkage, poverty became widespread. The wealthy, together with some in the middle class, managed to bolster their assets, with the result that social inequality increased. On the other hand, schoolgirls from poor families increasingly took wealthy, older lovers to pay school fees or exchanged sexual services for school grades. More significantly, structural adjustment programs forced the Ivoirian government to cut back public health expenditures and liberalize the health sector. Ivoirians, always avid consumers of modern (i.e., bio-) medicine, continued to seek out intravenous treatments as before, but in increasingly unsafe conditions: underfunded public hospitals and private injectionists alike often re-used needles to either save costs or maximize profits. Increased inequality and a culture of biomedical resort created a particularly volatile mix that would ignite easily once HIV was introduced.

Because Abidjan had been the hub of repeated large migratory flows, the epidemic registered quickly throughout the region, in part because of the extent of migration back to poorer countries. In good times, migrants returned from Abidjan yearly to observe holidays and to keep up social relations in their villages of origin;

in economically difficult times, reverse migration served as a safety valve for urban unemployment. By far the largest migratory flow of people was to northern Burkina Faso, a landlocked and arid country that had been integrated into the Ivoirian economy as a result of French colonial policies from the beginning of the twentieth century. HIV presumably crossed the border with Burkinabe migrants, igniting a major AIDS epidemic in that country.

Biological, Global, and Economic Factors Affecting HIV in West Africa

These social changes provide only part of the story, and biological factors must also be taken into consideration when accounting for the spread of epidemics. In the case of HIV, known biological factors that enhance disease spread are untreated sexually transmitted infections (STIs) and the absence of male circumcision. These factors enhance the risk of sexual transmission of HIV, and their contribution is thought to be more significant in explaining the spread of epidemics than are particular forms of sexual behaviors or practices.

The breadth of sexual networks is an important factor in determining the ability of an epidemic to spread through a large population. Broader sexual networks increase the likelihood that a sexually transmitted pathogen will be "seeded" into a critical number of groups of potentially susceptible individuals (who would otherwise not be linked to each other). For example, in North America, HIV was initially confined essentially to homosexual men because their sexual networks did not include heterosexuals. This pattern changed slowly at first through bisexual men's activities but then spread more rapidly once women became increasingly infected. The ability of a sexually transmitted pathogen to spread from such core groups depends on the efficiency of its transmission sexually. In other words, the risk of transmitting HIV per sexual act is also an important determinant of epidemic spread in a population, in addition to the density and extent of sexual networks.

Cultural factors alone do not offer robust explanations for epidemiological patterns of causation of HIV and its spread. Cultural beliefs may inform when people seek biomedical treatment and for what symptoms, thereby hindering or helping care-seeking behavior for STIs. However, the contribution of these beliefs is insignificant compared with economic constraints on access to biomedical care. Significantly, in the case of HIV, access to curative biomedicine represents an important route to treatment and to preventive intervention, making its availability crucial in curbing morbidity and mortality. A landmark Mwanza study showed that an intervention to improve diagnosis and treatment of STIs reduced the annual incidence of HIV by an astounding 40% (Grosskurth et al. 1995; Grosskurth et al. 2000). No behaviorally oriented intervention has been shown to achieve these results. Given this remarkable statistic, local differences in the public health system's capacity to diagnose and treat STIs, as well as that system's accessibility to patients, are highly robust determinants of health outcomes in epidemic settings.

To recapitulate, specific global and economic conditions are the most important contributors to HIV epidemics. They are implicated in the introduction of STIs into populations (as happened with colonialism and later migration influxes), as well as in a lack of facilities to diagnose and treat disease. Given that the availability and performance of biomedical facilities are largely functions of state capacity, the state's economic condition is a singularly important contributor in HIV spread. More diffuse cofactors, such as the nutritional condition of involved individuals, also play a role in conditioning susceptibility to infection, but these factors are usually independent of the state's ability to provide biomedical facilities. When, in addition to existing poverty, state cutbacks to curative biomedical services are instigated, a potential to greatly enhance HIV transmission exists in any given population.

A particular concatenation of sociohistorical and biological factors favored the spread of the HIV/AIDS epidemic in Côte d'Ivoire, and this contention can be tested by comparing the Ivoirian and Senegalese situations. Success at controlling the Senegalese epidemic has been attributed to the efforts of the national government, which deserves credit for mobilizing an early response. However, other factors must be considered. Senegal and Côte d'Ivoire were part of the same French colony and subject to the same economic and social policies designed to extract maximum economic return from the colonies. Dakar, the Senegalese capital, like Abidjan, was the terminus of a colonial railroad built to shuttle agricultural goods and migrant labor to and from the interior to the port. However, the migratory flows and the sociocultural transformations that accompanied them never materialized as they did in Côte d'Ivoire, largely because Senegal did not have a climate that permitted the development of a thriving plantation economy. As a result, the urban culture that developed during the late colonial period was not characterized by the ethnic heterogeneity characteristic of Côte d'Ivoire. Today Senegal is poor by macroeconomic indicators (almost as poor as Burkina Faso), but economic gradients are shallow compared with those in Côte d'Ivoire. In Senegal almost all the population is Muslim, whereas this proportion is less than 50% in Côte d'Ivoire and Burkina Faso.[3] Policies of strict control of STIs implemented in colonial times, particularly among soldiers and sex workers, continue today in Senegal, perhaps facilitated by its far longer colonial history and a greater degree of assimilation into a Westernized environment. In these respects Senegal is unique in postcolonial French West Africa. In Abidjan, sex and sexuality were more amenable to commodification in a city with a high level of socioeconomic inequality. The crisis of the 1970s led to an arrested modernity that simultaneously rendered large segments of the population socially vulnerable, encouraged a trade in sex, and decreased the availability of curative biomedical services.

Recent studies have indicated that HIV's genetic diversity is least in Senegal, indicating a relatively immature epidemic strongly marked, at the molecular level, by "founder effects." In other words, once HIV was introduced in Senegal, it saturated the most susceptible portion of the population in an initial burst, but then the epidemic did not go on to spread throughout the wider population. As a result, circulating HIV strains in that country resemble each other because they are the offspring of a common ancestor. There has not been enough on-going infection and reinfection to generate a significant emergence of recombinant strains, and genetic diversity is limited. This concurs with evidence that in settings of intense transmission, diversity increases and recombinant strains predominate.

Such contrasting webs of causality occurring side by side, in geographical proximity, point to the continuing pertinence of Virchow's view of medicine as a social science. However, molecular studies revealing accelerated rates of viral recombination under particular social conditions (e.g., when there is a rapid increase in intravenous drug use) have shown clearly that social behavior does not simply contribute to the incidence of disease but can actually change the pathogen itself. Given this situation, we can see how the notion of local biologies, introduced above, also captures the local and particularistic concatenations of biology, culture, and social organizations that condition disease distribution. This term has the advantage of emphasizing how biology and sociocultural phenomena, working in concert, differentially influence the incidence of disease across groups. Evidence that unequal access to treatment for HIV in West Africa may be contributing to the development of drug-resistant strains of HIV, a situation that will not stop at Côte d'Ivoire's borders, points to how global political and economic factors intersect with local forms of social organization to produce these local biologies. The need for a workably biosocial framework for understanding epidemics is underscored by mounting evidence that the HIV epidemic cannot be explained in terms of sexual behavior alone and by arguments that spread through unsafe injection practices may indeed be the major culprit in many parts of the world, including Africa.

This discussion of AIDS in West Africa reveals the extent to which biology, politics, economics, environment, and culture interact to differentially distribute disease risk. It also reveals the distance between conventional models—biomedical, epidemiological, or behavioral—and the much more complex reality of what takes place in specific locations. With this in mind, we turn to the final case study, which considers the difficulties of the cross-cultural application of several key concepts commonly used in population health research, and to the implications for policy making.

Refugee Experience and the Politics of Suffering

Refugees are the opposite of what we assume to be normal: They are on the move, they do not belong to any political jurisdiction, and they do not appear to have a stable environment, whether social or material. Yet one out of every hundred people worldwide is displaced, and displaced populations affect their host communities in manifold ways. Large-scale population movements affect local ecologies and economies, contribute to cultural change across wide areas, and, as is well recognized, are associated with important changes in patterns of disease and mortality. The fear of population movements triggers policies in Northern countries that influence both migrants and the host society—policies of interdiction, quarantine, protective custody, and arduous immigration procedures. These policies encourage millions of asylum seekers and migrants in Northern resettlement countries to live illegal lives that, even though hidden, nevertheless affect local labor and housing markets, social relations, and health conditions. For example, the spread of multidrug-resistant tuberculosis is, in part, a function of bureaucratic and financial obstacles to treatment, compounded by the rational reluctance of many asylum seekers to contact government officials. Almost all refugees and displaced populations come from and stay in poor countries. For example, 15 million of the 16.7 million refugees identified in 1991 were in "developing" or southern hemisphere countries. From the decolonization wars of the 1960s to the early 1990s, nine of the world's ten poorest countries each produced or received substantial numbers of refugees (Gorman 1993, 4).

Although most refugees stay in poor countries, they are significantly affected by the actions of the United Nations High Commissioner on Refugees (UNHCR), other actors in the refugee relief system, and Western countries in general. Refugee-producing and -receiving countries are connected to the world system through trade and aid. In the early 1990s, significant proportions of the gross national product of several such countries came from official development assistance: 31% in Tanzania, 43% in Somalia, and 70% in Mozambique (Gorman 1993). In the 1980s, when there were some 600,000 Ethiopian Somali and other Ethiopian refugees in Somalia, the World Health Organization (WHO) considered completely taking over the Somali Ministry of Health and contracting out services (Godfrey and Mursal 1990). Intergovernmental bodies such as UNHCR, the World Food Programme (WFP), the UN Development Program (UNDP), and Northern nongovernmental organizations (NGOs) stress the importance of collaborating with local governments and local NGOs and of consulting and empowering refugees (Forbes Martin 1992; Keen 1992; UNHCR 1990, 1991). However, most decisions about both immediate and long-term refugee assistance are made by Northern agencies, with little or no consultation (Allen and Turton 1996; Harrell-Bond 1986; Zetter 1999). This does not reflect deliberate exclusion of local governments but rather arises from a combination of ideological and administrative factors. These include assumptions about the nature of poverty, vulnerability, and conflict; unequal access among agencies and governments to funders and policy makers; bureaucratic inertia; the social consequences of initial technical interventions (de Waal 1995; Duffield 1992, 1999; Ferguson 1994; Summerfield 1999; Zetter 1999);[4] and the protection of individual NGOs' domains of influence.

The potential and real conflicts between institutional interests and humanitarian objectives have been recognized and trenchantly criticized from within the humanitarian field, particularly by individuals with extensive field experience (Minear and Weiss 1995; Keen 1992; Prendergast 1996; Rufin 1986), but the aid industry appears to be oblivious to its negative and even neocolonial effects (Rahnema 1997). The politics of pity are played out in many locations of the world today, and on-site action by donors and helpers is sculpted into remarkably similar forms. Regardless of local histories and dynamics, refugee camps and development projects in the "third world," plus mental health centers established in the West, are inevitably employed. It is therefore not surprising that superficially similar "refugee behaviors" are found around the world, but a closer look at refugee camps challenges generic models of refugee behavior and distress.

Trauma in Refugee Mental Health

Over the past two decades there has been increasing concern in the West about the suffering of refugees and victims of torture. This concern has most often been expressed in terms of these persons' mental health (Ager 1993; Agger 1994; Beiser 1991; Desjarlais et al. 1995). In a comprehensive review of the refugee mental health literature up to 1993, Ager (1993, 3) noted that "the first coherent attempt at the study of the psychosocial impact of becoming a refugee was represented by a number of researchers examining the psychiatric adjustment of refugees from central Europe following resettlement after World War II." This medical/psychiatric formulation of the psychosocial impact of forced migration has remained the predominant approach to research seeking to grasp the lived experience of refugees. The conflation of "psychosocial experience" with, ultimately, a psychiatric diagnosis has resulted largely from the institutional setting of most published research: psychiatric and other mental health centers in Western cities. As Ager (1993, 27) noted, "A coherent picture of mental health issues in refugee populations will only emerge when this imbalance has been redressed. There is an acute need for study of the psychological distress amongst those displaced *within* the developing world." Critical views have been expressed toward conventional refugee mental health research and practice (Becker 1995; Kornfeld 1995; Martín-Baró 1994), and the critiques have argued for a more politically engaged analysis and practice. Ager's review also supported a more social and political approach to refugee mental health issues.

However, such an expanded approach remains within the framework of psychiatry and psychology. It would not address the question of how the term *refugee experience* came to be virtually synonymous with *psychosocial* and, in turn, *mental health* and *post–traumatic stress disorder* (PTSD), and what the implications of this shift in phrasing and meaning might be for refugees and other involved peoples. Nor would it address the place of psychological distress and, indeed, the refugee experience in the lives of people who are or have been refugees, relative to other domains of experience and practice, including the enforced adoption of a refugee identity. Recent work has challenged the depoliticization, medicalization, and professional appropriation of misery that the expansion of the trauma model represents (Summerfield 1999; Bracken and Petty 1998; Zarowsky 2001).

For example, researchers studying two groups of refugees who had resettled in Sweden—one in a town with good employment prospects but no psychosocial services, and the other with good counseling and psychosocial support for refugees but no jobs—found that the employed refugees did much better not only economically but also psychologically, with less psychopathology (Eastmond 1998). This finding does not mean that work is more important than mental health, but rather it suggests that for the couples under study and their dependents, the relationship between meanings attributed to their experiences and individual psychopathology was influenced by fulfillment of expected gender and social roles and not through direct intervention on psychological processes. As the previous case studies in this chapter also demonstrated, attention must be paid to the various levels and relationships through which both meaning and biology are made.

Despite an acknowledgment of the structural pressures faced by asylum seekers (including uncertain legal status, poor economic conditions manifest in various domains, loss of social and interpersonal support, and discrimination) and an appreciation of cultural and individual variability, Western commentators focus on individual suffering in terms of the diagnosis and treatment of predictable symptoms of trauma and PTSD. Refugee advocates and mental health providers thus put into practice the frameworks implicit in most existing trauma research. A psychiatric model of human misery, disconnected from both interpersonal and macro political levels of understanding and analysis, has become dominant. Yet for Somali refugees and returnees in Ethiopia, these connections among individual experience, collective security, and political processes are critical. The trauma model is both scientifically inaccurate, in that it does not capture what is at stake, and of limited social and even individual value.

Medicine, Suffering, and Politics

Even as epidemiological thinking is becoming increasingly oriented to nonmedical "determinants of health" (e.g., health inequalities and the psychosocial environment [Marmot and Siegrist 2004]), political and moral debates in North America are increasingly being carried out in the language of medicine. This shift to medical language is reflected in the current Canadian anxiety about hospital waiting lists; in the history of PTSD; and in the ways in which medico-legal cases[5] are used to challenge the power of employers, large corporations, and the state. However, once in the domain of science and medicine, the use of scientific rules of evidence and the language of objectivity, neutrality, and facts are mandatory. Concepts such as PTSD that are the domain of medical experts become more important than the experience and voice of the sufferer; and political, moral, and social agendas are obscured (Tesh 1988). Although the outcomes of political contests fought in terms of medicine are not predetermined, inequalities of political and economic power are seldom inverted or eliminated. Among Somali returnees and refugees in Ethiopia, however, political legitimacy and power have not been sought through the medium of medicine but, rather, have been contested primarily in an openly political arena.

Somali refugees and returnees have taken it for granted that terrible life circumstances can cause individual unhappiness and even madness. To them, the obvious response is to do something about the circumstances or, failing that, to reinforce people's capacity to carry on. In the context of the re-creation of an ethnically federated Ethiopian state in the 1990s, Somalis found talking about their distress and their histories to be important, because it represented an attempt both to do something about their circumstances and to enhance people's capacity to carry on materially and emotionally: It reinforced local social networks and the community's political legitimacy in Somali, regional, national, and international arenas. Although many Somalis expressed anger and demoralization as the signature emotions of their "refugee experience," they did so without addressing those in a medical framework. In one small household survey ($n = 25$), for example, 73% of respondents indicated that at least one relative had died during the war, during the flight to refuge, or in the camps; and 61% had lost at least one first-degree relative (Zarowsky 2001). While a psychiatric model of suffering and the refugee experience would focus on the individual loss and trauma that such statistics indicate, in fact not one respondent identified these losses as the cause of the almost universal "poor morale" or, more strongly, demoralization *(niyed jab)*. Rather, they emphasized both the inability to envisage a sustained livelihood and the injustice of dispossession.

However, the increasing use of the language of development and humanitarianism in these communities suggests that the language of trauma could, in principle, become a new vehicle for expressing distress and pursuing political and moral objectives. Whether this language would be more effective in conveying lived experience and resolving the distress caused to these individuals and communities by war, dispossession, and destitution is another question. While a medicalizing approach to refugee distress may at times prove useful in providing a neutral territory for addressing what are often highly polarized issues, we need to examine much more closely the assumptions generally underlying the use of a medicalizing discourse. Recognition of the limitations of globally identifying refugees in terms of their mental (ill) health is important primarily because such discourse obscures the very real political, social, and economic stakes involved in refugee crises and refugee relief. Furthermore, this discourse erases the individual, as well as the collectivity, its history, and the power relations that are involved. Above all, it reinforces the commonsense view that individuals attribute meanings to their experiences and then direct those meanings inward and interpret them as personal, when in fact this individualistic type of meaning making is closely associated with European modernization (Taylor 1989).

The Somali refugee experience not only challenges many Western assumptions about mental health but also, perhaps more importantly, reveals some of the complexity of how meaning is created by involved individuals and with what implications for their well-being. The concepts of social capital, social cohesion, and community may well play the critical roles proposed for them in population health. But neither warm feelings nor modern Western civic-mindedness seems to be the key issue when attention is paid to the concerns of actual people in many of the populations under study. In Somalia, for example, security—of livelihood and of social and, hence, personal identity—appears to be much more important than community. Somali communities—geographically concentrated or mapped out over kinship networks throughout the Horn of Africa, the Middle East, and now Europe and North America—at first sight exhibit many of the characteristics to which the supposed good health of egalitarian societies is attributed. Yet the very cohesiveness of clan-based segments of Somali society makes it vulnerable to segmentation along clan lines. During and immediately after the cold war, in-group solidarity was manipulated for political and economic gain on a global stage. This manipulation exacerbated segmentary tendencies and culminated in the devastating civil war that destroyed the Somali state. Clearly, no simple lines can be drawn between social organization and apparent social cohesion, the meanings attributed to social life by local peoples, and the long-term viability of a population. Moreover, making linkages between the concepts used in population health research and local concepts of health are equally complex. On-site ethnographic research is probably the only way to bring some clarity to the situation.

Conclusion

Awareness of the complexity of biosocial configurations—the relationship among local biologies, social groupings, and dominant cultural values and concepts—can guide policy choices that are responsive to the particular dynamics of population health in any given location. Such an approach, one that takes contingency seriously, requires a knowledge of the relevant history and the application of an ethnographic approach in which the knowledge and meanings attributed by groups of people to specific events are recognized as indispensable data. For most survey research to be effective, it must be designed and carried out on the basis of local knowledge, language, and experience. Such knowledge is also crucial when interpreting quantitative findings. Without such an approach, there is a real danger of portraying a fictitious world after our own image, one that seriously distorts any efforts to introduce effective health policies.

Notes

1. Ethnic identities were ascribed by the colonial state as a strategy for managing the native population. Ethnic groups became associated with specific trades. Thus, who each individual was as a member of an ethnic group determined which strategies were available to people to survive in the new colonial economy. With the advent of an institutional modernity, who each person was as an individual replaced ethnicity as the primary determinant of how a person could productively participate in the economy.

2. At the time, Côte d'Ivoire was the world's first exporter of cocoa and its second of coffee; the country is still among the top three for both.

3. Many of our African informants have argued that Muslims may be less exposed to the disease because polygamy restricts sexual networks; such politically charged statements are understandably difficult to research.

4. For example, establishing emergency water-supply systems subsequently influences the social organization of getting and distributing water; providing medical care and food aid influences local economies and health care delivery systems (Abdulkadir 1994; Waldron and Hasci 1995; Zarowsky 2001).

5. This trend has been evident, for example, in efforts to secure compensation for PTSD, or the American class action suits against Dow Chemical on behalf of women whose leaking breast implants were considered the cause of extensive disability (CNN 1995).

References

Abdulkadir, A. 1994. *A Survey on the Repatriation of Somali Refugees to Northern Somalia from Eastern Ethiopia.* Addis Ababa: United Nations High Commissioner for Refugees.

Ager, A. 1993. Mental health issues in refugee populations: A review. Working paper for the Project on International Mental and Behavioral Health, Harvard Medical School, Department of Social Medicine, Cambridge, MA.

Agger, I. 1994. *The Blue Room: Trauma and Testimony among Refugee Women: A Psycho–Social Exploration.* London: Zed Books.

Allen, T., and D. Turton. 1996. Introduction: In search of cool ground. In *In Search of Cool Ground: War, Flight, and Homecoming in Northeast Africa,* ed. T. Allen. Trenton, NJ: Africa World Press.

Avis, N. E., and S. McKinlay. 1991. A longitudinal analysis of women's attitudes toward the menopause, results from the Massachusetts women's health study. *Maturitas* 13:65–79.

Becker, D. 1995. The deficiency of the concept of posttraumatic stress disorder when dealing with victims of human rights violations. In *Beyond Trauma: Cultural and Societal Dynamics,* ed. R. J. Kleber, C. R. Figley, and B. P. R. Gersons. New York: Plenum Press.

Beiser, M. 1991. The mental health of refugees in resettlement countries. In *Refugee Policy: Canada and the United States*, ed. H. Adelman. Toronto: York Lanes Press.

Beyene, Y. 1989. *From Menarche to Menopause: Reproductive Lives of Peasant Women in Two Cultures*. Albany: State University of New York Press.

Bracken, P. J., and C. Petty, eds. 1998. *Rethinking the Trauma of War*. London: Free Association Books.

Brown, P. J. 1987. Microparasites and macroparasites. *Cultural Anthropology* 2:155–171.

Burke, D. 1998. Evolvability of emerging viruses. In *Pathology of Emerging Infections 2*, ed. A. M. Nelson and C. R. Horsburgh Jr. Washington, DC: American Society for Microbiology.

Chen, Z., P. Telfier, A. Gettie, P. Reed, L. Zhang, D. D. Ho, and P. A. Marx. 1996. Genetic characterization of new West African simian immunodeficiency virus SIVsm: Geographic clustering of household-derived SIV strains with human immunodeficiency virus type 2 subtypes and genetically diverse viruses from a single feral sooty mangabey troop. *Journal of Virology* 70:3617–3627.

Chitnis, A., D. Rawls, and J. Moore. 2000. Origin of HIV type 1 in colonial French Equatorial Africa. *AIDS Research and Human Retroviruses* 16:5–8.

CNN. 1995. Jury awards $3.9 million in breast implant case. Accessed October 28, 1995, at http:/www.cnn.com/US/9510/implant_verdict.

De Cock, K. M., B. Barrere, L. Diaby, M. F. Lafontaine, E. Gnaore, A. Porter, D. Pantobe, G. C. Lafontant, A. Dago-Akribi, M. Ette, K. Odehouri, K., and W. L. Heyward. 1990. AIDS—the leading cause of adult death in the West African city of Abidjan, Ivory Coast. *Science* 249:793–796.

Desjarlais, R., L. Eisenberg, B. Good, and A. Kleinman. 1995. *World Mental Health: Problems and Priorities in Low-Income Countries*. Oxford: Oxford University Press.

de Waal, A. 1995. Response to William Demars' Waiting for early warning: Humanitarian action after the cold war. *Journal of Refugee Studies* 8(4):411–414.

Duffield, M. 1992. Famine, conflict, and public warfare. In *Beyond Conflict in the Horn: The Prospects for Peace, Recovery and Development in Ethiopia, Somalia, Eritrea and Sudan*, ed. M. Doornbos et al. (pp. 49–66). Trenton, NJ: Red Sea Press.

Duffield, M. 1999. *Aid Policy and Subjugation in Northern Sudan*. Unpublished manuscript.

Durham, W. 1991. *Coevolution: Genes, Culture and Human Diversity*. Stanford, CA: Stanford University Press.

Eastmond, M. 1998. Nationalist discourses and the construction of difference: Bosnian Muslim refugees in Sweden. *Journal of Refugee Studies* 11:161–181.

Farmer, P. 1999. *Infections and Inequalities: The Modern Plagues*. Berkeley: University of California Press.

Ferguson, J. 1994. *The Anti-Politics Machine: "Development," Depoliticization, and Bureaucratic Power in Lesotho*. Minneapolis: University of Minnesota Press.

Forbes Martin, S. 1992. *Refugee Women*. Women and World Development Series. London: Zed Books.

Garrett, L. 1994. *The Coming Plague: Newly Emerging Infectious Diseases in a World Out of Balance*. London: Penguin Books.

Godfrey, N., and H. M. Mursal. 1990. International aid and national health policies for refugees: Lessons from Somalia. *Journal of Refugee Studies* 3:110–135.

Gorman, R. F., ed. 1993. *Refugee Aid and Development: Theory and Practice*. Westport, CT: Greenwood Publishing Group.

Gould, P. 1993. *The Slow Plague: A Geography of the AIDS Pandemic*. London: Blackwell.

Grosskurth, H., R. Gray, R. Hayes, D. Mabey, and M. Wawer. 2000. Control of sexually transmitted diseases for HIV-1 prevention: Understanding the implications of the Mwanza and Rakai trials. *Lancet* 335:1981–1987.

Grosskurth, H., F. Mosha, J. Todd, E. Mwijarubi, A. Klokke, K. Senkoro, P. Mayaud, J. Changalucha, A. Nicoll, G. ka-Gina, J. Newell, K. Mugeye, D. Mabey, and R. Hayes. 1995. A community trial of the impact of improved treatment of sexually transmitted diseases on HIV infection in rural Tanzania: Randomised controlled trial. *Lancet* 346: 530–536.

Harrell-Bond, B. E. 1986. *Imposing Aid: Emergency Assistance to Refugees.* Oxford: Oxford University Press.

Headrick, R. 1994. *Colonialism, Health and Illness in French Equatorial Africa, 1885–1935.* Atlanta: African Studies Association Press.

Hill, D. A., N. S. Weiss, and A. Z. LaCroix. 1999. Adherence to postmenopausal hormone therapy during the year after the initial prescription: A population-based study. *American Journal of Obstetrics and Gynecology* 182:270–276.

Hooper, E. 1999. *The River: A Journey Back to the Source of HIV and AIDS.* Harmondworth: Penguin.

Kaufert, P., P. Gilbert, and R. Tate. 1992. The Manitoba Project: A reexamination of the link between menopause and depression. *Maturitas* 14:143–155.

Keen, D. 1992. *Refugees: Rationing the Right to Life. The Crisis in Emergency Relief.* London: Zed Books.

Kleinman, A. 1986. *Social Origins of Distress and Disease: Depression, Neurasthenia, and Pain in Modern China.* New Haven, CT: Yale University Press.

Kleinman, A., and B. Good, eds. 1985. *Culture and Depression: Studies in the Anthropology of Cross-Cultural Psychiatry of Affect and Disorder.* Berkeley: University of California Press.

Kornfeld, E. L. 1995. The development of treatment approaches for victims of human rights violations in Chile. In *Beyond Trauma: Cultural and Societal Dynamics,* ed. R. J. Kleber, C. R. Figley, and B. P. R. Gersons. New York: Plenum Press.

Lena, P., and P. Luciw. 2001. Polio vaccine and retroviruses. *Philosophical Transactions of the Royal Society of London,* series B 356:841–844.

Lock, M. 1980. *East Asian Medicine in Urban Japan: Varieties of Medical Experience.* Berkeley: University of California Press.

Lock, M. 1990. On being ethnic: The politics of identity breaking and making in Canada, or Nevra on Sunday. *Culture, Medicine and Psychiatry* 14:237–252.

Lock, M. 1993. *Encounters with Aging: Mythologies of Menopause in Japan and North America.* Berkeley: University of California Press.

Lock, M. 2002. Symptom reporting at menopause: A review of cross-cultural findings. *Journal of the British Menopause Society* 8:132–136.

Lock, M., and P. Kaufert. 2001. Menopause, local biologies and cultures of aging. *American Journal of Human Biology* 13:494–504.

Marmot, M., and J. Siegrist, eds. 2004. Health inequalities and the psychosocial environment. *Social Science and Medicine* 58:1461–1574.

Martín-Baró, I. 1994. *Writings for a Liberation Psychology,* ed. A. Aron and S. Corne. Cambridge, MA: Harvard University Press.

Marx, P. A, P. G. Alcabes, and E. Drucker. 2001. Serial human passage of simian immunodeficiency virus by unsterile injections and the emergence of epidemic human immunodeficiency virus in Africa. *Philosophical Transactions of the Royal Society of London,* series B 356:911–920.

Minear, L., and T. G. Weiss. 1995. *Mercy under Fire: War and the Global Humanitarian Community*. Boulder, CO: Westview Press.

National Institutes of Health (NIH). July 9, 2002. NHLBI stops trial of estrogen and progestin due to increased breast cancer risk, lack of overall benefit. [Press release] Available at http://www.nhlbi.nih.gov/new/press/02-07-09.htm.

Palumbi, S. R. 2001. Humans as the world's greatest evolutionary force. *Science* 293:1786–1790.

Prendergast, J. 1996. *Frontline Diplomacy: Humanitarian Aid and Conflict in Africa*. Boulder, CO: Lynne Rienner.

Rahnema, M (with V. Bawtree), ed. 1997. *The Post-Development Reader*. London: Zed Books.

Santoro, N. F., N. F. Col, M. H. Echman, J. B. Wong, S. G. Pauker, J. A. Cauley, J. Zmuda, S. Crawford, C. B. Johannes, J. E. Rossouw, and C. N. Bairey Merz. 1999. Hormone replacement therapy—where are we going? *Journal of Clinical Endocrinology and Metabolism* 84:1798–1812.

Summerfield, D. 1999. A critique of seven assumptions behind psychological trauma programs in war-affected areas. *Social Science and Medicine* 48:1449–1462.

Taylor, C. 1989. *Sources of the Self: The Making of the Modern Identity*. Cambridge, MA: Harvard University Press.

Tesh, S. 1988. *Hidden Arguments: Political Ideology and Disease Prevention Policy*. New Brunswick, NJ: Rutgers University Press.

United Nations High Commissioner for Refugees (UNHCR). 1990. *Guidelines for the Protection of Refugee Women*. Geneva: UNHCR.

UNHCR. 1991. *A Manual for People-Oriented Planning*. Geneva: UNHCR.

United Nations Program on HIV/AIDS (UNAIDS). 2004. AIDS epidemic update 2004. Available at http://www.unaids.org/wad2004/report.html.

Waldron, S., and N. Hasci. 1995. Somali refugees in the horn of Africa. State of the art literature review. *Studies on Emergencies and Disaster Relief, Report no. 3*. Uppsala, Sweden: Nordiska Afrikainstitutet.

Zarowsky, C. 2001. Refugee lives and the politics of suffering in Somali Ethiopia. Ph.D. dissertation, Department of Anthropology, McGill University, Canada.

Zetter, R. 1999. International perspectives on refugee assistance. In *Refugees: Perspectives on the Experience of Forced Migration*, ed. A. Ager (pp. 46–82). London: Cassell.

Chapter 4

A Life Course Approach to Health and Human Development

Clyde Hertzman and Chris Power

In wealthy societies, major disease in childhood is relatively rare, whereas adult chronic diseases are predominant. Thus, much attention is directed to factors in adult life that might predispose people to illness. This perspective, however, is seriously incomplete as an understanding of how disease manifests in humans. As we show in this chapter, many of the illnesses and disabilities that emerge in adult life, and the patterns of behavior and lifestyle that tend to be associated with them, have their roots in early life, even back to the fetal period. The health status of populations cannot, therefore, be adequately understood without recognizing health-determining influences across the life course. Without this longitudinal perspective, it is unlikely that we will be able to target the appropriate underlying mechanisms and, thus, design effective health-improving social or health care policies.

The field of population health has focused attention on socioeconomic gradients in health as a reflection of the powerful effects of differences in social and economic circumstances. Evidence is fairly consistent for socioeconomic gradients in health status among adults, with risk of poor health increasing from the highest to the lowest social positions. Yet, health gradients in childhood are less consistent. This observation may have obscured the life course contribution to gradients in adult health.

At the beginning of life there is a gradient in mortality in infancy, but some investigators believe that it disappears for health outcomes later in childhood, only to reemerge in adulthood.[1] In fact, the belief that the gradient disappears in childhood ignores a broad range of relevant measures of health and reflects a basic misunderstanding of the origins of the gradient that is resolved by adopting a life course perspective, as we later describe. The misunderstanding arises from the widespread use of conventional measures of health status—mortality and serious illness. Fortunately, mortality and serious illness are now relatively infrequent events, at least in developed countries; therefore, these do not fully capture either healthfulness or health potential in childhood. Alternative health measures—such as measures of physical growth, and cognitive and behavioral development—paint a much different picture. Furthermore, it turns out that these alternative measures in childhood predict health status, as traditionally measured, in adult life.

Social gradients may emerge during childhood as different levels of readiness to learn and of subsequent school performance; in adult life they emerge in differential rates of death, illness, and disability. Gradients in development reflect the influences of a broad range of factors in the family, neighborhood, and society, including the socioeconomic circumstances in which children develop. Socioeconomic gradients are evident for cognitive and behavioral development throughout childhood, from the earliest age at which they can be reliably measured in population studies—i.e., kindergarten age (Ross and Roberts 1999). Because cognitive and behavioral statuses are markers for brain development, these gradients have been interpreted as evidence of "differential access" to environments that provide adequate attachment, support, nurturance, and stimulation (McCain and Mustard 1999). In Canada, an Early Development Instrument (EDI) has been developed as a survey tool through which kindergarten teachers can assess children's readiness for school by using five scales: language and cognitive, social, emotional, physical health and well-being, and communication skills in English (Janus and Offord 2000). The EDI has demonstrated reliability and validity, and it is now being used in numerous communities, including Vancouver (Hertzman et al. 2002).

Figures 4.1 and 4.2 show Vancouver's neighborhood differences for language and cognitive development, as well as for social development. By the time children reach school age, large differences in the proportion of children who are vulnerable on each scale[2] (i.e., five- and sixfold differences) are apparent across the city's twenty-three planning neighborhoods, reflecting the geographic clustering of developmental and socioeconomic influences. These are very large differences, and their clustering has special significance. Children who are not ready for school obviously suffer a disadvantage in school performance. But it is also well known that the academic performance of a child with a given ability level will vary with the degree of academic readiness of the class as a whole (Willms 2002). Because children tend to go to school in their own residential neighborhoods, those from low-socioeconomic families will tend to experience both family-based risks at school entry, as well as "ecological risks" over time, based on the slower pace of academic progress in their neighborhood schools.

As the life course unfolds, gradients in cognitive and behavioral development in kindergarten are followed by gradients in school performance (Human Resources Development Canada and Statistics Canada 1995), which in turn are followed by gradients in literacy and numeracy in young adulthood (Statistics Canada and Organization for Economic Cooperation and Development 1995). This latter point deserves special attention because literacy and numeracy are important determinants of subsequent socioeconomic trajectories that have well-known relationships to subsequent health status. Furthermore, social gradients in adults' cognition, as indicated by literacy and numeracy skills, will influence the social and develop-

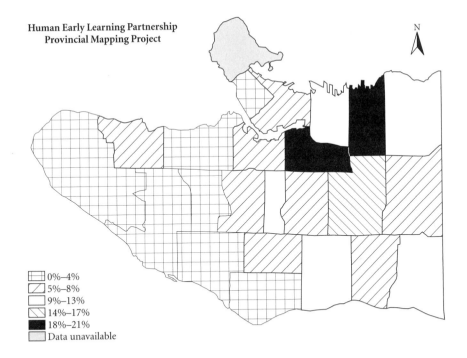

Figure 4.1. Language and cognitive development—percentage of vulnerable students in Vancouver, British Columbia

Note: Special-needs students not included; data from the Early Development Instrument, February 2000.

Source: Hertzman et al. 2002.

mental environments they provide their children, thus leading to the maintenance and reproduction of social differences in brain development across generations.

Other measures of child development are also illuminating. Physical measures, including birth weight and height during childhood, reflect patterns of growth in early life and hence are useful indicators of health status. These measures also show systematic social gradients; those living in more favorable circumstances are found to develop more rapidly and fully. For example, children in less advantaged socioeconomic groups are shorter, on average, than children from more advantaged groups: In the 1958 British birth cohort,[3] seven-year-olds from unskilled manual backgrounds were 3.3 centimeters shorter than similarly aged children from professional and managerial families (Goldstein 1971). Social gradients in height persist to adulthood, and these adult differences appear to be a worldwide phenomenon (Cavelaars et al. 2000). Shorter height in childhood predicts later coronary heart disease (Gunnell et al. 1998), as does shortness in adulthood (Marmot et al. 1984). The social gradients in physical development thus provide further evidence that socioeconomic circumstances in early life affect growing children, influencing their health potential throughout the life

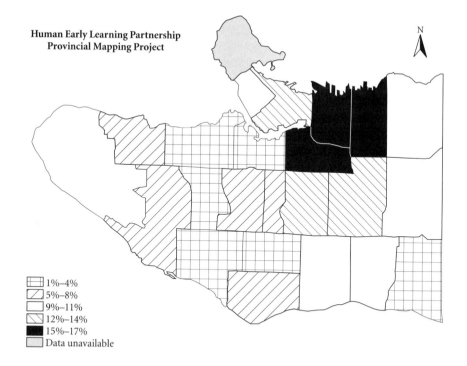

Figure 4.2. Social competence—percentage of vulnerable students in Vancouver, British Columbia

Note: Special-needs students not included; data from the Early Development Instrument, February 2000.

Source: Hertzman et al. 2002.

course. Moreover, socioeconomic conditions influence the health of individuals and, thereby, their offspring's physical development, once again reinforcing intergenerational patterns of social inequality (Emanuel 1992).

Gradients in child development may serve as success measures for whole societies. In 1995, Statistics Canada and the Organization for Economic Cooperation and Development International (OECD) conducted international comparisons and showed that, among wealthy countries, significant differences existed in young people's literacy and numeracy. In all countries surveyed, the offspring of well-educated parents showed, on average, high levels of literacy and numeracy. However, across the spectrum of parental education, large intercountry differences were evident among the offspring of the less educated. The slope of the gradient in literacy and numeracy among youth varied markedly from one wealthy country to another, as shown in figure 4.3 (Statistics Canada and OECD 1995). In some countries, such as Sweden, children of less-educated parents enjoyed literacy and numeracy skills similar to the children of well-educated parents. In other countries their skills were much more rudimentary. Overall differences in average literacy

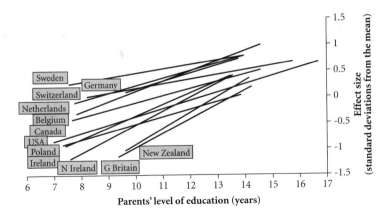

Figure 4.3. Numeracy scores for youth aged 16–25

Source: Data from International Adult Literacy Study, 1994, as reported in Statistics Canada and Organization for Economic Cooperation and Development 1995.

and numeracy in OECD countries were largely due to literacy and numeracy levels among the children of less-educated parents. The 1995 Statistics Canada and OECD study was significant because Sweden, the country with the flattest gradient and highest average competency scores, had invested much more heavily in programs and policies that supported early child development than the countries with the steepest gradients (Forssen 1998).

Understanding the Life Course

It is now well understood that life course factors affect a diverse range of outcomes, from general well-being to physical functioning and chronic diseases (Everson-Rose et al. 2003; Eriksson et al. 2003; Flouri 2004; Hypponen et al. 2003; Galobardes et al. 2004; Poulton et al. 2002; Keating and Hertzman 1999; Kuh and Ben-Shlomo 1997; Marmot and Wadsworth 1997). Exposure to both beneficial and adverse circumstances over the life course will vary for each individual and will constitute a unique "life exposure trajectory," which will manifest as different expressions of health and well-being. There are, of course, an infinite number of ways in which these exposure → expression relationships can unfold over time. In some instances, there will be contemporaneous exposure and expression. If, for example, a piano were to fall on someone's head, the exposure and the effects on that person's health and well-being would be simultaneous, unequivocal, and easily measured. But in most cases the connections from exposure to expression will be more subtle and will play out over long stretches of the life course.

The possible long-term exposure → expression relationships cluster into three generic models, which we label *latency, cumulative,* and *pathway.* By *latency* we mean relationships between an "exposure" at one point in the life course and the probability of health "expressions" years or decades later, regardless of intervening experience. One vivid example of such a relationship involves asbestos's elevation of the risk of various cancers decades after exposure to the substance has ceased. *Cumulative* refers to multiple exposures over the life course whose effects on health combine. These may be either multiple exposures to a single recurrent factor (e.g., chronic poverty or persistent smoking) or a series of exposures to different factors. An example of the latter would be the cumulative effects of exposure to respirable silica in the workplace with the tuberculosis bacillus, to produce the lethal silico-tuberculosis. Finally, the term *pathway* represents dependent sequences of exposures in which exposure at one stage of the life course influences the probability of other exposures later in the life course, as well as associated expressions. For example, the divorce of someone's parents in early childhood may reduce that child's readiness for school, which may in turn affect school performance, which would affect later employment opportunities and the socioeconomic trajectory throughout life.

Latent, pathway, and cumulative relationships will be present simultaneously in any individual's life course. The distinction between them is inherently difficult to establish. In what follows, we assemble evidence illustrating each relationship. Studies that collect data from the earliest stages of life and follow individuals over time provide the best lens on the relative importance of, and interaction among, these relationships. Accordingly, many of the examples used here to illustrate the ways in which the exposure → expression relationships can play out have been drawn from longitudinal studies. Prominent among these are the British birth cohorts that now extend from birth well into adult life. Although we have been foremost among those developing a life course approach, it is gaining currency among younger investigators as a way to approach the determinants of health (Pensola 2003).

The Latency Model

Perhaps the quintessential example of latency has arisen from longitudinal studies of rats, not humans. A series of experiments revealed that in several rat species, the degree of early suckling and licking of the newborn by its mother had a lifelong effect on a range of functions, most notably stress response, learning, and memory (Francis et al. 1999; Meaney 2001; Weaver et al. 2004; Szyf 2003). Maternal licking and suckling early in life influenced the expression of certain genes that regulate the development of the hypothalamic–pituitary–adrenal (HPA) axis. The HPA axis is critical to the regulation of the amount of cortisol, a hormone that a rat's body produces in response to stressful life circumstances. Cortisol has wide-ranging effects on body functioning. In the short term, it makes a rat more alert and ready to cope with danger. Over the long term, however, high levels of cortisol age various bodily organs. In the research, infrequently suckled baby rats tended to develop a permanently highly reactive HPA axis. Frequently suckled rats, however, developed a "downregulated" (that is, a less physiologically reactive) HPA axis. The implications of these differences were far-reaching. Having a downregulated HPA axis was associated with better decision-making functions, quicker task learning, and a slower rate of loss of learning and memory functions. Thus, the frequently suckled baby rats acquired a lifelong advantage (Francis et al. 1999).

Because of five features, this series of experiments stands as a quintessential example of latency. First, licking and suckling could influence HPA axis functioning only during a highly circumscribed critical period early in the development of the rat brain. Variations in licking and suckling later in life had no similar effects. Second, the effects of licking and suckling could be traced to the development of a biological system (i.e., the HPA axis) that functions throughout life. Third, the cortisol secretion pattern, once established, proved permanent; the effects on the biological system appeared to be irreversible. Fourth, the principal effects on health and well-being were expressed later in life, not when the exposure to licking and suckling occurred. Finally, the experimental rats were of common genetic heritage and had the same diet and surroundings. Confounding variables that might have influenced the effects on health and well-being had been excluded by design.

Such experimental control of human beings is, of course, rather more difficult, so that unambiguous latency relationships are inherently more difficult to demonstrate. There is, however, ample evidence that the human brain does have critical periods, during which experience shapes brain structure and affects brain function (Cynader and Frost 1999). And the brain may not be the only organ vulnerable to deprivation during critical periods. Nutritional deprivation in early life may compromise the development and function of other vital organs, thus affecting health in later life (Harding 2001).

There are, however, few longitudinal studies of humans that could unequivocally identify latency relationships, for reasons already noted. Instead, we rely on natural experiments, wherein the exposure, or "insult," is dramatic enough to stand out from normal human experience and, in some cases, can be ascertained retrospectively. Examples include the following:

- Serious congenital cataracts must be treated surgically within the first three months of life if eyesight is to be fully recovered. This is because the parts of the brain that process visual information and connect it to other sensing and cognitive functions need to be stimulated by visual input early in life to develop optimally (Cynader and Frost 1999). Depriving the individual of visual input later in life (i.e., after the critical period) does not give rise to visual defects (Taylor 1998).

- The last winter of World War II (1944–1945) was a time of acute food shortages for the people of the Netherlands and has come to be known as the Dutch Hunger Winter. Studies of offspring who were in gestation during the Dutch Hunger Winter showed that maternal nutritional deficiency in pregnancy was associated with an increased risk of antisocial personality disorder (ASPD) and schizophrenia among offspring in their adult life (Neugebauer et al. 1999; Susser et al. 1996). These effects appeared to depend on the timing of prenatal insult: Men exposed to severe maternal nutritional deficiency during the first and/or second trimesters of pregnancy had a risk of ASPD 2.5 times that of men who had not been exposed prenatally (Neugebauer et al. 1999).
- Individuals born during the harvest season in Gambia were found to have lower rates of premature mortality (i.e., by age fifty) by approximately one-third, compared with those born during the hungry season. These differences, which were especially marked for conditions dependent on immune responses, appeared to be due to prenatal, rather than postnatal, influences (Moore et al. 1999). In particular, those born during the hungry season were deprived of nutrition in utero during the sensitive period in the immune system's development, whereas those born during the harvest season, due to the timing of the sensitive period, were not.
- In the "fetal origins hypothesis," Barker (1990) posited that several chronic diseases in adult life originate from permanent changes in the structure, physiology, and metabolism of the fetal body as an adaptation to undernutrition. Studies of British records from early in the twentieth century have shown associations of birth weight, placenta size, and weight gain in the first year of life with cardiovascular disease in the fifth decade (Barker 1997). Evidence of the relationship between birth weight and cardiovascular risk factors, such as hypertension, has now been found in many populations (Huxley et al. 2000).

The Cumulative Model

Exposures to risk factors (and protective factors) may cumulate over the life course. In some cases, this cumulation will act in a dose-response manner. This is a common pattern in occupational and environmental health; the health effects of exposure to a toxic substance usually increase with the duration and intensity of exposure. Another variant would see different factors over the life course add to effects of factors from early life. This might be described as a "multiple factor additive" variant. Finally, we might also expect interactive effects, in which a particular health outcome depends on the coexistence of risk factors that are specific for the disease in question with life course factors that either reduce or exaggerate the disease-specific risk factors' influence on the disease outcome.

EVIDENCE ON THE EFFECTS OF EXPOSURE DURATION

Duration of exposure to particular socioeconomic circumstances has been shown to have a cumulative effect on several health outcomes in adulthood. For instance, in the 1958 British birth cohort, occupational class over the first three decades of life was found to be strongly predictive of health status in early adulthood (Power et al. 1999). Figure 4.4 shows a dramatic direct relationship between the risk of poor health and a score that is constructed by combining occupational status at four points in the life course (with the lowest scores indicating continuous high occupational status and vice versa). The lifetime score represents cumulative duration and intensity of material/social privilege or deprivation. Those always in the lowest occupational class were approximately four times as likely to report poor health as those who were always in the highest. "Lifetime" occupational class is a stronger predictor of poor health than occupational class at any single point in time, indicating that duration of exposure to poor socioeconomic circumstances matters a great deal. Moreover, for both men and women the risk increases monotonically with increasing lifetime scores (fig. 4.4). In other words, circumstances at each life stage build on one another.

Duration effects in midlife were found in the Alameda County Study in the

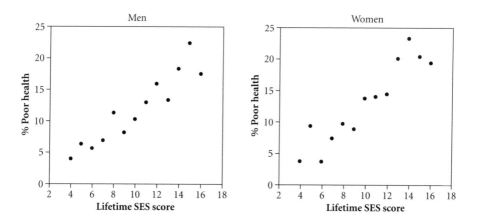

Figure 4.4. Poor health[a] at age 33 and cumulative socioeconomic circumstances (birth to age 33)
[a] includes subjects who rated their health as fair

Note: The lifetime socioeconomic score (SES) is derived from parental occupational class at birth and age 16 and from own occupational class at ages 23 and 33. A score of 4 represents the most favorable lifetime social position (i.e., classes I and II on all four occasions) and a score of 16 represents the least favorable circumstances (i.e., classes IV and V on all four occasions).

Source: Power et al. 1999.

United States (Lynch et al. 1997). Compared with subjects without economic hardship, low-income subjects were found on three occasions during an eighteen-year period (1965 to 1983) to have been more likely to have difficulties with instrumental activities of daily living (such as cooking, shopping, and managing money), with activities of daily living (such as walking, eating, dressing, and using the toilet), and with clinical depression. In each case the risk for people with sustained economic hardship was more than three times that of people without hardship (fig. 4.5). Other research showed that duration of exposure to adverse socioeconomic circumstances affected childhood growth, with persistent poverty increasing the risk of childhood stunting (low height for age) and wasting (low weight for age), whereas single-year income measures did not (Miller and Korenman 1994).

Duration of exposure to low income has also been shown to be related to mortality in adults. A seventeen-year follow-up of adults aged forty-five to sixty-four from the U.S. Panel Study of Income Dynamics showed that mortality rates gradually increased from top to bottom across the full range of income, using a measure of income persistence (McDonough et al. 1997). The odds for premature mortality were more than three times higher for those in persistent poverty than for those in persistent affluence (table 4.1). Also, the British Regional Heart Study found a significant relationship between the relative odds (adjusted for age) of myocardial infarction in men and a measure of lifetime occupational class. The odds ratio for men in the manual occupational class both at birth and in adulthood was 1.7

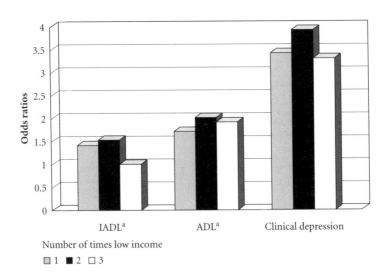

Figure 4.5. Odds ratios for reduced physical and psychological function and sustained hardship, 1965–1983

[a] = IADL: independent activities of daily living; ADL: activities of daily living.

Source: Lynch et al. 1997.

Table 4.1. All-cause mortality 45–64 years, by income persistence and income
level and drop: Panel Study of Income Dynamics, 1972–1989

Income persistence, 1993 $	Odds ratio[a] (n = 32,622)[b]	95% CI[c]
<20,000 4–5 y and never>70,000	3.54	2.34, 5.32
<20,000 1–3 y and never>70,000	2.51	1.45, 4.34
Always 20,000–70,000	1.51	0.96, 2.37
70,000 1–3 y and never <20,000	1.06	0.61, 1.84
>70,000 4–5 y and never <20,000	1.00	. . .

[a] Odds ratios (ORs) are adjusted for age, sex, race, family size, and period.
[b] Indicates number of persons, by 5-year periods.
[c] Confidence interval.
Source: McDonough et al. 1997.

(compared with 1.0 for men in nonmanual classes at both points in time (Wannamethee et al. 1996).

EVIDENCE ON MULTIPLE-FACTOR ADDITIVE EFFECTS

There is also evidence to suggest that factors from across the life course have independent but additive effects on health outcomes. The literature abounds with examples of multivariable studies in which several factors are seen to play a role in predicting a health outcome; typically these factors represent influences at different life stages. Several such analyses have shown that height, education, and adult life exposures (predominantly risky health behaviors) all contribute to cardiovascular risk status and disease outcome (Brunner et al. 1996; Marmot and Wadsworth 1997; Blane et al. 1996; Wannamethee et al. 1996). Similarly, in the 1958 British birth cohort, chronic illness and disability at age thirty-three were predicted by factors in early life (childhood socioeconomic disadvantage and height), in adolescence (behavioral adjustment), and in adult life (injury and underweight/overweight) (Power et al. 2000). Lifetime risks for middle-aged women in the 1946 birth cohort were also demonstrated for urinary incontinence. Having had childhood enuresis, having borne a child, and being overweight in adulthood each played an independent role in the women's risk of experiencing severe incontinence (Kuh et al. 1999).

EVIDENCE ON INTERACTIVE EFFECTS

In a third variant of cumulative life course patterns, health outcomes are affected by the interaction of factors at different life stages. The original formulation of the fetal origins hypothesis (noted earlier) emphasized poor nutrition that inhibited fetal growth as the primary influence on adult chronic disease (Barker 1990). However, we now understand that fetal growth is especially important when interacting with growth and weight gain during childhood. For example, in a cohort of men born in Helsinki between 1924 and 1933, death from coronary heart disease between 1971 and 1995 was related to size at birth (indicated by ponderal index [PI])[4] and body mass index (BMI) at age eleven. Compared with men with the highest PI at birth and lowest BMI at age eleven, men with the lowest PI at birth and highest BMI at age eleven had a 5.3-fold risk of coronary death (Eriksson et al. 1999). Table 4.2 shows that the effects of the risk factors were multiplicative rather than additive. Other work has shown that the risk of adult diseases such as diabetes and high blood pressure, which are associated with poor early growth, depends also on the presence of other conditions in adult life—in particular, obesity (Frankel et al. 1996; Leon et al. 1996). Rutter (1991) used the term "chains of risk," in which several intervening links in a chain are required before long-term sequelae become manifest. If any link in the chain is missing, adverse outcomes may not materialize. For example, one study showed that the adverse effects on psychosocial health of having been reared in an institution depended on whether individuals subsequently had supportive marriages. Such marriages were found to ameliorate the effects of childhood institutional care (Rutter et al. 1990).

The Pathways Model

In the pathways model, early events influence the life course trajectory leading to particular social destinations, and it is these destinations that influence health outcome. In other words, early events may have no particular significance for health outcome, other than in their role of affecting where an individual ends up in the socioeconomic hierarchy. Thus, early life influences in this model act, for example, through the development of cognitive and behavioral resources that are crucial at subsequent transitions, such as at the point of school or labor market entry. The following points describe a succession of events along the major pathways from early circumstances to adult health status, as illustrated in figure 4.6.

Table 4.2. Coronary heart disease in Finnish men born 1924–1933

PI[a] at birth	BMI[b] at age 11			
	≤15.5	−16.5	−17.5	>17.5
≤25	2.7	3.3	3.7	5.3
−27	1.5	3.2	4.0	2.7
−29	2.2	1.6	1.8	3.2
>29	1.0	1.7	1.5	1.9

Note: Coronary heart disease is reflected in terms of hazard ratios for death.
[a]PI = ponderal index, in terms of kg/m³.
[b]BMI = body mass index.
Source: Adapted from Eriksson et al. 1999.

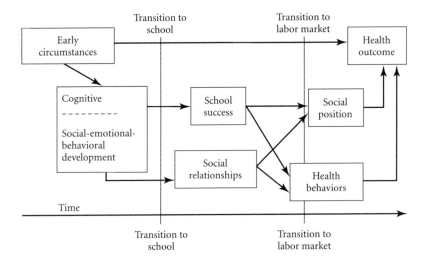

Figure 4.6. **Latency and pathway effects**

- At first, early life social origins influence readiness for school. Studies among preschool-aged children in Canada and the United States have demonstrated that early circumstances of the family (income, education, single parenthood, and parenting style), neighborhood (safety, cohesion, and socioeconomic ghettoization), and social institutions (access to "quality" child care arrangements) are powerful determinants of cognitive and behavioral development (Kohen et al. 2002; Duncan and Brooks-Gunn 1997; Leventhal and Brooks-Gunn 2003; Curtis et al. 2004).
- Cognitive, emotional, and behavioral readiness for school have consequences for school success and social adjustment. School readiness, as measured by cognitive and social–emotional competencies, is important because children who are not ready for school are more likely to experience school failure, conditions of unemployment, criminality (Tremblay et al. 1992), and psychological morbidity in young adulthood (Power et al. 1991). Longitudinal studies of behavioral development (Tremblay et al. 1992) show that physically aggressive behavior in situations of social conflict is at its most prevalent by age two. Thereafter, most, but not all, children learn to control their physically aggressive impulses and transform them into verbal negotiations. Tremblay (1999) has demonstrated that those who have not completed this developmental task by school age are at high risk of both grade failure and antisocial behavior by adolescence. Intervention studies demonstrate that improvements in the childhood environment can have a long-lasting benefit on an individual's life course trajectory (Hertzman and Wiens 1996). The Perry Preschool Project, a randomized controlled trial in a poor ghettoized neighborhood in the Detroit area, demonstrated that an intensive child-care and home-visiting

intervention at ages three and four could improve high school graduation rates, reduce teenage pregnancy, increase income, reduce dependence on social services, and reduce criminal activity by age twenty-seven among socially disadvantaged children (Schweinhart et al. 1993). From the standpoint of the pathway model, the most interesting observation was that the long-term benefits seemed to accrue from the manner in which the intervention improved the children's transition to school (Schweinhart et al. 1993).

- Next along the pathway, there is abundant evidence that people with a poorer education have more harmful health-related behaviors than those with a better education. Evidence for this pattern has been found in relation to smoking, diet, seat belt use, and use of preventive health care, such as immunizations and Pap smears (Federal, Provincial and Territorial Advisory Committee on Population Health 1999; Winkleby 1992; Davey Smith et al. 1998).
- Adult socioeconomic circumstances, in turn, have an impact on health in adult life (Drever and Whitehead 1997; Kunst et al. 1998; Evans et al. 1994). International studies of European, U.S., and Canadian populations have demonstrated poorer self-reported health and mortality among the least-educated groups (Kunst et al. 1995; Feldman et al. 1989; Pappas et al. 1993; Federal, Provincial and Territorial Advisory Committee 1999).

The sequence beginning with social origins and progressing through educational attainment to adult outcome has been shown to lead to differential mortality. Thus, social origins have their effect through their influence on social destinations.

Latency/Pathway/Cumulative Effects

Whereas latency and pathway effects are easy to differentiate in the abstract, evidence from observational studies is difficult to interpret as being unequivocally indicative of one or the other. Nonetheless, in relative terms, some pieces of evidence appear to support one type of relationship more than another. For example, recent studies on the long-term effects of parental divorce, based on the 1958 British birth cohort, have shown contrasting patterns for symptoms of psychological distress (indicated by the malaise score) and for heavy drinking (Rodgers et al. 1997; Hope et al. 1998). Table 4.3 presents odds ratios for study subjects whose parents divorced during their childhood (i.e., before age sixteen). As these data show, the effects of parental divorce on psychological distress were apparent before age twenty-three and persisted to age thirty-three. For heavy drinking, on the other hand, associations with parental divorce were weak at age twenty-three but emerged ten years later. These findings suggest that the relationship between parental divorce and heavy drinking is, in relative terms, more of a latency effect than the relationship between parental divorce and psychological distress.

It is possible for an early life exposure simultaneously to have latent, cumulative, and pathway relationships to health in adulthood. For example, environmental lead

Table 4.3. Odds ratios (95% confidence interval) of psychological distress and heavy drinking and at ages 23 and 33 by parental separation

	N	Age 23	Age 33
Men			
Psychological distress			
No separation	3,818	1.00	1.00
Separation	390	2.54 (1.80–3.60)	2.03 (1.43–2.89)
Heavy drinking			
No separation	3,813	1.00	
Separation	387	1.28 (1.00–1.63)	1.59 (1.21–2.10)
Women			
Psychological distress			
No separation	3,947	1.00	1.00
Separation	480	1.69 (1.34–2.14)	1.82 (1.41–2.35)
Heavy drinking			
No separation	3,945	1.00	1.00
Separation	483	1.18 (0.82–1.70)	1.85 (1.21–2.82)

Note: Odds ratios are presented in terms of 95% CI. Psychological distress is indicated by a "malaise score" of more than 7. Heavy drinking is defined as more than 35 units of alcohol for men and more than 20 for women.

Sources: Rodgers et al. 1997; Hope et al. 1998.

exposure may be one of several factors that cumulate to affect health, since lead is retained in the body and causes greater health risks as more of it is retained. Yet, lead exposure in utero may also have a latent effect on subsequent health and well-being (Needleman and Bellinger 1991) through inhibiting the production of brain cells. In addition, there may be a pathway effect, since socioeconomic position will affect the probability of exposure to lead in utero and in childhood, which in turn, may result in academic underachievement as reflected in lower educational attainment and subsequent adult mortality.

In some instances, effects that appear to be exclusively latent may in fact be mediated by subsequent life course exposure—that is, they form part of cumulating exposures. For example, in the Dutch Hunger Winter Study, early gestational exposure to famine during the winter of 1944–1945 was found to increase women's risk of obesity at age fifty (Ravelli et al. 1999); in addition, prenatal exposure to famine in *late* gestation was associated with an increased risk of diabetes among the offspring (Ravelli et al. 1976). Hence, nutritional deprivation in fetal life is suspected of having long-term consequences for the metabolism of sugars. However, individuals exposed in utero to the Dutch famine experienced a time of increasing affluence in the postwar period, with plentiful food supplies. The study was therefore one not simply of prenatal famine exposure (latent effect) but of prenatal famine combined with an abundant diet after initial exposure (cumulative effect). This life course pattern contrasted with that associated with the Leningrad famine of 1941 to 1944, since people born between those years endured a longer period of food shortage (approximately 2.5 years versus 6 months) during early life and a less abundant diet thereafter. Among the newborn survivors from Leningrad, no association was found between famine exposure and obesity at age fifty-two to fifty-three (Stanner et al. 1997). These contrasting "natural experiments" suggest that the latent effect (gestational nutritional deprivation) is expressed under certain subsequent life course conditions (plentiful food) and not others, representing a cumulative effect.[5]

The coexistence of latency and cumulative effects was also suggested by the findings from a study of participants born in Newcastle-upon-Tyne, England, in 1947, for whom information was collected in infancy, childhood, and adult life (Lamont et al. 2000). This population was examined in middle age to determine their cardiovascular health status, as indicated by the thickness of the wall of a key artery supplying blood to the brain. This "thickness" measure, an important indicator of cardiovascular health, predicts coronary heart disease and stroke because thickened blood vessels are less able to transport blood and are highly susceptible to blockage. Early life factors (birth weight, socioeconomic position at birth and in childhood, adverse life events, illness, and growth pattern), explained 9.15% of the total variance in thickness for men and 4.73% for women, whereas adult socioeconomic position and lifestyle (smoking and alcohol consumption, exercise level, physical inactivity, and dietary fat intake) explained 3.42% and 7.56%, respectively. This study provided evidence for latency, in that early life factors exerted an independent effect on artery thickness and a cumulative effect because factors from different life stages further contributed to the thickness of the arterial walls.

Life Course and Society

Life course trajectories do not unfold in a vacuum but are defined by broad societal influences that determine both the barriers and the opportunities that individuals will confront at important times in their lives. This fact is most visible during times of social cataclysm, when well-established trajectories may be deflected. For instance, the Great Depression in the United States altered the social development of the generation of children born at or immediately prior to its onset (Elder 1986). Later, America's economic revival with the mass mobilization for World War II created an environment that compensated for the earlier developmental effects of the Depression in this generation (Elder 1986). Such cataclysms affect everyone, but their effects may be positive or negative, and moreover, their impact will vary depending on the stage of life at which they are experienced.

During major social cataclysms, everyone within the society is affected by societal changes that, among other things, have implications for health, but the relationship between life course and social context is not confined to social cataclysm. Indeed, such events may be viewed as the extreme end of a continuum of macrolevel influences on an individual's health and well-being. Less dramatic variations in the socioeconomic environments that populations encounter over time could also be expected to influence life course trajectories and health, albeit in ways more subtle and more difficult to measure. The levels of potential influence are illustrated in figure 4.7. At the macro level are such societywide influences as levels and fluctuations of national income, particularly patterns of distribution, and policies intended to affect these (e.g., income–support, education, health care, or employment policies). At an intermediate, or "meso" level, are the characteristics of one's immediate community or workplace. Influences here would include, among other things, the ways people interact with each other, as well as the levels of local trust and civility in the community and the workplace. These will be reflected, in part, in the nature and availability of schools, libraries, newspapers, policing, and parks, and also in the nature of work characteristics and environments (Putnam et al. 1993; Rose 1995; Kaplan et al. 1996; Kawachi et al. 1997). At the minutest level, there are the influences on health associated with private life, such as the nature and quality of personal social support: intimate relationships, friendships, and the availability of personal help when needed (Berkman 1995). Not all relevant influences fit neatly into one level of social aggregation. For example, job insecurity and sense of control are perhaps best understood as resulting from the interaction between mesolevel and microlevel influences on the individual at a particular stage in the life course (Hertzman et al. 2001).

We have examined the life course in the context of broad social influences by incorporating the concept of macro-, meso-, and microlevels of social aggregation to create a parsimonious predictive model of health in early adulthood in the 1958

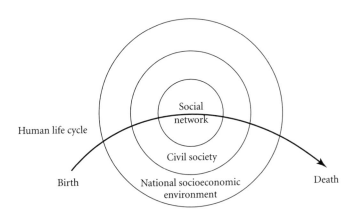

Figure 4.7. Framework for human development and the social determinants of health

birth cohort. Table 4.4 presents the model for self-rated health at age thirty-three. In our research the effects of childhood factors—latent, pathway, or cumulative— were not "explained" statistically by including society-level factors, and conversely, society-level effects were not "explained" by life course factors (Hertzman et al. 2001). Behavioral adjustment to school at age seven, whether or not parents were reading to their children regularly by that age, and atypical growth were all independent predictors of health status by age thirty-three, even after subsequent life course and societal factors were taken into account (Hertzman et al. 2001). Cognitive, behavioral, and physical aspects of development are all important links between early life and adult health. The recent findings have supported our contention that both life course and societal factors need to be considered together to fully understand adult health.

Conclusions

In wealthy societies, almost all health problems that consume medical services have their clinical onset in middle and old age. Accordingly, there is a strong tendency for the health care system, and health policy more generally, to focus on factors in adulthood that influence the onset or modify the clinical course of disease. Yet the life course perspective reveals that the focus on adult disease is limited. Without

Table 4.4. Life course and society influences on self-rated health (age 33) ($n = 6,463$)

Factors	β	SE (β)	P	$r(r^2)$
Early life				
Behavior score, age 7	.016	.007	.017	
Parents read to child at age 7	−.022	.006	<.001	.30 (.09)
Height, age 7/height, age 33	.006	.002	.012	
Cumulative				
Social class, age 0, 7, 11, 16	.011	.002	<.001	
Behavior scores, ages 11 and 16	.013	.004	.003	
Qualifications at school graduation	.042	.009	<.001	
Socioeconomic				
Material circumstances, age 33	.066	.012	<.001	
Civil society				
Most people can be trusted	.054	.018	.003	
Level of control at work	.025	.009	.007	
Intersecting				
Job insecurity, age 33	.033	.008	<.001	
Level of control in life	.127	.012	<.001	

Source: Hertzman et al. 2001.

a consideration of both childhood and adult life experiences, policies designed to improve health status will tend to overlook root causes. This is not to say that all disease has its origin in early childhood. We would not challenge the notion that there may be major influences, with late-life onset, that affect health and functioning in old age. Nor do we claim that each life stage is equally relevant to all health outcomes. Yet, we argue that health policies should be based on the understanding that problems emerging today may be related to life experiences years and decades earlier. More important, the range of social and economic policy decisions made today will affect future health profiles. For instance, investments in child development now should improve outcomes for children in the short term, and in addition, they can be viewed as investments in health over the long term.

For policy makers, distinctions between latency, pathway, and cumulative may seem unnecessary. Would it not be enough to know that life course matters, without being asked to think through the details of how it matters? Yet, it turns out that each life course pattern carries with it a strategic message for policies and interventions to improve population health. The message of latency is "the earlier the better." Gradients in cognitive and behavioral development are early manifestations of the brain's plasticity as it responds to the child's early environment. Gradients in readiness for school, although based on broader constructs, are early "health" indicators and should be the focus of intervention for reasons of long-term health, as well as for other social objectives. The message of pathways is "intervene at strategic points in time." For example, strategies designed to facilitate the transition from education to labor market may give individuals a second chance to achieve a life trajectory with better health expectations. The message of the cumulative model is "intervene wherever there is an effective intervention." For example, the home-visiting program for vulnerable families, the hot-meal program at school, and the Big Brothers/Big Sisters program for children of broken families all have the potential to reduce the rate at which disadvantages accumulate.

The time frame for the health benefits of these strategies may be very long. For instance, we may expect that school nutrition programs now would reduce the incidence of low birth weight in the offspring of girls who are themselves program recipients. This intervention could break the cycle of the intergenerational transmission of low-weight births (Emanuel 1992). If the evidence from animal studies is any guide (Suomi 1999; Francis et al. 1999), then improvements in parenting styles may not only lead to better developmental outcomes among cohorts of today's children but also be passed from one generation of parents to the next, leading to sustainable improvements in human well-being.

Notes

1. This has fueled speculation that the gradient in health status in adulthood is attributable to "reverse causality" (i.e., that differences in health status lead to different socioec-

onomic circumstances) (West 1991), although little support for this has emerged from studies that directly examine socioeconomic mobility (Manor et al. 2003; Blane et al. 1993).

2. Although we present only two of the five scales here, the neighborhood differences were similar for the others (Hertzman et al. 2002).

3. The 1958 British birth cohort is a study of everyone born in England, Scotland, and Wales during one week in March in 1958. Information has been collected at birth, during childhood (ages 7, 11, and 16), and in adulthood (ages 23, 33, and 41) on social, economic, family, and health characteristics (Ferri 1993).

4. The ponderal index measures the degree of fatness at birth and is calculated by dividing birth weight by the height, cubed, of the newborn (kg/m3).

5. Earlier we referred to the Dutch Hunger Winter Study as an example of the latent effect of famine on antisocial personality disorder and schizophrenia. These outcomes may also be moderated by subsequent life experience, though this remains to be clarified. This illustrates an important general point that life course patterns cannot necessarily be generalized from one health outcome to another.

References

Barker, D. J. P. 1990. The fetal and infant origins of adult disease. *British Medical Journal* 301:1111.

———. 1997. Fetal nutrition and cardiovascular disease in later life. *British Medical Bulletin* 51:96–108.

Berkman, L. F. 1995. The role of social relations in health promotion. *Psychosomatic Medicine* 57:245–254.

Blane, D., G. Davey Smith, and M. Bartley. 1993. Social selection: What does it contribute to social class differences in health? *Sociology of Health and Illness* 1:1–15.

Blane, D., C. L. Hart, G. Davey Smith, C. R. Gillis, D. J. Hole, and V. M. Hawthorne. 1996. Association of cardiovascular disease risk factors with socioeconomic position during childhood and during adulthood. *British Medical Journal* 313:1434–1438.

Brunner, E., G. Davey Smith, M. Marmot, R. Canner, M. Beksinska, and J. O'Brien. 1996. Childhood social circumstances and psychosocial and behavioral factors as determinants of plasma fibrinogen. *Lancet* 347:1008–1013.

Cavelaars, A. E. J. M., A. E. Kunst, J. J. M. Geurts, R. Crialesi, L. Grötvedt, U. Helmert, E. Lahelma, O. Lundberg, A. Mielck, N. K. Rasmussen, E. Regidor, T. H. Spuhler, and J. P. Mackenbach. 2000. Persistent variations in average height between countries and between socio-economic groups: An overview of 10 European countries. *Annals of Human Biology* 27:407–421.

Curtis, L. J., M. D. Dooley, and S. A. Phipps. 2004. Child well-being and neighbourhood quality: Evidence from the Canadian National Longitudinal Survey of Children and Youth. *Social Science and Medicine* 58:1917–1927.

Cynader, M. S., and B. J. Frost. 1999. Mechanisms of brain development: Neuronal sculpting by the physical and social environment. In *Developmental Health and the Wealth of Nations*, ed. D. Keating and C. Hertzman. New York: Guilford.

Davey Smith, G., C. Hart, D. Hole, P. MacKinnon, C. Gillis, G. Watt, D. Blane, and V. Hawthorne. 1998. Education and occupational social class: Which is the more important indicator of mortality risk? *Journal of Epidemiology and Community Health* 52:153–160.

Drever, F., and M. Whitehead. 1997. *Health Inequalities*. London: Office for National Statistics.

Duncan, G. J., and J. Brooks-Gunn, eds. 1997. *Consequences of Growing Up Poor.* New York: Russell Sage Foundation.

Elder, G. H. 1986. Military times and turning points in men's lives. *Developmental Psychology* 22:233–245.

Emanuel, I. 1992. Intergenerational studies of human birthweight from the 1958 birth cohort. 1. Evidence for a multigenerational effect. *British Journal of Obstetrics and Gynaecology* 99:67–74.

Eriksson, J. G., T. J. Forsen, C. Osmond, and D. J. Barker. 2003. Pathways of infant and childhood growth that lead to type 2 diabetes. *Diabetes Care* 26:3006–3010.

Eriksson, J. G., T. Forsen, J. Tuomilehto, P. D. Winter, C. Osmond, and D. J. P. Barker. 1999. Catch-up growth in childhood and death from coronary heart disease: Longitudinal study. *British Medical Journal* 318:427–431.

Evans, R. G., M. L. Barer, and T. R. Marmor, eds. 1994. *Why Are Some People Healthy and Others Not? The Determinants of Health of Populations.* New York: Aldine de Gruyter.

Everson-Rose, S. A., C. F. Mendes de Leon, J. L. Bienias, R. S. Wilson, and D. A. Evans. 2003. Early life conditions and cognitive functioning in later life. *American Journal of Epidemiology* 158:1083–1089.

Federal, Provincial and Territorial Advisory Committee on Population Health. 1999. *Statistical Report on the Health of Canadians.* Ottawa: Health Canada.

Feldman, J. J., D. M. Makuc, J. C. Kleinman, and J. Cornoni-Huntley. 1989. National trends in educational differentials in mortality. *American Journal of Epidemiology* 129:919–933.

Ferri, E. 1993. *Life at 33: The Fifth Follow-up of the National Child Development Study.* London: National Children's Bureau.

Flouri, E. 2004. Psychological outcomes in midadulthood associated with mother's childrearing attitudes in early childhood—evidence from the 1970 British Birth Cohort. *European Child and Adolescent Psychiatry* 13 (1):35–41.

Forssen, K. 1998. *Child Poverty and Family Policy in OECD Countries.* Study no. 178. Syracuse, NY: Luxembourg Income Study.

Francis, D., J. Diorio, D. Liu, and M. J. Meaney. 1999. Nongenomic transmission across generations of maternal behavior and stress responses in the rat. *Science* 286:1155–1158.

Frankel, S., P. Elwood, P. Sweetnam, J. Yarnell, and G. Davey Smith. 1996. Birthweight, body-mass index in middle age, and incident coronary heart disease. *Lancet* 348:1478–1480.

Galobardes, B., J. W. Lynch, and G. Davey Smith. 2004. Childhood socioeconomic circumstances and cause-specific mortality in adulthood: Systematic review and interpretation. *Epidemiology Reviews* 261:7–21.

Goldstein, H. 1971. Factors influencing the height of seven-year-old children—results from the National Child Development Study. *Human Biology* 43:92–111.

Gunnell, D. J., G. Davey Smith, S. Frankel, K. Nanchahal, F. E. M. Braddon, J. Pemberton, T. J. Peters. 1998. Childhood leg length and adult mortality: Follow up of the Carnegie (Boyd Orr) Survey of Diet and Health in pre-war Britain. *Journal of Epidemiology and Community Health* 52:142–152.

Harding, J. E. 2001. The nutritional basis of the fetal origins of adult disease. *International Journal of Epidemiology* 30:15–23.

Hertzman, C., S. A. McLean, D. E. Kohen, J. Dunn, and T. Evans. 2002. *Early Development in Vancouver: Report of the Community Asset Mapping Project (CAMP).* Canadian Institute for Health Information, Ottawa. Reproduced with permission from the Human Early Learning Partnership (HELP).

Hertzman, C., C. Power, S. Matthews, and O. Manor. 2001. Using an interactive framework of society and lifecourse to explain self-rated health in early adulthood. *Social Science and Medicine* 53:1575–1585.

Hertzman, C., and M. Wiens. 1996. Child development and long-term outcomes: A population health perspective and summary of successful interventions. *Social Science and Medicine* 43:1083–1095.

Hope, S., C. Power, and B. Rodgers. 1998. The relationship between parental separation in childhood and problem drinking in adulthood. *Addiction* 93:505–514.

Human Resources Development Canada and Statistics Canada. 1995. *Growing Up in Canada: National Longitudinal Survey of Children and Youth.* Ottawa: Minister of Industry.

Huxley, R. R., A. W. Shiell, and C. M. Law. 2000. The role of size at birth and postnatal catch-up growth in determining systolic blood pressure: A systematic review of the literature. *Journal of Hypertension* 18:815–831.

Hypponen, E., C. Power, and G. Davey Smith. 2003. Prenatal growth, BMI, and risk of type 2 diabetes by early midlife. *Diabetes Care* 26:2512–2517.

Janus, M., and D. R. Offord. 2000. Reporting on readiness to learn in Canada. *ISUMA Canadian Journal of Policy Research* 1:71–75.

Kaplan, G. A., W. J. Strawbridge, R. D. Cohen, and L. R. Hungerford. 1996. Natural history of leisure-time physical activity and its correlates: Associations with mortality from all-causes and cardiovascular disease over 28 years. *American Journal of Epidemiology* 144:793–797.

Kawachi, I., B. P. Kennedy, K. Lochner, and D. Prothrow-Smith. 1997. Social capital, income inequality, and mortality. *American Journal of Public Health* 87:1491–1498.

Keating, D., and C. Hertzman, eds. 1999. *Developmental Health and the Wealth of Nations.* New York: Guilford Press.

Kohen, D. E., Brooks-Gunn, J., Leventhal T., and C. Hertzman. 2002. Neighborhood income and physical and social disorder in Canada: Associations with young children's competencies. *Child Development* 73:1844–1860.

Kuh, D. L., and Y. Ben-Shlomo. 1997. *A Life Course Approach to Chronic Disease Epidemiology: Tracing the Origins of Ill Health from Early to Adult Life.* Oxford: Oxford University Press.

Kuh, D., L. Cardozo, and R. Hardy. 1999. Urinary incontinence in middle aged women: Childhood enuresis and other lifetime risk factors in a British prospective cohort. *Journal of Epidemiology and Community Health* 53:453–458.

Kunst, A. E., J. J. M. Geurts, and J. van den Berg. 1995. International variation in socioeconomic inequalities in self-reported health. *Journal of Epidemiology and Community Health* 49:117–123.

Kunst, A. E., F. Groenhof, J. P. Mackenbach, and E. W. Health. 1998. Occupational class and cause specific mortality in middle aged men in 11 European countries: Comparison of population-based studies. *British Medical Journal* 316:1636–1642.

Lamont, D., L. Parker, M. White, N. Unwin, S. M. Bennett, M. Cohen, D. Richardson, H. O. Dickinson, A. Adamson, K. G. Alberti, and A. W. Craft. 2000. Risk of cardiovascular disease measured by carotid intima-media thickness at age 49–51: Lifecourse study. *British Medical Journal* 320:273–278.

Leon, D. A., J. Koupilova, H. O. Lithell, L. Berglund, R. Mohsen, D. Vagero. 1996. Failure to realise growth potential in utero and adult obesity in relation to blood pressure in 50 year old Swedish men. *British Medical Journal* 312:401–406.

Leventhal, T., and J. Brooks-Gunn. 2003. Moving to opportunity: An experimental study of neighborhood effects on mental health. *American Journal of Public Health.* 93:1576–1582.

Lynch, J. W., G. A. Kaplan, and S. J. Shema. 1997. Cumulative impact of sustained economic hardship on physical, cognitive, psychological, and social functioning. *New England Journal of Medicine* 337:1889–1895.

Manor, O., S. Matthews, and C. Power. 2001. Health selection: The role of inter- and intra-generational mobility on social inequalities in health. *Social Science and Medicine* 57: 2217–2227.

Marmot, M. G., M. J. Shipley, and G. Rose. 1984. Inequalities in death-specific explanations of a general pattern. *Lancet* 1:1003–1006.

Marmot, M. G., and M. E. J. Wadsworth, eds. 1997. Fetal and early childhood environment: Long-term health implications. *British Medical Bulletin* 53.

McCain, M. N., and J. F. Mustard. 1999. *Reversing the Real Brain Drain: Early Years Study Final Report*. Toronto: Ontario Children's Secretariat.

McDonough, P., G. J. Duncan, D. Williams, and J. House. 1997. Income dynamics and adult mortality in the United States, 1972 through 1989. *American Journal of Public Health* 87:1476–1483.

Meaney, M. J. 2001. Maternal care, gene expression, and the transmission of individual differences in stress reactivity across generations. *Annual Review of Neuroscience* 24:1161– 1192.

Miller, J., and S. Korenman. 1994. Poverty and children's nutritional status in the United States. *American Journal of Epidemiology* 140:233–243.

Moore, S. E., T. J. Cole, A. C. Collinson, E. M. E. Poskitt, I. A. McGregor, and A. M. Prentice. 1999. Prenatal or early postnatal events predict infectious deaths in young adulthood in rural Africa. *International Journal of Epidemiology* 28:1088–1095.

Needleman, H. L., and D. Bellinger. 1991. The health effects of low level exposure to lead. *Annual Review of Public Health* 12:111–140.

Neugebauer, R., H. W. Hoek, and E. Susser. 1999. Prenatal exposure to wartime famine and development of antisocial personality disorder in early adulthood. *Journal of the American Medical Association* 282:455–462.

Pappas, G., S. Queen, W. Hadden, and G. Fisher. 1993. The increasing disparity in mortality between socio-economic groups in the United States, 1960 and 1986. *New England Journal of Medicine* 329:103–108.

Pensola, T. 2003. From past to present: Effect of lifecourse on mortality, and social class differences in mortality in middle adulthood. *Yearbook of Population Research in Finland, XXXIX Supplement*. Helsinki: The Population Research Institute.

Poulton, R., A. Caspi, B. J. Milne, W. M. Thomson, A. Taylor, M. R. Sears, T. E. Moffitt. 2002. Association between children's experience of socioeconomic disadvantage and adult health: A life-course study. *Lancet* 360:1640–1645.

Power, C., L. Li, and O. Manor. 2000. A prospective study of limiting longstanding illness in early adulthood. *International Journal of Epidemiology* 29:131–139.

Power, C., O. Manor, and A. J. Fox. 1991. *Health and Class: The Early Years*. London: Chapman Hall.

Power, C., O. Manor, and S. Matthews. 1999. The duration and timing of exposure: Effects of socioeconomic environment on adult health. *American Journal of Public Health* 89: 1059–1066.

Putnam, R. D., R. Leonardi, and R. Y. Nanetti. 1993. *Making Democracy Work: Civic Traditions in Modern Italy*. Princeton, NJ: Princeton University Press.

Ravelli, A. C., J. H. Der Meulen, C. Osmond, D. J. Barker, O. P. Bleker. 1999. Obesity at the age of 50 y. in men and women exposed to famine prenatally. *American Journal of Clinical Nutrition* 70:811–816.

Ravelli, G. P., Z. A. Stein, and M. W. Susser. 1976. Obesity in young men after famine exposure in utero and early infancy. *New England Journal of Medicine* 295:349–353.

Rodgers, B., C. Power, and S. Hope. 1997. Parental divorce and adult psychological distress: Evidence from a national birth cohort: A research note. *Journal of Child Psychology and Psychiatry* 38:867–872.

Rose, R. 1995. Russia as an hour-glass society: A construction without citizens. *East European Constitutional Review* (summer): 34–42.

Ross, D. P., and P. Roberts. 1999. *Income and Child Well-being: A New Perspective on the Poverty Debate.* Ottawa: Canadian Council on Social Development.

Rutter, M. 1991. Childhood experiences and adult psychosocial functioning. In *The Childhood Environment and Adult Disease,* ed. G. R. Bock and J. Whelan. Chichester, UK: J. Wiley and Ciba Foundation.

Rutter, M., D. Quinton, and J. Hill. 1990. Adult outcome of institution-reared children: Males and females compared. In *Straight and Devious Pathways from Childhood to Adulthood,* ed. L. N. Robins and M. Rutter. Cambridge: Cambridge University Press.

Schweinhart, L. J., H. V. Barnes, and D. P. Weikart. 1993. Significant benefits: The High/Scope Perry preschool study through age 27. *Monographs of the High/Scope Educational Research Foundation* 10.

Stanner, S. A., K. Bulmer, C. Andres, O. E. Lantseva, V. Borodina, V. V. Poteen, and J. S. Yudkin. 1997. Does malnutrition in utero determine diabetes and coronary heart disease in adulthood? Results from the Leningrad Siege Study, a cross sectional study. *British Medical Journal* 315:1342–1348.

Statistics Canada and Organization for Economic Cooperation and Development (OECD). 1995. *Literacy, Economy and Society.* Paris: OECD.

Suomi, S. J. 1999. Developmental trajectories, early experiences, and community consequences: Lessons from studies with rhesus monkeys. In *Developmental Health and the Wealth of Nations,* ed. D. Keating and C. Hertzman. New York: Guilford.

Susser, E., R. Neugebauer, and H. W. Hoek. 1996. Schizophrenia after prenatal famine: Further evidence. *Archives of General Psychiatry* 53:25–31.

Szyf, M. 2003. DNA methylation enzymology. In *Encyclopedia of the Human Genome.* New York: Macmillan Publishers Ltd, Nature Publishing Group.

Taylor, D. 1998. Congenital cataract: The history, the nature, and the practice. *Eye* 12:9–36.

Tremblay, R. E. 1999. When children's development fails. In *Developmental Health and the Wealth of Nations,* ed. D. Keating and C. Hertzman. New York: Guilford.

Tremblay, R. E., B. Masse, D. Perron, and M. LeBlanc. 1992. Disruptive behavior, poor school achievement, delinquent behavior, and delinquent personality: Longitudinal analyses. *Journal of Consulting and Clinical Psychology* 60:64–72.

Wannamethee, G., P. Whincup, G. Shaper, and M. Walker. 1996. Influence of father's social class on cardiovascular disease in middle-aged men. *Lancet* 348:1259–1263.

Weaver, I. C. G., N. Cervoni, F. A. Champagne, A. C. D. Alessio, S. Sharma, J. R. Seckl, S. Dymov, M. Szyf, and M. J. Meaney. 2004. Epigenetic programming by maternal behavior. *Nature Neuroscience* 7:847–854.

West, P. 1991. Rethinking the health selection explanation for health inequalities. *Social Sciences and Medicine* 32:373–384.

Willms, D. 2002. *Vulnerable Children: Findings from Canada's National Longitudinal Survey of Children and Youth.* Edmonton: University of Alberta Press.

Winkleby, M. A. 1992. Socioeconomic status and health: How education, income, and occupation contribute to risk factors for cardiovascular disease. *American Journal of Public Health* 82:816–820.

Chapter 5

Universal Medical Care and Health Inequalities: Right Objectives, Insufficient Tools

Noralou P. Roos, Marni Brownell, and
Verena Menec

Central to any understanding of the social and biological determinants of health is the answer to this question: What role does medical care play in determining population health? Several approaches have been taken in finding an answer. Cross-national comparisons of expenditures on health care have shown that there is little relationship between the amount of money spent on health care and longevity in high-income countries. The United States, for example, has the world's highest medical care expenditures but performs poorly on most measures of health status relative to countries spending much less. Yet, these studies leave open the question of what difference health care can make when it is universally available—and typically have not examined how care is delivered relative to need or how health status changes over time relate at the individual level to the receipt of health care.

The Canadian health care system, with its universal medical care coverage, provides an important opportunity for assessing the impact of medical care on health. This chapter presents research that examines the question in the province of Manitoba, where an exceptional population-based database including detailed information on both health outcomes and medical care utilization is available.

For more than a decade, a group of researchers at the Manitoba Centre for Health Policy has been examining how the population uses the health care system. Most recently, we have focused on who uses how much care (Forget et al. 2002) and how this differs by health and socioeconomic status (N. Roos et al. 2003). We have been particularly interested in whether health care is an effective policy tool for reducing inequalities in health. In this chapter we present findings of a study that spans ten years—and review existing evidence—on the relation between socioeconomic disparities, health care use, and health.

Personal health care experiences, along with policy changes likely to affect those experiences, are of great interest to Canadians. Across Canada, front-page stories about "hallway" medicine (medical patients waiting for beds), waits for surgery, and new schemes for letting the wealthy "buy" their way to the front of queues have become routine. This constant barrage takes its toll: In one survey (Hindle 2000), only 20% of Canadians reported having confidence in the system, even though more than 50% said that the medical care they and their family had personally received in the last year had been very good or excellent.

In Manitoba the 1999 provincial election was largely fought (and won) around opposition accusations that the ruling party failed to solve the problems of surgical waiting lists and hallway medicine. The Conservative government lost, despite the fact that when Conservatives entered office, Manitoba was spending 31% of its budget on health care, and when they left, health care was taking 38% of the budget. The current fascination with all things related to health care creates a challenge for those trying to communicate evidence about the role that health care plays as a determinant of health. On the one hand, it is clear that individual patients benefit greatly from medical interventions: the pneumonia patient treated with antibiotics, the Pap test that identifies cervical cancer at an early stage, the elderly patient who can see clearly again with a new lens or walk pain free with a new hip. But paradoxically, the benefits that an individual receives from a specific treatment do not seem to be reflected in the benefits that populations receive from health care investments. This discrepancy between what benefits an individual versus what benefits the population is often difficult to convey to the public and policy makers. For example, what extra health improvement does the United States buy by spending 4% to 6% more of its gross national product (GNP) on health care than other countries including Canada and many members of the European Union (Reinhardt et al. 2004)? On indicators of population health such as life expectancy and infant mortality, Americans score poorly, in the bottom quartile of industrialized countries (Hussey et al. 2004). On nineteen quality-of-care measures Americans scored highest on three and lowest on two when the care they received was compared with that received by Canadians, Australians, the English, and New Zealanders (Hussey et al. 2004). There is conflicting evidence on whether even affluent Americans show marginal benefits from their expensive system. (In 2001 Americans spent $4,887 per person on health care relative to Canadians' $2,792 [see Reinhardt et al. 2004]). For example, although one study found some cancer survival advantage for American residents of high-income communities compared with Canadian residents of such communities (Boyd et al. 1999), several others find no such advantage (Gorey et al. 1998; Gorey et al. 2000; Gorey at al. 2003).

Reflecting on his year as president of the Association of Health Services Research,

David Kindig (1999, p. 209) said, "We know . . . that all health improvement does not come from individual medical care interventions, and we say we act on it, but it is almost inevitable that the money and status in medical care overwhelms other considerations most of the time." Perhaps the problem is that we do not target health care to those who would benefit most, and if we did, the health status inequities could be reduced.

What type of evidence would, therefore, be useful in clarifying the potential of health care to reduce health status disparities and the relative role of such care as a determinant of population health? And are there data on which we can draw to address these important questions? Can such data help distinguish among hypotheses about the relationship and direction of causality linking the quantity and quality of health care, on the one hand, and health status, on the other? After all, if health care were an important determinant of a population's health, then an unhealthy population might be explained by its receipt of low levels of medical care relative to its needs, whereas healthier populations might be a reflection of high levels of health-improving care. In this chapter we examine analyses of data from Manitoba that have provided some insights into the relationship between health care and population health.

Specifically, we examine three main areas. First, we examine 1986 health care use by residents of neighborhoods differing in socioeconomic characteristics in Winnipeg, Canada, as well as the health care use by those same individuals alive and residing in the province ten years later (in 1996). Individuals' rates and types of physician contact, as well as their hospital use, their rates of surgery, their use of pharmaceuticals (in 1996 only), and their use of nursing homes, are reviewed. Second, we examine the health characteristics of these neighborhoods' residents in 1986; their mortality rates between 1986 and 1996; and for those who survived and remained in the province, their health status ten years later (1996). Several widely used indicators of population health, including premature mortality, life expectancy, and prevalence of serious chronic disease (e.g., diabetes), are examined. Rates of "avoidable" hospitalization (i.e., for conditions for which medical treatment is believed to be effective in preventing the condition, finding and treating the condition in an early phase to avoid major consequences, or treating the condition in a late phase, thereby avoiding death or disability) and for ambulatory-care–sensitive conditions (e.g., asthma, diabetes, congestive heart failure) are also presented. Third, to take an alternative approach to assessing the role of medical care as a determinant of health, we review how the marked downsizing of the Winnipeg acute hospital system (closure of 24% of the acute-care beds and cuts to budgets during this period) affected the area residents' health status.

How We Approached These Questions

Our analyses focused on the population of Winnipeg, Manitoba, a city of 650,000, and home to the province's only medical school and seven hospitals. The province is similar to other provinces with respect to physician supply and other key health care resources. Manitoba has somewhat fewer physicians per capita than the average for Canadian provinces (132 full-time–equivalent physicians per 100,000 population) but a relatively rich supply of specialists (60 per 100,000 population), with only one Canadian province, Ontario, having a substantially greater specialist supply (N. Roos et al. 1999). Comparing hospital use across areas is always difficult because of how these institutions are used. However, our analyses suggested that the Winnipeg acute hospital system would have been considered tight by North American standards before downsizing, and hence, the bed closures represented a significant challenge for the system.

Assessing Socioeconomic Status

Residents of Winnipeg were divided into five socioeconomic groups. The first set of analyses tracking health care use and health of individuals through time focused on educational levels,[1] using data on the percentage of residents in the neighborhood aged twenty-five to forty-four with at least a high school education. The data on educational attainment were taken from the 1986 Canadian census public use database. Data describing characteristics of neighborhood residents, including the percentage of households headed by females, income levels, and unemployment rates, were also taken from the 1986 census. Census data were aggregated at the geographic unit of the enumeration area; an enumeration area has an average population of 700 people.

The Manitoba urban (Winnipeg and Brandon) enumeration areas were ranked from least to most educated and then grouped into five population quintiles; each quintile contained approximately 20% of the urban population.[2] Each Winnipeg resident was linked to an enumeration area by residential postal code, and thus for each resident a quintile education rank was assigned. The same process was followed for creating the neighborhood income quintiles, using mean household income as the grouping measure.[3]

For the analyses tracking the health and health care use of individuals through time, a cohort was defined on the basis of relative education in the neighborhood of residence in 1986. (This means that 1996 use patterns were recorded under the individual's 1986 neighborhood of residence, regardless of the actual neighborhood of residence in 1996.)[4]

Since the Canadian census does not report income or education for institutionalized individuals (and thus not for residents of nursing homes), nursing home

residents were excluded from the 1986 study population. Everyone else was assigned to education or income quintiles. Those entering a nursing home over the
subsequent ten-year period were so identified.

Age- and sex-standardized mortality rates, as well as hospital, surgical, and physician visit rates, were calculated and standardized to the 1996 population. De-
nominators were based on counts of individuals in each educational quintile (as
of December 1986), with numerators based on event counts (i.e., hospitalizations
or deaths) for individuals identified as members of a quintile.

Health Care Utilization Measures

The health care utilization measures were obtained from the Population Health
Research Data Repository. These data originated from Manitoba Health, the provincial agency that administers Manitoba's universal health insurance program.[5]
These data consisted of encounter-based, anonymous records of Manitobans' interactions with the health care system, housed at the University of Manitoba. These
administrative databases have been repeatedly established to be both reliable and
valid for examining health and health care use (L. Roos et al. 1993; L. Roos et al.
1996; Kozyrskyj and Mustard 1998).

HOSPITAL USE

All hospital separations (and hospital days) were analyzed regardless of where in
Manitoba the hospitalization had taken place (out-of-province hospitalizations reimbursed by the province including those involving emergencies were also included).

SURGICAL USE

Manitoba Health data on both inpatient and outpatient surgery, including emergency procedures performed outside the province, were analyzed. This represented
almost all surgical care provided to Manitobans. According to the Canadian National Population Health Survey, only 0.1% of Canadians reported having gone to
the United States in the previous twelve months specifically for medical treatment
(Naylor 1999), and even fewer would have received surgery in a country other
than the United States.

NURSING HOME USE

The number of individuals who entered a nursing home after 1986 and still resided
there in 1996 was tracked. Well over 90% of individuals who enter nursing homes
in Manitoba remain there until death (DeCoster et al. 1995). Access to nursing
homes (both for-profit and not-for-profit) is through a standardized assessment

based on need, with copayments assessed on the basis of income. We report the number of individuals aged seventy-five or older in nursing homes in 1996 per 1,000 residents in that age range.

PHYSICIAN CONTACTS

Data describing physician visits were taken from claims payment data, which captured approximately 90% of all ambulatory medical care, including visits to nursing home residents and visits in hospital emergency departments and outpatient departments. Most Winnipeg physicians are reimbursed through fees for specific services, according to a uniform provincial payment schedule. Salaried physicians are typically required to submit "evaluation claims," and these were included in our analyses. There is no copayment associated with any type of physician visit. In this study we focused on all physician visits, including specialist consultations; only visits to hospital inpatients were excluded. Three measures were included: (1) the per capita rate of referred visits, in which one physician was seeking another physician's opinion (although almost all paid referrals are to specialists, there is no requirement that such a referral precede patient contact with a specialist), (2) the percentage of patients having at least one physician contact during the year, and (3) the per capita rate of physician contacts (including those to specialists and family practitioners).

PHARMACEUTICAL USE

In 1994 Manitoba began collecting point-of-sale information on pharmaceuticals. In 1996 the province provided 100% coverage for most pharmaceuticals once the deductible was reached (2% of incomes up to $15,000; 3% of incomes $15,000 and above). Social allowance recipients have no deductible on pharmaceuticals. Using the database of the Drug Programs Information Network (DPIN), two indicators of pharmaceutical use were obtained: the percentage of residents with one or more prescriptions received during the year and the number of prescriptions per resident. DPIN is administered through real-time computer links with every community-based pharmacy in the province and includes all prescriptions dispensed for out-of-hospital use in Manitoba and most prescriptions for outpatient use dispensed by hospitals. Patterns exhibited by these two measures across socioeconomic groups have been shown to be highly correlated with those of more comprehensive or specific measures of pharmaceutical use, including expenditures per resident and use of specific agents (Metge et al. 1999). This computerized tracking system was not in place in 1986, so only 1996 data were analyzed.

Health Status Indicators

Health status indicators were developed from provincially reported Vital Statistics death information (a single cause of death is routinely recorded in Manitoba) and from utilization data employing previously validated measures. Overall mortality rates and mortality rates for newborns to seventy-four-year-olds are reported separately for males and females. British (Carstairs and Morris 1989), Canadian (Birch and Eyles 1991), and American (U.S. General Accounting Office 1996; Kindig 1997) researchers have suggested that the standardized mortality ratio for birth to age seventy-four years (reflecting what is commonly regarded as premature mortality) is one of the most valid health status indicators reflecting a population's need for health care. Life expectancy, which is defined as the average years of life an individual of a given age is expected to live if current age-specific mortality rates remain stable, is another commonly used measure of health status (Hansluwka 1985). In our study, life expectancy was calculated from age ten separately for males and females using Manitoba Vital Statistics data.

Two additional indicators of health status were constructed using information on conditions for which health care is believed to be particularly effective. These were developed from hospital discharge data: rates of hospitalization for ambulatory-care–sensitive conditions (Falik et al. 2001) and for avoidable hospitalizations (Weissman et al. 1992). We also examined the prevalence of diabetes, defined as those having one or more physician contacts over the three-year period in which the disease was reported. Manitoba physician claims data have been shown to produce valid estimates of prevalence of this disease (Robinson et al. 1997).

What We Found

In the following section we describe changes in health care use and health status from 1986 to 1996 among Winnipeg residents who differed in terms of the relative education level of residents in the neighborhood in which they lived. We then discuss evidence related to socioeconomic disparities in quality of care and conclude by examining what impact the permanent closure of acute hospital beds, which occurred in Winnipeg in the early 1990s, had on the health of population.

Relationship between Health Care Use and Health over a Ten-year Period

Table 5.1 identifies key characteristics of individuals residing in each group of neighborhoods. As indicated, 89% of the residents aged twenty-five to thirty-four of the highest educational quintile neighborhoods (Q5) had at least a high school education, compared with 51.8% of residents in the least-educated neighborhoods. Mean household income and the unemployment rate also varied almost twofold across these neighborhood groupings, and 22.8% of the families in the least-educated neighborhoods were headed by a single mother, compared with 4.6% in the most-educated neighborhoods. Approximately three-quarters of the residents remained in the province ten years later (i.e., they had not died or left the prov-

Table 5.1. Characteristics of Winnipeg residents, by relative educational level of neighborhood residents

Variable	Q1 Least educated	Q2	Q3	Q4	Q5 Most educated	Ratio
Residents aged 25–34 with at least high school education (%)	51.8	64.8	72.8	79.9	89.0	0.58
Mean household income ($)	24,434	29,520	32,469	36,052	44,432	0.55
Female-headed households (%)	22.8	14.0	9.5	6.2	4.6	4.9
Unemployment rate ages 45–54 (%)	7.8	5.8	5.2	4.0	3.8	2.0
Treaty status aboriginals (%)	3.9	1.1	0.7	0.6	0.3	13.0
Number of residents (1986)	136,153	117,407	102,986	113,688	118,798	
Age 10+	116,036	101,464	87,176	97,893	104,858	
Age 0–9	20,117	15,943	15,810	15,795	13,940	
Died, left province between 1986–1996	30,553	24,920	20,476	26,052	29,100	
Number of cohort in province (1996)	105,600	92,487	82,510	87,636	89,698	

Sources: Data for the first four indicators come from the 1996 Canadian Public Use Census tapes. Data for the other indicators come from the Population Health Research Data Repository, Manitoba Centre for Health Policy.

ince), ranging from 77.5% of the residents of the least-educated neighborhoods to 75.5% of the most-educated neighborhoods' residents.[6]

Table 5.2 identifies the health care use patterns of the individuals in the cohort in 1986 and then ten years later. As explained earlier, an individual's use was reported by 1986 neighborhood of residence.[7] As of 1986, more health care, of almost every type, was delivered to residents of the least-educated neighborhoods, compared with that delivered to residents of the neighborhoods with the highest educational levels. Also, residents of the least-educated neighborhoods in 1986 who remained in the province also received more health care of almost every type in 1996. The differences were particularly profound with regard to hospital use, where those in the least-educated group spent approximately 40% more days in hospital and had about one-third more admissions than did those in the most-educated group.[8] However, residents of the least-educated neighborhoods also received more surgery (12%), were much more likely by 1996 (28%) to have been cared for in a nursing home (as noted before, none of the cohort resided in a nursing home in 1986), and received more pharmaceuticals (27%) than did residents of the neighborhoods with higher levels of education (although a similar proportion of each group received at least one prescription). The patterns of physician contact

Table 5.2. Medical care use rates (1986 and 1996), by relative educational level of individuals' neighborhoods in 1986 (age and sex standardized to the 1996 population)

Variable	Q1 Least educated	Q2	Q3	Q4	Q5 Most educated	Q1/ Q5
Hospital use (days)						
1986	2,003.86	1,773.24	1,617.61	1,563.89	1,439.82	1.40
1996	1,394.13	1,210.67	1,104.83	1,138.45	1,011.41	1.38
Admissions (per 1,000)						
1986	141.16	126.55	121.32	118.58	107.92	1.31
1996	118.08	102.03	96.50	95.29	89.25	1.32
Surgical rate (per 1,000)						
1986	85.67	82.24	80.95	80.99	76.59	1.12
1996	87.17	84.96	86.53	87.15	83.72	1.04
Nursing home residents per 1,000 aged 75+						
1996	143.78	133.21	136.26	137.04	112.53	1.28
Physician contacts						
One or more visits (%)						
1986	77.40	79.64	80.07	80.62	80.25	0.96
1996	82.02	82.34	82.50	82.53	81.56	1.01
Visits per person						
1986	4.70	4.66	467	4.66	4.57	1.03
1996	5.30	4.98	4.91	4.91	4.80	1.10
Referrals per person						
1986	0.19	0.19	0.20	0.20	0.20	0.94
1996	0.27	0.27	0.28	0.28	0.28	0.96
One or more prescriptions (%)						
1996	68.88	68.24	67.92	68.21	66.99	1.03
Prescriptions per person						
1996	77.88	70.25	65.61	65.11	61.30	1.27

Source: The Population Health Research Data Repository, Manitoba Centre for Health Policy.

were somewhat mixed: a similar proportion of residents with at least one physician contact during the year, with residents of neighborhoods with lower levels of education having a somewhat higher physician visit rate but a somewhat lower rate at which they were referred to a specialist for consultation.

The gradient characteristic of this relationship proved remarkable: In 1986 for most types of care where residents of the least-educated neighborhoods received more than did residents of the most-educated neighborhoods, those in the fourth quintile received more than those in the fifth, those in the third more than those in the fourth, those in the second more than those in the third, and so on. Thus, it was not just that those in the least-educated groups received the most care; it was that the lower the education level of the neighborhood, the more health care its residents received. Even in 1996, when some of the individuals had moved to neighborhoods of different socioeconomic characteristics, with a few exceptions, this pattern persisted.

Approximately 20% of each group had no physician contact in 1986. In earlier work with the Manitoba elderly linking interview and utilization data, we had found that those with no physician contact tended to be healthy, with few hospitalizations (Shapiro and Roos 1985). These characteristics were also true of our 1986 nonusers. Analyses (not presented here) found that no-contact individuals of all ages, regardless of socioeconomic background, continued to be low users in 1996: 60% to 62% made one or more contacts with a physician in 1996 (in contrast, among 1986 users, 81% to 82% made contact with physicians in 1996). The nonusers were also healthier; those who had no physician contact in 1986 were less likely to die over the period 1986–1987 than were those in their socioeconomic group who contacted physicians. Their mortality rates were also lower in 1996.

Table 5.3 reviews a set of health status indicators for each group in 1986 and 1996, pertinent to answering the following question: Is receiving more medical care over long periods of time related to improved health or decreasing inequalities in health? In both 1986 and 1996 there was a much higher mortality rate among residents of the least-educated neighborhoods, and the gap had widened substantially by 1996. Life expectancy was also considerably longer for residents of the most-educated neighborhoods in both years, and by 1996 that advantage, too, had increased.[9] Put somewhat differently, the greatest improvements in health status over this period occurred in precisely those groups who received the least medical care, and the least improvement occurred in those who received the most.

Although the previous measures were based on mortality, we also found that the prevalence of diabetes was higher among residents of low-education neighborhoods. The remaining two health status measures in table 5.3 focused on conditions for which timely medical intervention had been found effective in reducing the likelihood of hospitalization, either through preventing the condition (e.g., cervical cancer), finding and treating the condition in an early phase to avoid major consequences (e.g., iron deficiency anemia or peptic ulcer), or through controlling an acute episode (e.g., asthma) or managing a chronic disease (e.g., diabetes). Despite their somewhat higher rates of contact with physicians (visits per person) and higher drug-use rates, residents of the low- and middle-education neighborhoods had much higher rates of hospitalizations for these conditions than did residents of high-education neighborhoods. We again noted a gradient relationship between these indicators and education level: It was not just that the residents of the least-educated neighborhoods fared less well by these indicators—all suffered relative to those in the most-educated neighborhoods, and all, as noted in table 5.2, received at least as many physician contacts in both 1986 and 1996 as did the residents of the high-education neighborhoods. The comparison across quintiles

Table 5.3. Health status (1986 and 1996), by relative educational level of individuals' neighborhoods in 1986 (age and sex standardized to the 1996 population)

Variable	Q1 Least educated	Q2	Q3	Q4	Q5 Most educated	Q1/Q5
Mortality						
All-cause deaths per 1,000						
1986	11.40	10.55	10.14	9.58	9.41	1.21
1996	11.62	10.05	9.77	9.47	8.18	1.42
Premature deaths per 1,000 (Age 0–74)						
1986	6.07	5.37	4.69	4.60	4.38	1.39
1996	6.01	4.55	4.45	4.14	3.25	1.85
Life expectancy (age 10) in years						
Males						
1986	66.49	68.23	69.65	69.75	70.14	0.95
1996	66.38	69.04	69.82	71.20	73.69	0.90
Females						
1986	73.71	74.83	75.52	76.04	76.50	0.96
1996	72.65	75.99	75.87	75.50	76.59	0.95
Disease prevalence cases per 1,000						
Diabetes (ages 20–79)						
1986	53.08	45.36	42.20	39.00	34.37	1.54
1996	72.35	59.05	53.18	48.94	42.20	1.71
Hospitalization for:						
Avoidable conditions						
1986	7.67	5.97	5.33	5.25	4.12	1.86
1996	7.74	6.19	5.81	4.74	4.69	1.65
Ambulatory sensitive						
1986	17.09	14.61	12.89	13.04	10.22	1.67
1996	16.49	13.09	12.69	12.03	10.86	1.51

Source: The Population Health Research Data Repository, Manitoba Centre for Health Policy.

of rates of hospitalization for these two sets of conditions over time presented a somewhat different pattern: In 1996, compared to 1986, there was some narrowing of the gradient, produced by a decrease in rates of hospitalization for these conditions in the lowest-education group and an increase in the highest-education group, although this pattern was not consistent across the socioeconomic groups.[10]

Indicators of Quality of Care Received

Although the quantity of medical care received may have been higher for residents of low-education neighborhoods, is it possible that they showed relatively little improvement in health over time because of the poor quality of care received?

Inferential evidence from examining selected types of procedures or places where care had been received was not definitive. Whereas in 1986 residents of low-education neighborhoods spent 40% more days in the hospital than residents of high-education neighborhoods (after age–sex adjustment, see table 5.2), they spent more than twice as many of those days in teaching hospitals (908 versus 433 days per capita) as did residents of high-education neighborhoods. Teaching hospitals are generally found to provide higher quality care[11] (Ayanian and Weissman 2002; Dimick et al. 2004).

Residents of low-education neighborhoods did have a somewhat lower rate of referral to specialists, as well as a lower contact rate with specialists, than that of residents of high-education neighborhoods (although not reported in the tables, their specialist contact rate was approximately 15% lower in 1986 and 1996). However, access to specialist care seems unlikely to explain the better health of residents of the higher socioeconomic status neighborhoods. Indeed, residents of the healthiest areas of rural Manitoba had much lower specialist contact rates than did the unhealthy residents of low-education Winnipeg neighborhoods.[12] Previous research also shows that women in Winnipeg's more affluent neighborhoods were somewhat more likely than residents of the poorest neighborhoods to have had at least one Pap test over a three-year period (74% versus 65%) and were more likely to have undergone mammography screening (70% versus 48%). Children of both groups were very likely to have received their immunizations (85% and 91% in Q1 and Q5, respectively) (L. Roos et al. 1999; Gupta et al. 2003).

Evidence on whether access to procedures that often markedly improve quality of life (e.g., hip and knee replacement, percutaneous transluminal coronary angioplasty, pacemaker implant) varies with socioeconomic status has been mixed. For example, Roos and Mustard (1997) found that although those in the highest-income quintiles had higher rates of coronary artery bypass surgery than residents of low-income neighborhoods, the highest rates were experienced by those in the middle-income neighborhoods. For cataract surgery, we found higher rates among those in the lowest-income groups (7.6 versus 6.1 procedures per 1,000 residents, after age and sex adjustment). More recent analyses (Frohlich et al. 2002) have compared rates of many of the quality of life procedures across areas of Winnipeg organized by the relative health status of area residents. The ranking of areas on health status (premature mortality rates) correlates 0.98 and 0.96 with community and neighborhood scores on a measure of socioeconomic status (the socioeconomic factors index). No relationship between age–sex-standardized rates of care and relative health status of area residents was found for any of the following procedures: cardiac catheterization, angioplasty, coronary artery bypass, hip and knee replacement, cataract surgery. There were higher rates of computed tomography (CT) scans among residents of the least healthy areas, as well as higher rates of magnetic resonance imaging among residents of the healthier areas.

In Manitoba, there were generally no differences in waiting times for surgery based on socioeconomic status, and, if anything, median waiting times for residents of the lowest-income neighborhoods for hernia repairs, carpal tunnel surgeries, prostatectomies, and carotid endarterectomies was shorter than the Winnipeg median wait (DeCoster et al. 1999). Thus, although we have little direct evidence on the quality of care received by groups, across a variety of quasi-indicators, we have found no consistent socioeconomic status–related differences in the type of health care received.

Hospital Bed Closures and Health of the Population

As noted in table 5.2, between 1986 and 1996 a remarkable drop occurred in inpatient hospital use (days and admissions) by Winnipeg residents.[13] This finding is explained by the fact that in the late 1980s and early 1990s Manitoba, along with other Canadian provinces, began to restrain health care spending, mainly by downsizing the acute hospital sector. By the end of fiscal year 1996, a total of 731 acute beds (or 24% of the supply in 1992) had been closed in Winnipeg hospitals. Between 1991 and 1994 hospital expenditures per capita (after adjusting for inflation) declined by 7.2%. This downsizing created enormous anxiety among health professionals and the public. Hospital cutbacks were (and continue to be) associated with front-page coverage portraying a health care system in distress—even crisis. But how has downsizing affected Manitobans' health status?

In a study of several cross-sectional groups of Winnipeg residents, we (Brownell et al. 1999; Brownell et al. 2001) used mortality rates to track the impact of this downsizing on the Winnipeg population's health status. All-age mortality indicators for males and females, cause-specific mortality measures (deaths from chronic disease, cancer, and injuries), and premature-death rates (among residents from birth to seventy-four years) were essentially unchanged over the period of downsizing (between 1990 and 1996). Indeed, overall mortality rates, as well as mortality rates for males and for deaths due to chronic diseases, actually decreased between 1991 and 1996 (the largest decrease, for deaths due to chronic diseases, was 6.4%).[14] Because older adults tend, on average, to be sicker than the rest of the population and are consequently the heaviest users of hospitals, we also tracked age-specific mortality rates for those aged seventy-five and older. The data showed that only for residents ninety and older was there an increase in mortality rates between 1990 and 1996, but this increase occurred between 1990 and 1991, prior to the bed closures. This increase is likely due to the increase in life expectancy; as individuals live longer, more can be expected to die at very old age.

Of course these overall trends in mortality might have masked increases in certain socioeconomic strata. But similar to the findings we presented earlier in table 5.3, in fact all deaths (6.7%) and deaths for those between birth and seventy-four years (premature mortality, 12%) increased between 1991 and 1996 for residents of neighborhoods in the lowest-income group. Residents of neighborhoods in the other four income groups did not show similar increases. And for those from the wealthiest neighborhoods, the mortality rate actually decreased, by 15% (in 1991, 2.47 deaths per 1,000; in 1996, 2.08).

These results, too, send mixed messages about the role of health care as a determinant of health. We found that the downsizing of the acute hospital sector had no detectable negative impact on the health status of the vulnerable elderly (as measured through mortality rates, at least) or on the overall population. If anything, the overall health status of Winnipeg residents appears to have improved over this period. But might the apparent decline in health status among the poor and the improved health status among wealthy Winnipeg residents be explained by differential impacts of health reform? Were the wealthy better able to maintain access to beds as the system downsized? In fact, quite the opposite appears to have happened. All income groups used fewer days of hospital care in 1996 than in 1991, with the lowest-income group having the smallest proportional decrease overall (fig. 5.1). Once again it is important to note the marked differences in hospital use across income groups. In 1996, low-income residents were still spending 83% more days in hospital (per 1,000 population) than those living in the

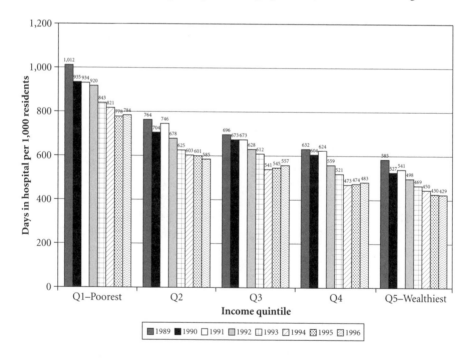

Figure 5.1. **Days in hospital by Income Quintile: Winnipeg Residents (Short Stay < 60 days) 1989–1996. Q1–Q5 each represents 20% of population residing in Winnipeg neighborhoods.**

Source: The Population Health Research Data Repository, Manitoba Centre for Health Policy.

wealthiest neighborhoods.[15] These findings parallel those we showed earlier in table 5.2, where we compared 1986 to 1996.

We also specifically examined the hospital use patterns of the poor to see if there were any detectable changes in quality of care that might have contributed to the health declines (Brownell et al. 1999). Using the data at our disposal, again we were unable to identify any such changes. When mortality rates and readmission rates for several common conditions were examined separately for those from the lowest-income group, no increases were found, with the exception of an increased readmission rate for those with digestive disorders. We checked deaths within thirty days of discharge from hospitals for digestive disorders and found that the numbers were very small (thirty deaths in 1991 and twenty-nine deaths in 1996) and therefore would not have had an impact on changes in population mortality rates.

Health Care and Population Health— Reconsidering the Evidence

The health care system in Manitoba appears to be doing a good job of allocating medical care on the basis of relative need. Even a 24% reduction in acute hospital bed supply, combined with a real decrease in hospital spending, was implemented in Manitoba in such a way that socioeconomically disadvantaged groups whose health is poorer continued to receive relatively more care than advantaged groups whose health is better. Furthermore, the bed closures had no detectable impact on the measures of health status that we examined.

These analyses, however, also suggest that medical care is the wrong policy tool if the objective is to reduce inequalities in the health of a population. Ample evidence exists that those in lower socioeconomic groups are less healthy. What is less widely understood, however, is that this poor health persists despite their high use of most types of health care. In Manitoba we found that, over time, health status worsened in those groups who received the most medical care and improved in those who received the least. Some researchers tend to assume that the differential accessibility of health care to different socioeconomic strata within a society may "partially explain" the social gradient in avoidable mortality (Wood et al. 1999). Thus, Macintyre (1989, p. 329) has argued that not only do we not know how to produce "equalities in health" but also that attempting to reach this goal would potentially involve "very unequal distributions of (health-care) resources."[16] Mackenbach, Stronks, and Kunst (1989) have also argued that a truly egalitarian health care policy aimed at the equalization of health status in the population would require a radical redistribution of medical care in favor of those most in need. The Manitoba data showed that even where markedly unequal distributions of medical care had been achieved and maintained over time, sharp inequalities in health continued to exist.

Could our documented lack of relationship between medical care consumption and health outcomes be explained by the fact that Manitoba invests too little in its health care system? Not likely. The province has spent almost twice as much delivering health care to Manitoba's least-healthy populations (Winnipeg's inner-core residents and residents of the remote northern regions) as it has spent on other Manitobans (Shanahan and Gousseau 1999); and the health of these least healthy groups has fallen, both absolutely and relative to that of residents of more affluent areas of the province (Mustard et al. 1999; Brownell et al. 2001). In 1996, Manitoba ranked among the upper half of Canadian provinces in terms of per capita expenditure on health care, depending on which costs (e.g., provincial, federal, private) were included (Shanahan et al. 1999), and Canadian per capita expenditures, though lower than American, are higher than those of many European countries including France, Austria, Belgium, Denmark, and Italy (Anderson et al. 2003). Furthermore, it is likely that the unhealthy, lower socioeconomic groups consume much more health care than higher socioeconomic groups wherever public insurance plays a major role (Mackenbach, 2003; van Doorslaer et al. 2000).

Even in the United States, those in the lowest income group (i.e., people with annual incomes less than $15,000) have 2.3 times the hospital admissions of those in the highest income group (with incomes over $50,000) and make 30% more contacts with physicians (7.4 visits per year versus 5.6) (Pamuk et al. 1998).[17]

We found no consistent socioeconomic status–related differences in the type of health care received, but our indicators were crude. Did we likely miss something? Starfield (1992) and others (Shi et al. 2000; Shi and Starfield 2000) have provided evidence, first, that strengthening primary care can ameliorate some of the adverse health outcomes of income inequalities and, second, that the availability of primary care physicians is more strongly related to positive health outcomes at the population level than is the total physician supply. Residents of low socioeconomic status neighborhoods in Manitoba already make higher use of primary care physicians than do residents of high socioeconomic status neighborhoods (Roos and Mustard 1997), and a greater proportion of their care is delivered by primary care physicians. The quality of care they receive obviously could be improved: Residents of less affluent neighborhoods receive fewer recommended preventive services and have poorer continuity of care (Mustard et al. 1996; L. Roos et al. 1999) than those of more advantaged neighborhoods.

Others might argue that the lower rates of specialist contact and specialist-derived services (e.g., scans, cardiac procedures), particularly relative to the high health needs of Winnipeg's lower socioeconomic groups, might help explain the poor health we have documented among those residents. However, the real contribution of specialized, high-tech care to population health status is difficult to estimate. For example, Alter and colleagues (1999) reported that the higher the neighborhood income level of Ontario residents, the higher the use of coronary angiography, the shorter the waiting times for catheterization, and the lower the mortality one year after acute myocardial infarction. Nevertheless, they concluded that "reduced access to coronary revascularization does not account for income-related differences in one-year mortality" (p. 1365). Lower income was a significant and *independent* predictor of higher one-year mortality in all the multivariate analyses.

Even studies showing some benefit from more intensive and arguably higher-quality medical care have suggested that the health benefits are modest and short-acting, relative to the effect sizes of other non–health-care determinants. For example, in a comparison of the use of invasive cardiac procedures and mortality outcomes after acute myocardial infarction in elderly U.S. and Canadian patients (Tu et al. 1997), U.S. patients were found to have been much more likely than Canadian patients to have received cardiac procedures such as coronary angiography, percutaneous transluminal coronary angioplasty, and coronary artery bypass graft surgery after their heart attacks. Thirty-day mortality rates were slightly but significantly lower for U.S. patients than for Canadian patients, but one-year mortality rates were virtually identical for the two groups. The authors concluded that much higher rates of use of cardiac procedures in the United States did not appear to result in better long-term survival rates.

In contrast, systematic relationships between socioeconomic characteristics and health status have been observed for roughly a hundred years in England and France (Liberatos et al. 1988), and they became a focus of research in North America in the 1990s (Pamuk et al. 1998; Pappas et al. 1993; Durch et al. 1997). An examination of data from the U.S. Longitudinal Study of Aging showed clearly that the more educated were not only living longer but also doing so without disabilities (Olshansky and Wilkins 1998). Studies from the Netherlands, Finland, Belgium, and Britain have also found both longer life and better health expectancy for the higher socioeconomic groups. That is, people of higher socioeconomic status spend a smaller proportion of their longer lives in poor health (Bone et al. 1998; Van Lenthe et al. 2004). Although some conditions may be more related to socioeconomic circumstances than others, a strong gradient in health status has been shown to exist across socioeconomic groups for most types of diseases (Vagero 1991; Millman 1993) and for most types of morbidity. This holds for morbidity defined using clinical measures (Stamler and Hardy 1987; Payne and Saul 1997), self-reports of functional status, self-perceived health, symptoms, pain levels, days spent ill in bed, and reports of long-standing illness (Keskimaki et al. 1995; Lundberg 1991). In contrast, despite decades of research documenting that some areas of most countries, states and provinces have twice as many physicians per capita as other areas (or hospital beds or hip replacements), there is little or no evidence that "more care" actually results in improved health in the high use populations.

If, as suggested by the large and growing body of evidence alluded to above, socioeconomic conditions per se drive the development of disease and its complications, then effective medical care can be expected at most to reduce or minimize the gradients in negative outcomes. The underlying gradient in poor health is likely to persist, even with effective, efficiently delivered, and equitably distributed medical care.

In summary, knowing the level of health-care provision, at least in a developed society, can tell us little about the health of the population (though at least in Manitoba, understanding the distribution of health care provision permits us to refute claims that, under universal health insurance, health care resources are not distributed on the basis of relative health needs). In sharp contrast, if we know a population's relative education, income, or socioeconomic level, we have key information about how likely that population is to be healthy, and the relationship is a remarkably sensitive one: those in the lower-middle class are healthier than those in the poorest groups, and those in the upper-middle class are less healthy than those in the wealthiest group.

But health care does matter. Ask anyone who has received a knee replacement or successful chemotherapy, either of which obviously can be an effective medical intervention.[18] So why do two- to fourfold variations in the provision of health care not seem to produce detectable differences in health status at the population level (Fisher et al. 2003a, 2003b)? It has been argued that the higher rates of care are not delivered to people who need, and could benefit from, them most. It may simply be that those most in need of care face multiple symptom or illness complexes against which "reactive" medical care is relatively impotent. Studies identifying medical interventions that have helped reduce socioeconomic inequalities in health have stressed the importance of targeting high-risk populations, combined with providing systematic and intensive interventions (Arblaster et al. 1996).

Health insurance also matters. The series of reports from the Institute of Medicine (National Academies of Science 2001, 2002, 2004) make a persuasive case that America's uninsured are undertreated and receive poorer care. The Manitoba results provide strong support for universal health care such as the Canadian Medicare program, with the allocation of many types of care appearing to be remarkably needs-driven.[19] In other research we and others have also shown that the relatively high use of hospitals by patients from lower socioeconomic groups does in fact represent needs-driven servicing patterns, not "social admissions" (DeCoster et al. 1997; Billings et al. 1993). The acuity levels of hospitalized patients in the lowest socioeconomic group have proven just as high as the acuity levels of hospitalized patients in the highest socioeconomic group. Individuals in poorer health have more conditions for which the health care system can offer pain relief, a supportive environment, and palliative care.

If much of what we receive from the health-care system provides care rather than cure, then policy makers must confront the fundamental choices implied by the data presented in this chapter. The health care system will, as Wildavsky (1977) so astutely noted a couple of decades ago, absorb any and all resources thrown its way. But this infinite absorptive capacity comes at a cost. Thus, for example, Labonte (1992) estimated that for the $350 million that Ontario hospitals received above a previous year's budget, the province could have funded 70,000 more rent-geared-to-income housing units, 450,000 more subsidized day-care spaces, and 12,000 transitional shelter beds. The research suggesting which of these investments might have done the most for Ontario residents' health has not yet been done, but the evidence suggesting that the biggest health bang for those bucks came from that hospital sector investment is not strong. Yet with a continuing preoccupation with crowded emergency rooms and waiting lists for surgery, that is the sector in which the Canadian government is directing most of its renewed social investment.

Britain, in contrast, has set National Health Inequalities Targets, an approach that holds considerable promise for real improvement in population health (Mitchell et al. 2000). Although the jury is still out on whether the British initiative will make a real impact (Exworthy et al. 2003), both the Netherlands and Sweden are also taking steps in this direction, including potential initiatives in labor markets and working conditions (Mackenbach and Bakker, 2003). Graham (2004) argues that it is these inequalities in health determinants that societies must tackle if they are to reduce inequalities in health.

To conclude, a universal health care system is definitely the right policy tool for delivering care to those in need, and for this it must be respected and supported. However, investments in health care should never be confused with, or sold as, policies whose primary intent is to improve population health or to reduce inequalities in health. Claims to that effect are misleading at best, dangerous and highly wasteful at worst.

Acknowledgment

Funding from the Canada Research Chair in Population Health held by Noralou Roos supported this study. The results and conclusions are those of the authors; we are indebted to Health Information Services, Manitoba Health, and the Office of Vital Statistics in the Agency of Consumer and Corporate Affairs for providing data. No official endorsement by Manitoba Health or the Office of Vital Statistics is intended or implied.

Notes

1. Of the various nominal measures of socioeconomic status (income, occupation, education) education is the most stable over the life course and is the best reflection of an individual's earlier life developmental history. This history itself is a powerful determinant of health (see chapter 4).

2. Since the quintiles were developed using total urban population, each Winnipeg quintile did not necessarily contain 20% of the population.

3. Although some data were reported by education quintiles and some by income quintiles, all analyses based on educational quintiles were also repeated using income quintiles, and the results were very similar.

4. Of those alive and residing in Winnipeg in 1996, 68% continued to live in a neighborhood ranked within 1 quintile above or below their neighborhood of residence in 1986. This comparison was made only for those who remained in Winnipeg over the entire period; however, individuals' health care use over the ten years was tracked regardless of where in the province they moved.

5. The provincial health program, known as the Manitoba Health Services Insurance Plan, provides universal first-dollar coverage (i.e., no deductibles, no copayments) for hospital care and most physician services. Prescription drugs are covered, subject to an income-based deductible.

6. The sample size in each group was large, with 102,986 to 136,153 available for analysis in 1986 and from 82,510 to 105,600 alive and remaining in the province in 1996.

7. Of those alive and residing in Winnipeg in 1996, 68% continued to live in a neighborhood ranked within 1 quintile above or below their neighborhood of residence in 1986. This comparison was made only for those who remained in Winnipeg over the entire period, since quintiles were calculated separately for urban and rural areas; however, health care use by those remaining in Manitoba was reported, regardless of where the use occurred.

8. The days per capita fell markedly over the period. The rates have been adjusted by age and sex, so the impact of aging has been removed. This was a period of substantial bed closures in the Winnipeg hospitals; the impact of these on the various groups is reviewed in upcoming portions of the chapter.

9. Although the difference in life expectancy between residents of the low- and high-education neighborhoods appears small, it is nevertheless impressive. That is, in 1986 males in the high-education neighborhoods had a life expectancy that was 3.65 years longer than the life expectancy of males in the low-education neighborhoods; by 1996 the advantage for males in high-education neighborhoods had grown to 7.3 years. Manton (1991) has estimated that the gain in American life expectancy from eliminating all types of cancer at birth would be 2.8 years; from eliminating cardiovascular disease, 5.5 years.

10. Since ambulatory care, particularly specialist contact and referrals to specialists, was the one type of medical care for which the higher-socioeconomic group had, if anything, equal or better access at both points in time than the lower-socioeconomic group, the increase in hospital admissions for these ambulatory-care–sensitive or avoidable conditions is difficult to explain by changing patterns of access to ambulatory care.

11. Kahn, Pearson, and Harrison (1994) found in the United States that poor and black Medicare patients received worse care at specific hospitals than did others. But because Medicare patients were twice as likely to use teaching hospitals where care tended to be better, the study showed that Medicare patients received as high a quality of care as others, regardless of race or financial status.

12. Unhealthy residents of the low-education neighborhoods have specialist contact rates two to three times as high as do residents of some of Manitoba's very healthy rural areas (N. Roos et al. 1999).

13. All rates are age- and sex-adjusted using the December 1992 Manitoba population and a direct method of standardization. This approach provides an indication of the use of care and health status relative to that of another year after the effects of changes in population structure—most importantly, over these years, the aging of the population—have been removed.

14. In the province of Saskatchewan, where fifty-two rural hospitals stopped delivering acute care, mortality rates also declined after bed closures, with the largest declines occurring in those communities that either converted their hospitals to other uses or closed them. Residents' perceptions of their health were consistent with the mortality data; respondents

"overwhelmingly reported that the loss of acute care funding did not adversely affect their own or their family's health" (Health Services Utilization and Research Commission [HSURC] 1999, 16).

15. As the full report shows, Winnipeg hospitals have managed health reform very well; while total days that residents spent in hospitals fell markedly, this was essentially achieved by shortening lengths of stay and moving to outpatient surgery. Overall access to hospitals (when outpatient surgery and inpatient admissions are combined) did not change significantly between 1991 and 1996 for any income group. That is, even after controlling for the aging of the population, access to hospitals was similar before and after downsizing.

16. To be fair, however, Macintyre (1989, p. 329) also recognized that "rarely . . . is the magnitude of the disparities in health care sufficient to explain the disparities in health or death rates." She also states, "it is difficult to conclude that disparities in health care are a, or the, cause of the disparities in health."

17. Importantly, in 1964, before Medicare, the U.S. hospitalization gradient was reversed, with those in the lowest income group reporting 102 admissions per capita (compared with 141 in 1995), and those in the highest income group reporting 111 admissions per capita (compared with 62 in 1995) (Pamuk et al. 1998). These patterns of usage are likely driven by the elderly who have access to Medicare. In contrast, wealthy American children have more contacts with physicians than do middle-class children, and poor American children have the lowest rate of physician contact (Pamuk et al. 1998). In Manitoba, all children, regardless of socioeconomic status, show similar rates of contact with physicians, with those from the poorest neighborhoods having somewhat higher contact rates.

18. Bunker, Frazier, and Mosteller (1994) and Bunker (1995) have provided some of the most thoughtful attempts to summarize the contributions of specific medical interventions to life expectancy and quality of life.

19. This conceptualization of need is quite consistent with the concept of relative fairness (Fox and Carr-Hill 1989), grounded in data that focus on access and use relative to health status, and combined with a sense of the key role of other determinants of health.

References

Alter, D. A., C. D. Naylor, P. Austin, and J. V. Tu. 1999. Effects of socioeconomic status on access to invasive cardiac procedures and on mortality after acute myocardial infarction. *New England Journal of Medicine* 341:1359–1367.

Anderson, G. F., U. E. Reinhard, P. S. Hussey, and V. Petrosyan. 2003. It's the prices, stupid: Why the United States is so different from other countries. *Health Affairs (Millwood)* 22 (3):89–105.

Arblaster, L., M. Lambert, V. Entwistle, M. Forster, D. Fullerton, T. Sheldon, and I. Watt. 1996. A systematic review of the effectiveness of health service interventions aimed at reducing inequalities in health. *Journal of Health Services Research Policy* 1 (2):93–103.

Ayanian, J. Z., and J. S. Weissman. 2002. Teaching hospitals and quality of care: A review of the literature. *Milbank Memorial Fund Quarterly* 80:569–593.

Billings, J., L. Zeitel, J. Lukomnik, T. S. Carey, A. E. Blank, and L. Newman. 1993. Data watch: Impact of socioeconomic status on hospital use in New York City. *Health Affairs* 12:162–173.

Birch, S., and J. Eyles. 1991. Needs-based planning of health care: A critical appraisal of the literature. Working paper no. 91-5, Centre for Health Economics and Policy Analysis, Hamilton, Ontario.

Bone, M. R., A. C. Bebbington, and G. Nicolas. 1998. Policy applications of health expectancy. *Journal of Aging Health* 10:136.

Boyd, C., J. Y. Zhang-Salomons, P. A. Groome, and W. J. Mackillop. 1999. Associations between community income and cancer survival in Ontario, Canada, and the United States. *Journal of Clinical Oncology* 17:2244–2255.

Brownell, M., N. P. Roos, and C. Burchill. 1999. Monitoring the impact of hospital downsizing on access to care and quality of care. *Medical Care* 37 (suppl. 6):JS135–S150.

Brownell, M. D., N. P. Roos, and L. L. Roos. 2001. Monitoring health reform: A report card approach. *Social Science Medicine* 52:657–670.

Bunker, J. 1995. Medicine matters after all. *Journal of the Royal College of Physicians of London* 29:105–112.

Bunker, J., H. Frazier, and F. Mosteller. 1994. Improving health: Measuring effects of medical care. *Milbank Memorial Fund Quarterly* 72:225–258.

Carstairs, V., and R. Morris. 1989. Deprivation: Explaining differences in mortality between Scotland and England and Wales. *British Medical Journal* 229:866–889.

DeCoster C., N. Roos, and B. Bogdanovic. 1995. Utilization of nursing home resources. *Medical Care* 33 (suppl 12):DS73–DS83.

DeCoster, C., K. C. Carriere, S. Peterson, R. Walld, and L. MacWilliam. 1999. Waiting times for surgical procedures. *Medical Care* 37 (suppl. 6):JS187–JS205.

DeCoster, C., N. P. Roos, K. C. Carriere, and S. Peterson. 1997. Inappropriate hospital use by patients receiving care for medical conditions: Targeting utilization review. *Canadian Medical Association Journal* 157:889–896.

Dimick, J. B., J. A. Cowan Jr., L. M. Colletti, and G. R. Upchurch Jr. 2004. Hospital teaching status and outcomes of complex surgical procedures in the United States. *Archives of Surgery* 139:137–141.

Durch, J. S., L. A. Bailey, and M. A. Stoto, eds. 1997. *Improving the Health in the Community: A Role for Performance Monitoring.* Washington, DC: National Academy Press.

Exworthy, M., D. Blane, and M. Marmot. 2003. Tackling health inequalities in the United Kingdom: The progress and pitfalls of policy. *Health Services Research* 38.6 (II):1905–1921.

Falik, M., J. Needleman, B. L. Wells, and J. Korb. 2001. Ambulatory care sensitive hospitalizations and emergency visits: Experiences of Medicaid patients using federally qualified health centres. *Medical Care* 39:551–561.

Fisher, E. S., D. E. Wennberg, T. A. Stukel, D. J. Gottlieb, F. L. Lucas, and E. L. Pinder. 2003a. The implications of regional variations in Medicare spending. Part 1: The content, quality, and accessibility of care. *Annals of Internal Medicine* 138:273–287.

Fisher, E. S., D. E. Wennberg, T. A. Stukel, D. J. Gottlieb, F. L. Lucas, and E. L. Pinder. 2003b. The implications of regional variations in Medicare spending. Part 2: Health outcomes and satisfaction with care. *Annals of Internal Medicine* 138:288–298.

Forget E., R. B. Deber, and L. L. Roos. 2002. Medical savings accounts: Will they reduce costs? *Canadian Medical Association Journal* 167:143–147.

Fox, J., and R. Carr-Hill. 1989. Introduction. In *Health Inequalities in European Countries*, ed. J. Fox. Aldershot: Gower.

Frohlich, N., R. Fransoo, and N. Roos. 2002. Health service use in the Winnipeg Regional Health Authority; variations across areas in relation to health and socioeconomic status. *Health Care Management Forum* (Winter):9–14.

Gorey, K. M., E. J. Holowaty, E. Laukkanen, G. Fehringer, and N. L. Richter. 1998. An international comparison of cancer survival: Advantage of Toronto's poor over the near poor of Detroit. *Canadian Journal of Public Health* 89:102–103.

Gorey K. M., E. J. Holowaty, G. Fehringer, E. Laukkanen, N. L. Richter, and C. M. Meyer. 2000. An international comparison of cancer survival: Metropolitan Toronto, Ontario, and Honolulu, Hawaii. *American Journal of Public Health* 90:1866–1872.

Gorey, K. M., E. Kliewer, E. J. Holowaty, E. Laukkanen, and Y. Edwin. 2003. An international comparison of breast cancer survival: Winnipeg, Manitoba and Des Moines, Iowa, metropolitan areas. *Annals of Epidemiology* 13:32–41.

Graham, H. 2004. Social determinants and their unequal distribution: Clarifying policy understandings. *Milbank Memorial Fund Quarterly* 82:101–124.

Gupta, S., L. Roos, R. Walld, D. Traverse, and M. Dahl. 2003. Delivering equitable care: Comparing preventive services in Manitoba. *American Journal of Public Health* 93:2086–2092.

Hansluwka, H. E. 1985. Measuring the health of populations: Indicators and interpretations. *Social Science and Medicine* 20:1207–1224.

Health Services Utilization and Research Commission (HSURC). 1999. Assessing the impact of the 1993 acute care funding cuts to rural Saskatchewan hospitals. Summary report no. 13. Saskatoon. Hindle, D. 2000. Health care in Canada: A first annual report. *Canadian Institute for Health Information (CIHI)*, Ottawa.

Hussey, P. S., G. F. Anderson, R. O. C. Feek, V. McLaughlin, J. Millar, and A. Epstein. 2004. How does the quality of care compare in five countries? *Health Affairs* 23:89–99.

Kahn, I., M. Pearson, and E. Harrison. 1994. Health care for black and poor hospitalized Medicare patients. *Journal of the American Medical Association* 271:1169–1174.

Keskimaki, I., M. Salinto, and S. Aro. 1995. Socioeconomic equity in Finnish hospital care in relation to need. *Social Science and Medicine* 41:425.

Kindig, D. 1997. *Purchasing Population Health Paying for Results.* Ann Arbor: University of Michigan Press.

Kindig, D. A. 1999. Beyond health services research. *Health Services Research* 34:205–214. Kozyrskyj A., and C. A. Mustard. 1998. Validation of an electronic, population-based prescription database. *Annals of Pharmacotherapy* 32:1152–1157.

Labonte, R. 1992. Health care spending as a risk to health. *Canadian Journal of Public Health* 81:251–252.

Liberatos, P., B. Link, and J. Kelsey. 1988. The measurement of social class in epidemiology. *Epidemiological Reviews* 10:87–121.

Lundberg, O. 1991. Causal explanations for class inequality and health: An empirical analysis. *Social Science and Medicine* 32:385–393.

Macintyre, S. 1989. The role of health services in relation to inequalities in health in Europe. In *Health Inequalities in European Countries*, ed. J. Fox. Brookfield, UK: Gower.

Mackenbach, J. 2003. An analysis of the role of health care in reducing socioeconomic inequalities in health: The case of The Netherlands. *International Journal of Health Services* 33:523–541.

Mackenbach J. P., and M. J. Bakker. 2003. European network on interventions and policies to reduce inequalities in health. Tackling socioeconomic inequalities in health: Analysis of European experiences. *Lancet* 362:1409–1414.

Mackenbach, J. P., K. Stronks, and A. Kunst. 1989. The contribution of medical care to inequalities in health: Differences between socioeconomic groups in decline of mortality from conditions amenable to medical interventions. *Social Science and Medicine* 29:369–376.

Manton, K. G. 1991. The dynamics of population aging: Demography and policy analysis. *Milbank Memorial Fund Quarterly* 69:309–340.

Metge, C., C. Black, S. Peterson, and A. L. Kozyrskyj. 1999. The population's use of pharmaceuticals. *Medical Care* 37 (suppl. 6):JS42–JS59.

Millman, M. 1993. *Using Indicators to Monitor National Objectives for Health Care.* Washington, DC: National Academy Press.

Mitchell, R., D. Dorling, and M. Shaw. 2000. *Inequalities in Life and Death: What If Britain Were More Equal?* Bristol: Policy Press.

Mustard, C., S. Derksen, and C. Black. 1999. Widening regional inequality in premature mortality rates in Manitoba. *Canadian Journal of Public Health* 90:372–376.

Mustard, C., T. Mayers, C. D. Black, and B. Postl. 1996. Continuity of pediatric ambulatory care in a universally insured population. *Pediatrics* 98:1028–1034.

National Academies of Science. Committee on the Consequences of Uninsurance, Board on Health Care Services, Institute of Medicine. 2001. *Coverage Matters: Insurance and Health Care.* Washington, DC: National Academies Press.

National Academies of Science. Committee on the Consequences of Uninsurance, Board on Health Care Services, Institute of Medicine. 2002. *Care without Coverage: Too Little, Too Late.* Washington, DC: National Academies Press.

National Academies of Science. Committee on the Consequences of Uninsurance, Board on Health Care Services, Institute of Medicine. 2004. *Insuring America's Health: Principles and Recommendations.* Washington, DC: National Academies Press.

Naylor, D. 1999. Health care in Canada: Incrementalism under fiscal duress. *Health Affairs* (May–June):9–26.

Olshansky, S. J., and R. Wilkins. 1998. Introduction. *Journal of Aging Health* 10:123.

Pamuk, E., D. Makuc, K. Heck, C. Reuben, and K. Lochner. 1998. *Health, United States, 1998, with Socioeconomic Status and Health Chartbook.* Hyattsville, MD: National Center for Health Statistics.

Pappas, G., S. Queen, W. Hadden, and G. Fisher. 1993. The increasing disparity in mortality between socioeconomic groups in the United States, 1960 and 1986. *New England Journal of Medicine* 329:103–109.

Payne, N., and C. Saul. 1997. Variations in use of cardiology services in a health authority; Comparison of coronary artery revascularization rates with prevalence of angina and coronary mortality. *British Medical Journal* 314:257–261.

Reinhardt, U., P. S. Hussey, and G. F. Anderson. 2004. Health care spending in an international context. *Health Affairs* 23 (3):10–25.

Robinson, J. R., T. K. Young, L. L. Roos, and D. Gelskey. 1997. Estimating the burden of disease comparing administrative data and self-reports. *Medical Care* 35:932–947.

Roos, L., C. Mustard, J. Nicol, D. F. McLerran, D. Malenka, K. Young, and M. Cohen. 1993. Registries and administrative data: Organization and accuracy. *Medical Care* 31:201–212.

Roos, L., D. Traverse, and D. Turner. 1999. Delivering prevention: The role of public programs in delivering care to high-risk populations. *Medical Care* 37 (suppl. 6):JS264–JS278.

Roos, L., R. Walld, A. Wajda, R. Bond, and K. Hartford. 1996. Record linkage strategies, outpatient procedures, and administrative data. *Medical Care* 34:570–582.

Roos N. P., E. Forget, R. Walld, and L. MacWilliam. 2003. Does universal comprehensive insurance encourage unnecessary use? Evidence from Manitoba says "no." *Canadian Medical Association Journal* 170:209–214.

Roos, N., R. Fransoo, B. Bogdanovic, K. C. Carriere, N. Frohlich, D. Friesen, and L. MacWilliam. 1999. Issues in planning for specialist physicians. *Medical Care* 37 (suppl. 6):JS229–JS253.

Roos, N. P., and C. A. Mustard. 1997. Variation in health and health care use by socioeconomic status in Winnipeg, Canada: Does the system work well? Yes and no. *Milbank Memorial Fund Quarterly* 75:89.

Shanahan, M., and C. Gousseau. 1999. Using the POPULIS framework for interprovincial comparisons of expenditures on health care. *Medical Care* 37 (suppl. 6):JS83–JS100.

Shanahan, M., C. Steinbach, C. Burchill, D. Friesen, and C. Black. 1999. Adding up provincial expenditures on health care for Manitobans. A POPULIS project. *Medical Care* 37 (suppl. 6):JS60–JS82.

Shapiro, E., and N. P. Roos. 1985. Elderly non-users of health care services: Their characteristics and their health outcomes. *Medical Care* 23 (3):247–257.

Shi, L., and B. Starfield. 2000. Primary care, income inequality, and self-rated health in the United States: A mixed-level analysis. *International Journal of Health Services* 30 (3):541–555.

Shi, L., B. Starfield, B. Kennedy, and I. Kawachi. 2000. Income inequality, primary care, and health indicators. *Journal of Family Practice* 48 (4):275–284.

Simpson, J. 2000. That nasty health-care-spending monster. *Globe and Mail*, April 17, A14.

Stamler, R., and R. J. Hardy. 1987. Educational level and 5-year all-cause mortality in the hypertension detection and follow-up program. *Hypertension* 9:641.

Starfield, B. 1992. *Primary Care: Concept, Evaluation, and Policy*. New York: Oxford University Press.

Tu, J. V., C. L. Pashos, C. D. Naylor, E. Chen, S. L. Normand, J. P. Newhouse, and B. J. McNeil. 1997. Use of cardiac procedures and outcomes in elderly patients with myocardial infarction in the United States and Canada. *New England Journal of Medicine* 336:1500–1505.

U.S. General Accounting Office. 1996. *Public Health: A Health Status Indicator for Targeting Federal Aid to States*. GAO/HEHS-97-13.

Vagero, D. 1991. Inequality in health—some theoretical and empirical problems. *Social Science and Medicine* 32:367–371.

van Doorslaer, E., A. Wagstaff, H. VanDerBerg, T. Christiansen, D. DeGraeve, I. Duchesne, U. G. Gerdtham, M. Gerfin, J. Geurts, L. Gross, U. Hakkinen, J. John, J. Klavus, R. E. Leu, B. Nolan, O. O'Donnell, C. Propper, F. Puffer, M. Schellhorn, G. Sundberg, and O. Winkelhake. 2000. Equity in the delivery of health care in Europe and the U.S. *Journal of Health Economics* 19:553–583.

Van Lenthe, F. J., C. Schrijvers, M. Droomers, I. M. A. Joung, M. J. Louwman, and J. Mackenbach. 2004. Investigating explanations of socio-economic inequalities in health: The Dutch globe study. *European Journal of Public Health* 14:63–70.

Weissman, J. S., C. Gatsonis, and A. M. Epstein. 1992. Rates of avoidable hospitalization by insurance status in Massachusetts and Maryland. *Journal of the American Medical Association* 268:2388–2394.

Wildavsky, A. 1977. Doing better and feeling worse: The political pathology of health policy. *Daedalus* 106 (1):107–13.

Wood, E., A. M. Saller, M. T. Schecter, and R. S. Hogg. 1999. Social inequalities in male mortality amenable to medical intervention in British Columbia. *Social Science and Medicine* 48:1751–58.

Part II

An In-depth Look at Several Determinants of Health

Chapter 6

Food, Nutrition, and Population Health: From Scarcity to Social Inequalities

Lise Dubois

Food is a basic necessity for individuals' day-to-day survival and, therefore, for human populations. Even if, globally, food production is not a problem in the world today, the distribution of food remains a problem in developing and developed countries. It is therefore important to study the social distribution of nutritional inequalities in different populations. Is access to food restricted among materially deprived groups living in rich countries? If there are disparities among socioeconomic groups in wealthy countries, are they increasing or decreasing over time? And what role do socioeconomic differences in access to food play in producing health inequalities? My general intention in this chapter is to suggest some answers to these questions. Figure 6.1 presents a general Nutrition and Population Health Framework of understanding guiding the chapter. Broadly, I describe the effect of food and nutrition on different health outcomes at the population level, examine the relationship between different social determinants and nutrition, and then consider what is not known but would be important to know to diminish nutritional and related health inequalities within and between nations in the years to come.

Food, Nutrition, and Health: A Population Perspective

Providing food for everyone is one of the most complex and fundamental activities that societies always have to fulfill to ensure their survival, yet it is so fundamental that it is banalized. At the individual level, a lack of food can cause growth retardation and nutrient deficiency diseases resulting in goiters, blindness, weakness,

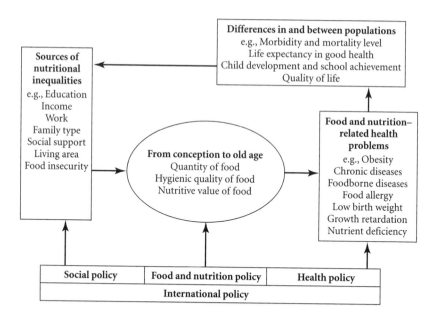

Figure 6.1. Food, nutrition, and population health framework

and death. Poor nutrition can also affect the immune system, making it easier for infectious diseases to develop and harder for someone to recuperate after an infection. Moreover, in a period of food restriction, people often eat poor-quality or contaminated food for immediate survival (Hamlin 1995; Tanner 1992). These observations point to three important attributes of food for population health: the quantity of food, the hygienic quality of food, and the nutritive value of food.

For a nation, a lack of food can lead to less productivity, high mortality rates in infancy and childhood, limited life expectancy, massive emigration (as during Ireland's nineteenth-century potato famine), revolution (as during the French Revolution), and war (Fogel 1994; Flandrin and Montanari 1996). Over the years, urbanized societies developed social structures to ensure the right quantity of widely varied, hygienic foods for all their citizens (McIntosh 1996). This results in the development of complex social organizations adapted to each nation, in which market forces and international trade agreements play an important role. These social organizations include the public sector, the private sector, and the community sector. These sectors regroup public health programs, community-based philanthropic interventions, agriculture and food industries, laws and regulations, and policy interventions at the national and international levels. All of these elements can affect the social distribution of nutritional inequalities in and between countries.

Nutritional Improvement: From Environment to Public Health

McKeown (1988) argued that since the nineteenth century, medicine in Great Britain has had less to do with the decline of infectious disease than broad environmental improvements, including those involving food access and diet quality. The importance of food availability for population health has been confirmed through Fogel's (1994) work on population height and through many other studies in the developing nations. Fogel argued that a better nutritional status—following food supply improvement and the development of nutritional science relating nutrient deficiency to specific diseases and infection—has driven the British population's national productivity and wealth in the past 200 years. Szreter (1986) concluded that, during the period studied by McKeown, public health interventions contributed to 25% of the mortality rate's decline, whereas nutritional improvement contributed to 50% of this decline. Many major public health programs were—and still are—related to nutrition: hygienic interventions (milk pasteurization, meat inspection), food programs for the poor, nutrition education for pregnant women, and dietetic advice for the population (Mackenbach 1993; Guidotti 1997).

Modern public health was born between 1830 and 1840 in Great Britain. As early as 1834, public policies were implemented to improve the nutritional status of the poor (Hamlin 1995). The first food regulations followed when it was understood that rotten meat and contaminated milk were causing disease and death, especially among infants and children. Municipal meat inspection was put in place with the creation of the Adulteration of Food Act in 1870 and the Safety of Food and Drugs Act in 1899 (Szreter 1986). On medical advice, the British government also abolished the tariff on imported food to improve food availability during the same period (Hamlin 1995). In the United States, the first milk stations were put in place in 1895, and school lunch programs for the poor of New York City were begun in 1889 (Egan 1994). In Canada, the first public health interventions began with the creation of the Conseil d'hygiène de la province de Québec in 1887, for the hygienic control of food, including meat inspection by municipalities (Guérard 1996).

The Epidemiological Transition: From Nutritional Deficiency to Nutritional Quality

Industrialization triggered major social transformations that improved food availability, variety, and hygienic quality as never before in the history of humankind. In the United States, vast new lands were available for wheat cultivation, fruit and vegetable growing, and cattle development (Levenstein 1988). Concurrently, life expectancy increased greatly. The nutritional transition from food restriction and lack of hygienic control to better access to a large variety of foods made available by industrialization (which improved transportation and food processing and conservation, and introduced food enrichment in vitamins and minerals) preceded the epidemiological transition, the period in which chronic diseases replaced infectious diseases as the main causes of death in populations. At the beginning of the twentieth century, the general living conditions in North America were better than in Europe, and the first consumer society was developed (Levenstein 1993, 1996). Medical practitioners and dieticians developed nutritional rules to improve the "morality" of people from the lower working classes who were spending their wages on alcohol and other pleasures (Levenstein 1996). This period of nutritional education oriented toward the population's increase of energy and protein consumption has been called the new nutrition period. It was followed by the so-called newer nutrition era, when the role of vitamins and minerals began to be understood, and by the negative nutrition era after the second World War, when it was believed that the population had to learn about the health-harming effects of too much fat, salt, and sugar (Levenstein 1996).

Since the second World War, society has come to think of nutrition as a health-related behavior. To think this way conceals the more fundamental aspect of nutrition—survival. To stay in good health, all people must daily consume enough energy to cover their bodily needs for work and leisure, and they must get an appropriate variety and quantity of different nutrients (World Health Organization [WHO] Study Group on Diet, Nutrition and Prevention of Noncommunicable Disease 1991). A study of nutrition in relation to population health is more relevant if cultural, socioeconomic, and political factors related to food production and consumption are added to dietetic preoccupations for the prevention of chronic diseases. Countries such as Norway have developed food policies targeting the food industry to improve the population's nutritional habits (Norum et al. 1997). It was different in the United States, where the production of low-price, nutritious foods has been countered by the fast-food industry and where the food industry seems to exert a big influence on the development of food policies (Levenstein 1993; Nestle 2002). The efficient production and distribution of plentiful, hygienic, nutritious food in a society is related to the importance accorded to health more generally. Food and nutrition policy are driven by scientific knowledge, as well as by the lobby of the food industry. On the other hand, food industry companies use claims about health benefits to promote their products (Levenstein 1988), forcing governments to restrain the use of health claims on food products (Hurt 2002; Marquart et al. 2003). For the consumer, food has always been used as a tool for disease prevention and cure, and the development of high-tech food especially designed to prevent or cure diseases (e.g., orange juice with added calcium for the prevention of osteoporosis, milk products with added probiotic bacteria to prevent allergy) has added to the complexity of choosing the "right" diet (Dubois 1996).

Table 6.1 illustrates the diversity of governmental food and nutrition policies,

Table 6.1. Canadian governmental policies and programs related to food and nutrition, from the early 1600s to the present

Key health approaches, by time period implementation	Some characteristics of the policies, programs, and interventions put in place at each time period	Main preoccupations guiding the development of the policy
Survival Since the beginning of the colony	Food laws and regulations Land property control Food price control Food importation/exportation control	*Food availability* Food quantity Food diversity
Public health Since mid-18th century	Milk pasteurization and meat inspection programs Act to prevent adulteration of foods, drinks, and drugs Food hygiene control and food conservation standards Public health nutrition education (mothers and children)	*Food safety* Hygienic quality of food Foodborne diseases
Nutrient deficiencies and disease prevention Since first half of 20th century	Food enrichment and fortification programs (first in 1942) Food labeling—nutrient content of food Canadian Dietary Standards (first in 1937) Canadian Food Guide (first in 1942) Nutrition education programs	*Food nutritional quality* "New nutrition": caloric and protein needs "Newer nutrition": nutrient content of food (vitamins and minerals)
Health promotion and chronic diseases prevention Since second half of 20th century	Nutrition recommendations including prevention of chronic diseases (first in 1983) Health promotion programs Food labeling—health claims control Harmonization of Canada—U.S. nutrition recommendations (end of the 1990s)	*Diet nutritional quality* "Negative nutrition": too much fat, sugar, salt, animal products; not enough fiber, fruits, vegetables, etc. "Health food": industry development
Population health Since the mid-1990s	Canada National Nutrition Plan Canada's Action Plan for Food Security Nutrition during pregnancy, breastfeeding, and infant feeding recommendations Action plan of the Canadian government for the future of biotechnology	*Social nutritional inequalities* Poverty and food insecurity Healthy child development Integration of nutrition consideration into health, agriculture, education, social and economic policies and programs *Food safety for novel foods* Novel foods (e.g., *nutraceuticals*) and genetically modified foods

Source: Adapted from Tarlov 1996, p. 76.

programs, and interventions put in place in Canada since the beginning of the colony in the 1600s. These types of programs and interventions still coexist to ensure food availability, food safety, and diet nutritional quality for the population. Policy interventions aimed at reducing nutritional inequalities caused by social inequalities would have to be developed in line with the population health approach used by the Canadian Government since the mid-1990s.

The Social Costs of Food- and Nutrition-related Diseases in Developed Countries

To eat a diversity of food every day is a risky endeavor. Humans learned empirically, by trial and error, which animal and vegetable substances found in their environment were suitable for consumption. Edible foods can nevertheless be contaminated by nonnutritional contaminants (e.g., mercury, lead, pesticides) or by improper conservation. Moreover, some individuals are allergic to foods commonly eaten by the rest of the population (e.g., peanuts, milk, seafood). Finally, food choices need to be in accordance with body needs, which vary over life. Different food constituents (e.g., nutrients) present different long-term health risks to humans in terms of chronic diseases. For example, an excess of saturated fat over the years may lead to cardiovascular diseases, a lack of calcium may lead to osteoporosis, and an excess of stored energy may lead to obesity. Societies develop many strategies to minimize the social and health care costs related to these risks.

Food Contamination and Food Poisoning

Food contamination and food poisoning are not a new source of preoccupation at the population level, and food safety is clearly a public health issue. Foodborne diseases vary from temporary discomfort to disease and death, thus imposing costs to the states, and a food poisoning incident can quickly cause sickness or death for many people. Furthermore, contaminants in foods can be either biological or chemical (e.g., pesticides, toxic elements, naturally occurring toxins, antibiotic residuals in animal products, trace substances in food) (U.S. Department of Health and Human Services [USDHHS] 2000). Public health agencies work closely with agriculture, environment, and other government agencies to ensure food safety. To protect the population, many nations developed over the years food laws and regulations covering the production, transformation, distribution, and conservation of foods.

Even with the best system in the world, however, the risk of food poisoning never equals zero. In Denmark, for example, it has been estimated that 160,000 to 200,000 cases of illness caused by microorganisms in food occur annually, and the figure has been growing in recent years (Danish Ministry of Health 1999). The U.S. government determined that between 1988 and 1992 the microbial contamination of food resulted in 325,000 hospitalizations and 5,000 deaths annually, for a cost in hospitalization of $3 billion and a cost in lost productivity of $20 billion to $40 billion (USDHHS 2000). In Canada, it has been estimated that 2.2 million cases of foodborne infection occur every year. Overall, however, rates of foodborne illness are seriously underreported even in developed countries (Warwick 2004; Tamblyn 2000). A survey done in the United States in 1996–1997 indicated that during a four-week period, only 8% of people with acute diarrhea had sought medical care and that physicians had tested only half of them to determine the cause (Tamblyn 2000). In addition to causing acute illnesses, some microorganisms can cause delayed or chronic diseases (USDHHS 2000). Because the food system and food safety are becoming more and more complex due to global trade and new food products, such as those made through biotechnology, the problems associated with foodborne illnesses may also grow more complex (Robertson et al. 2004). The international policy implication of the mad cow disease appeared in Britain in the mid-1980s represents a good illustration of this phenomenon.

Nutrition and Chronic Diseases

The relationship between the quality of the diet and chronic diseases is now well documented (Glanz 1997; Anand and Basiotis 1998; Organisation Mondiale de la Santé 1999; Buss 1999; WHO 2003; Yang et al. 2003). Diet is related to four of the ten leading causes of death for Americans, especially cardiovascular diseases, stroke, some cancers, and type 2 diabetes (USDHHS 2000). Osteoporosis, also related to nutrition, affects 25 million Americans and is an important cause of bone fracture in postmenopausal women and the elderly (USDHHS 2000). It has been shown that 65% to 70% of the main premature mortality causes and at least a third of annual deaths from cancer are related to the quality of the diet in North America and Great Britain (Milio 1991; Buss 1999; Bal and Forester 1993; Scottish Office Department of Health. 1998). For the United States alone, the cost—in medical expenses and lack of productivity—of diet-related diseases has been estimated to be more than $200 billion a year (USDHHS 2000).

Concurrent with other social changes, nutrition is a modifiable risk factor at the population level, indicating that these social costs could be lowered. Improvement of diet quality has been associated with a decrease in cardiovascular disease and some cancers in various developed countries. A third of the 28% diminution of cardiovascular diseases in the United States since 1970 has been attributed to better food habits, and a quarter has been attributed to the reduction of smoking (Crawford 1988). The decrease in coronary heart disease in Great Britain over time has followed decreases in the proportion of energy that Britons have consumed from saturated fatty acids and increases in consumption of polyunsaturated fat (Committee on Medical Aspects of Food Policy 1994). In Finland, the 73% decline in mortality from cardiovascular disease in the past twenty-five years has also been attributed to the modification of eating habits in that country (Organisation Mondiale de la Santé 1999).

Since the late 1980s, long-term follow-up studies covering periods between twelve and twenty-five years in various developed countries have analyzed the relationship between nutrition and population health. Independent of other risk factors, these studies have revealed associations between the quality of the diet (measured by its content in nutrients or in foods or by its overall quality) and different population health indicators (morbidity level, mortality from coronary heart disease and some cancers, or all causes of mortality) for different countries (Kushi et al. 1985; Keys et al. 1986; Morrison et al. 1996; Farchi et al. 1994; Farchi et al. 1995; Gunnell et al. 1996; Huijbregts et al. 1997; Nube et al. 1987; Strandhagen et al. 2000; Johansen et al. 1987). However, the roots of dietary differences are complex, since they refer to historical, cultural, and geographical factors, and social transformations can impair the benefit of the epidemiological transition. For example, for years, the Mediterranean diet high in fruits and vegetables and low in animal products has been associated with a decreased risk of premature death and morbidity (Wahlqvist et al. 1997; De Lorgeril et al. 1999; Barzi et al. 2003; Panagiotakos et al. 2003; Fortes et al. 2003; Trichopoulou et al. 2003). But in southern European countries, people have been slowly but surely converting from the Mediterranean diet to the higher-fat diet of northern European countries (Helsing 1993). Studies of the Italian food supply indicated a steady rise from 2,838 to 3,309 kilocalories per day from 1961 to 1992, mainly due to a rise in fat consumption as a proportion of daily caloric intake (from 25% to 39%) and a decrease in carbohydrates (from 66% to 51%) (Zizza 1997). This example shows how changing to a "globalized" diet can undermine certain healthy local traditions.

Even in countries reporting an improvement in diet quality between 1970 and 1990 in food consumption and nutrition data, there also are indicators of shifts that could negatively affect chronic diseases in the years to come. These trends are the opposite of the ones showing a U.S. diminution of caloric and fat consumption in the 1980s (Kennedy and Goldberg 1995; Stephen and Sieber 1994). In the United States, recent nutrition surveys have indicated that total caloric intake rose rapidly between 1990 and 1995. This trend involved an increase in absolute fat and saturated fat consumption, even though the relative fat consumption (i.e., the percentage of total calories from fat) was declining (especially in men) and the global quality of the diet was improving slightly (Anand and Basiotis 1998; Katz et al. 1998; Bowman et al. 1998; Centers for Disease Control and Prevention 2004). The same trends have been observed for children two to seventeen years old, between 1989 to 1991 and 1994 to 1995 (Morton and Guthrie 1998). In Great Britain, a reduction in the percentage of calories from fat consumed by all income groups since 1980 has been observed (Committee on Medical Aspects of Food Policy

1994), but little progress has been made in reducing total fat and saturated fat consumption (Bourn 1996). Even in Finland, where important nutritional improvements had been made after the second World War, the decline of risk factors has slowed since the mid-1980s (Milio 1998).

Nutrition and Obesity: The Modern "Epidemic"

Social transformations that lead countries to solve age-old nutrition deficiency problems by improving the access to a wide variety of affordable foods are now creating new nutrition-related problems. One of these problems is the rise of a new epidemic: obesity in rich countries. Obesity has always been considered an important risk factor for chronic diseases, such as non—insulin-dependent diabetes, stroke, respiratory problems, arthritis, cancers, and psychiatric disorders (Pérusse et al. 1998; Launer et al. 1994; Hamm et al. 1989; Semenciw et al. 1988). Being overweight, even in the absence of obesity, is a factor for premature mortality (Organisation Mondiale de la Santé 1999). A moderate but steady weight gain from age twenty on is strongly associated with an increase of coronary death and nonfatal myocardial infarction later in life (Rosengren et al. 1999). A genetic predisposition is said to account for 10% to 50% of obesity (Pérusse et al. 1998), whereas the rest is a matter of poor diet quality (too many calories, too much fat and sugar, etc.) and lack of physical activity (International Obesity Task Force 2001). Hence, the recent increase in total caloric intake probably has played a role in the increase in overweight and obesity observed in developed countries (WHO 2003; Organisation Mondiale de la Santé 1999; Committee on Medical Aspects of Food Policy 1994; Drummond et al. 1996).

Fewer than half of all Europeans are within a normal weight range (Martinez et al. 1999). One of Denmark's population health targets is stopping the increase of obesity (Danish Ministry of Health 1999), and overweight and obesity in the United States are seen by the federal government as the biggest challenge for that nation's health policy (U.S. Food and Drug Administration and National Institutes of Health 2000). The total annual cost of obesity alone (medical cost plus loss of productivity) in the United States in 1995 was evaluated at $99 billion (USDHHS 2000). Rates of overweight and obesity have reached approximately 40% to 60% in adults and between 5% to 10% in children and adolescents in different developed countries (U.K. Department of Health 1999b; Danish Ministry of Health 1999; USDHHS 2000; New Zealand Ministry of Health 1999). The rapidity of the increase in the past several decades has been impressive in some of these countries (table 6.2).

The rise in overweightness and obesity among adolescents and children as observed in most developed countries is of particular concern (USDHHS 2000; Australian Institute of Health and Welfare 2000; Danish Ministry of Health 1999; McCreary Centre Society 1993; Lobstein et al. 2004; Yoshinaga et al. 2004; Heude

Table 6.2. Rise in overweight and obese persons in different countries

Country	Period	Rise
United Kingdom[1]	1993–1996	Obesity Men: from 13% to 16% Women: from 16% to 18%
Denmark[2]	1987–1994	Young men: up by 90% Young women: up by 66%
Belgium[3]	Past 20 years	Overweight: from 16% to 21% Obesity: from 2% to 4%
Canada[4]	1985–1996/1997	Overweight Men: from 22% to 24% Women: from 14% to 24%
United States[5]	1976–1994	Obesity: up by 50%
New Zealand[6]	1989–1997	Obesity: from 11% to 17%

Notes: [1] UK Department of Health 1999b.
[2] Danish Ministry of Health 1999.
[3] Lorant and Tonglet 2000.
[4] Comité consultatif fédéral, provincial, territorial sur la santé de la population 1999b.
[5] U.S. Department of Health and Human Services 2000.
[6] New Zealand Ministry of Health 1999b.

et al. 2003), because these conditions have long-term health impacts (Power et al. 1997). Even moderate overweight at adolescence can cause excess mortality in adulthood (Must 1996), and obesity at adolescence can be more harmful than adult obesity for chronic diseases (Kennedy and Goldberg 1995). Weight gains that lead to overweight and obesity in various populations of adolescents result from both a lack of physical activity and bad eating habits (Anand et al. 1999; Organisation Mondiale de la Santé 1999; Schneider 2000). In one fifty-seven-year follow-up study, higher childhood body mass index (BMI)[1] was associated later in life with higher rates of mortality from all causes and cardiovascular mortality (Gunnell et al. 1998). Other research has shown that from age three on, obesity in children is linked with obesity in adults (Parsons et al. 1999, Danish Ministry of Health 1999; Guo et al. 1994). Since obesity in adults is, in turn, transmitted to the next generation (Parsons et al 1999), the weight increases could be cumulating for more than one generation.

Adding to the health impact, obesity at adolescence can alter self-esteem and cause discrimination (Danish Ministry of Health 1999). Surveys conducted in different European countries and the United States examined adolescents' body images and showed that between a quarter and a half of children and adolescents wanted to lose weight and that approximately a tenth were dieting or taking pills to control their weight (McCreary Centre Society 1993; Choquet and Ledoux 1994;

Irish Department of Health and Children 2000). Schneider (2000), studying international trends in adolescent nutrition, called this phenomenon "malnutrition of affluence." Some adolescents are eating too much and gaining weight, whereas others are eating less than enough to stay thin, thus putting themselves at risk for delayed puberty, growth retardation, or osteoporosis. This phenomenon is important because as these cohorts of adolescents live longer, they will have increased rates of chronic disease (Schneider 2000).

Earliest Nutritional Effects and Later Outcomes during the Life Span

Getting enough energy and nutrients to restore those lost in day-to-day life is complex for adults, but the situation is much more critical in periods of rapid human body growth and development. The first intensive period of development in life takes place in utero, followed by infancy and childhood. Rapid changes in caloric and nutrient needs must be fulfilled in accordance with different intensive developmental phases (e.g., body physical growth, specific organ development, brain wiring). The quality of this experience—the adequate response to all nutritional needs in early life—is essential to give every child the possibility of living a long and healthy life with a good social status.

Prenatal and Infant Nutrition

The impact of nutrition on later outcomes begins in utero. Malnutrition in the third trimester of pregnancy, for example, has been shown to be related to low birth weight and other negative health outcomes (Harris 1997; Hautvast 1997). Damage to genetic potential also can begin with fetal malnutrition, which is a reflection of the mother's nutritional status and health. For example, iodine or folic acid deficiency can alter the brain and nervous system development (Scrimshaw 1995). Between 1991 and 1994, only 21% of U.S. women of childbearing age had adequate levels of folic acid (USDHHS 2000). Prenatal exposure to famine is related to decreased glucose tolerance in adults, which is an especially important factor in the onset of obesity (Ravelli et al. 1998). A variety of other long-term health consequences of prenatal nutrition have been studied. For instance, Barker and colleagues (1997) found growth in fetal life to be associated with fat distribution for babies and for adolescent girls, as well as with the risk of dying from cardiovascular disease at age fifty to sixty (which is specifically related to the placenta development and to weight gain in the first year of life). In England, Acheson and colleagues (1998) studied health inequalities and identified small size at birth, obesity in childhood, mother's nutrition during pregnancy, mother's prepregnancy weight, and birth weight as factors related to coronary heart disease, diabetes, and hypertension later in life. Birth weight has been one of the most widely used indicators to monitor a population's health status, and birth weight and weight gain in the first year of life have been negatively associated with cardiovascular diseases in adulthood (Barker et al. 1997; Alberman 1991; Fall et al. 1992). A low weight for a one-year-old, probably related to caloric restriction in utero and after birth, influences blood pressure, BMI and waist-to-hips ratio, serum lipid levels, fibrinogen, and glucose tolerance as an adult, and this effect is independent of other factors such as tobacco, obesity, or poverty (Fall et al. 1992).

Breast Milk: The First Food in Life

Breastfeeding is an important factor to consider for infants, for a wide variety of reasons. It has been associated with lower blood cholesterol levels among prepubertal French children (Plancoulaine et al. 2000) and with a reduction of infections such as Haemophilus influenza, even after the cessation of breastfeeding, in Swedish preschoolers (Silfverdal et al. 1997). Breastfeeding has been described as contributing to the development of a close mother-child relationship, as well as to the reinforcement of the immune system and the protection against otitis media, urinary tract infections, and allergy development throughout infancy and childhood (Organisation Mondiale de la Santé 1999; Société canadienne de pédiatrie et al. 1998). In addition, breastfeeding has been associated with a lower risk of juvenile diabetes, inflammatory bowel disease, some childhood cancers, and a delayed onset of celiac disease for children, while protecting mothers against premenopausal breast cancer and osteoporosis (Australian Institute of Health and Welfare 2000). Breastfeeding initiation and duration, as well as the delayed introduction of solid food (to four to six months), could also be inversely related to childhood obesity (Kennedy and Goldberg 1995), and this relationship could be associated with the lower growth rate in the first months of life of breastfed children (Dubois et al. 2000a; Dewey et al. 1992; Oski 1993; Yoneyama et al. 1994). Breastfeeding also has been shown to benefit cognitive development and contribute to the reduction of respiratory illness (Société canadienne de pédiatrie et al. 1998).

The World Health Organization (WHO) recommendation is to give children breast milk exclusively (no water, juice, food, formulas, milk) up to six months and to continue breastfeeding up to two years (2001). Analysis we have done with the data of the Longitudinal Study of Child Development in Québec indicates that in 1998, fewer than half of the Québec children were breastfed (exclusively or not) up to three months, and only 6% received breast milk exclusively during their first four months (Dubois and Girard 2003). In this study, the duration of breastfeeding increased with a better socioeconomic status, and a longer duration was associated with lower rates of infection and antibiotic consumption between ages one and three (Dubois and Girard 2003). Breastfeeding rates vary from one country to another, indicating that public health programs could be developed to improve the situation.

Long-term Consequences of Nutrition in Childhood

Poor childhood nutrition can alter children's physical and cognitive development and affect chronic diseases later in life, and even mild undernutrition may have lifelong effects (Brown and Sherman 1995). Nutrition in childhood has been studied for its long-term impact on health conditions, such as arteriosclerosis, some cancers, osteoporosis, and diabetes (WHO 2003; Frankel et al. 1998; Gallo 1996). In the late 1990s, Lino and colleagues (1998b) found that in the United States a good diet was being eaten by only 35% of two- to three-year-olds (males and females), dropping by 6% for fifteen- to eighteen-year-old males. In the United Kingdom, only 10% of a sample of children aged 1.5 to 4.5 were found to be fulfilling the recommendations for more than three of the five most important nutrients for their age group (iron, zinc, and vitamins A, D, and C) (Watt et al. 2001). The average height of a population is also a good guide to the net nutritional status and a visible record of food availability in infancy, childhood, and adolescence (Fogel 1994; Carr-Hill 1990; Tanner 1992; Illsley 1990). In industrialized countries, lower average height of a population has been associated with higher rate of cardiovascular diseases and lower life expectancy, indicating that deprivation in the growing years has consequences throughout life (Tanner 1992; Barker et al. 1992).

Anemia remains the most prevalent nutritional deficiency in both developing and developed countries (Rose et al. 1998). Malnourished children or children with repeated infections due to nutrient deficiency can suffer from altered growth and delayed puberty (Harris 1997). In Britain, evidence has been found of suboptimal iron status among one- to four-year-olds (Buss 1999), and up to 34% of otherwise healthy preschool children may have levels of hemoglobin consistent with iron deficiency (Watt et al. 2001). In the United States during the mid-1990s, 3.4% of younger children were suffering from iron deficiency anemia, while a poor iron status was more prevalent (U.S. Department of Agriculture [USDA] 1996). A study of nine-month-olds in Vancouver reported that 7% had iron deficiency anemia and 24% had low iron stores (Millar 1998). Such conditions can alter children's physical and cognitive development, as well as their school achievement (Walter 1993; Lozoff et al. 1991; Lawson 1995).

Social Inequalities, Nutrition, and Health

To study the relationship between social position and health, Adler and colleagues (1994) have suggested focusing on variables for which there is empirical evidence of a link with socioeconomic status and with important health problems in a society. Nutrition is one variable that is strongly related to the main causes of disease and death in developed countries, and evidence has been accumulating on a link between nutrition and socioeconomic status, as measured by income, education, and/or occupation. This is not to say that a clinical approach based on the modification of specific nutrients is not pertinent to nutrition, but for individuals, the tasks of buying and preparing food and of finding the time to eat it are becoming more complex every day. For instance, in 1951, 1,500 food products were sold in the United States. Today, the middle-class consumer has to choose between 30,000 different food products (Kessler 1995). It is only one of the social factors exerting their influence on different aspects of food choices and thereby nutritional status.

Social Position and Quality of Diet: A Gradient Relationship

For many years, researchers studied social inequalities by contrasting the diets of poor families with those of the rest of the population. Various studies showed that people in the lower social classes were consuming fewer fruits and vegetables, more fat, and less fiber than the rest of the population (Smith and Baghurst 1992; Dunkin et al. 1998; Acheson et al. 1998; USDHHS 2000). In addition to having more limited financial resources, poor people are often less educated and may lack important knowledge regarding nutrition (Little et al. 2002; Parmenter et al. 2000). But nutrition education alone is insufficient to ensure positive change. In developed nations, for example, only a small proportion of the population are eating in accordance with nutritional recommendations, even if the majority are aware of them (Australian Institute of Health and Welfare 2000; Danish Ministry of Health 1999; Lino et al. 1998a). The fact that people are aware of nutritional recommendations but not following them indicates that other factors in the social environment are affecting food choices.

Recent studies in developed countries have indicated that diet changes gradually from one social position to the next—that is, there is a gradient in diet across the socioeconomic spectrum. In the United States and Canada, we showed that the socioeconomic gradient exists for almost all nutrients and different types of food consumption, such that, as one goes up the socioeconomic spectrum, a higher proportion of diets conform to current dietary recommendations (Dubois and Girard 2001). Finnish and Norwegian research has indicated similar patterns of difference in food consumption between social groups. These results add to the studies showing that the quality of the diet tends to be closer to nutritional recommendations among better-educated people, higher-income families, and people working in more prestigious jobs (Hulshof et al. 1991; Bowman et al. 1998; Bolton-Smith et al. 1991; Roos et al. 1998; Shi 1998; Lino et al. 1998a; Woo et al. 1999; Dubois and Girard 2001; New Zealand Ministry of Health 2000). A recent review of the studies done in fifteen European countries on disparities in food habits also concluded that people in higher social classes generally were eating healthier diets (Roos and Prättällä 1999). We found that in North America socioeconomic differences were more often related with food consumption than with the nutrient content of the diet, but we also observed gradual social disparities in nutrient consumption (Dubois and Girard 2001). Some of the major health risk factors influenced by diet also follow a gradient with different social position indicators. Obesity is inversely associated with different indicators of social position in North America, some European countries, and Hong Kong (Power et al. 1991; Anand et al. 1999; Martinez et al. 1999; Acheson et al. 1998; Kubzansky et al. 1998; Woo et al. 1999; Danish Ministry of Health 1999; New Zealand Ministry of Health 2000; USDHHS 2000). Underweight, however, increases with education level (Martinez et al. 1999; Vaz de Almeida et al. 1999).

Social Status: The Influence from Infancy

Various researchers have demonstrated that the relationship between nutrition and social status begins in childhood. For example, investigators found that in the United States in 1991 to 1994, adequate levels of folic acid in women of childbearing age varied with education, leading to different health risks for children to be born (USDHHS 2000). Different social position indicators have been found to be positively related to the initiation and duration of breastfeeding in developed countries (USDHHS 2000; Pande et al. 1997; Crost and Kaminski 1998; Dubois et al. 2000a; Williams et al. 1996; Ryan 1997; Acheson et al. 1998). Doan (1989) observed a positive relationship between child nutritional status (measured by weight by age) and parents' degree of autonomy in the workplace, mother's education, and household income. A positive relationship was also observed between mother's educational level and more favorable children's eating patterns in the Alspac Study in the United Kingdom (North et al. 2000). Power, Manor, and Fox (1991) found that height (an indicator of dietary quality during infancy) was also positively related to social class among the young, as well as inversely related to some chronic diseases or mortality among adults. In Québec, we found family socioeconomic status to be related to some elements of the quality of the diet in preschoolers as young as 1.5 years, as illustrated in figure 6.2 (Dubois et al. 2000b).

Social Inequalities and Nutrition: Positive or Negative Trend?

In developed nations, the diseases of abundance (called white-collar diseases in the 1960s) are now more prevalent in the lower social classes than in the higher ones (Fall et al. 1992). The prevalence of obesity also experienced a social class inversion in the twentieth century. Food consumption models have always been an object of social distinction (Bourdieu 1979)—that is, a popular type of food in the upper

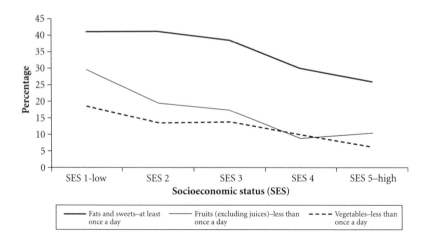

Figure 6.2. Proportion (%) of Québec children (1.5 years) eating fruits and vegetables less than once a day and fats and sweets at least once a day, by family socioeconomic status, 1999

Source: Data are from the Longitudinal Study of Child Development in Québec (LSCDQ), 1998–2002, conducted by Santé Québec, a division of the Institut de la Statistique du Québec.

class is adopted by the lower class, forcing the upper class to find something else to differentiate themselves from the "masses." It has been shown that the lower social class has been following the higher social class's eating model with a ten-year lag (Prättälä et al. 1991).

If social inequalities were narrowing and if the upper social class were doing better and better in terms of diet quality, then better nutritional health for all could be achieved in the next several decades. But social transformations induce eating-habit transformations that are not always in accordance with nutritional and health improvements (Milio 1991). The emergence of new groups of poor, the transformation in the workforce and in families, and the aging of the population make it hard to predict the nutritional and population health benefits in the years to come. For example, single-parent households are more prone to poverty than two-parent households (Dubois et al. 2000b). Being married rather than single is also positively associated with a better diet (Roos et al. 1998; Dunkin et al. 1998) and negatively associated with BMI (Martinez et al. 1999; Vaz de Almeida et al. 1999). The number of one-person households rose in England from 25% in 1984 to 28% in 1995 and 1996 (Acheson et al. 1998). Changes in the workforce could also affect these trends, not necessarily in a positive way. For example, working women in Norway eat a diet similar to that of young men (with more fast food). Couples without children and unmarried people eat more prepared meals with a high fat and salt content than do couples with children or married people (Milio 1991). In Québec, we found that people living alone, even those of a higher social status, had a lower self-reported diet quality, parallel to eating out more often or buying more pre-pared food than couples did (Dubois et al. 2000b).

Food eaten away from home also has been described as an increasing problem in the United States, because these foods are generally higher in total fat, saturated fat, cholesterol, and sodium and lower in fiber and calcium than foods prepared and eaten at home (USDHHS 2000). As of 1995, as much as 40% of the average U.S. family's food budget was spent in restaurants and on carryout meals, and children were eating an increasing number of meals prepared away from home (Kennedy and Goldberg 1995). The Finnish, as of 1996, consumed about 125 meals outside their homes every year (Finland Ministry of Health and Social Affairs 1996). Over the past thirty years, a rise in the number of meals eaten outside the home has also been observed in France (Poulain 1998). In Great Britain, basic cooking skills have been declining, and processed foods have been making up more of the average diet (Caraher and Dixon 1996; Godlee 1996). In Québec (fig. 6.3), we found that toddlers of lower socioeconomic status were eating less often outside and that their diets contained fewer fruits and vegetables than those of children from higher socioeconomic status. For this age group, meals taken outside the home were mainly due to day-care attendance generally offering diet-balanced meals, which is less frequented by poor children than by the others (Dubois et al. 2000a).

For elderly people, mealtime may diminish social isolation, which is a risk factor for mortality from different causes (House et al. 1988). In general, a lack of social support is related to obesity and lower diet quality (Ford et al. 2000; Sanders-Phillips 1994; House et al. 1988). In Canada, we observed that social isolation of

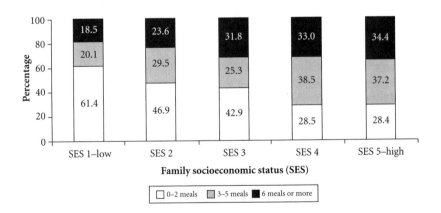

Figure 6.3. Proportion (%) of Québec children aged 1.5 years eating meals outside the home in a week, by family socioeconomic status, 1999

Source: Data are from the Longitudinal Study of Child Development in Québec (LSCDQ), 1998–2002, conducted by Santé Québec, a division of the Institut de la Statistique du Québec.

the elderly generates more nutritional inequalities than economic disparities (Dubois et al. 1999). Gathering elderly people together at lunchtime has been shown to help them feel less isolated and to improve their appetite and nutritional status (Dubois et al. 1999). House, Landis, and Umberson (1988) found that collective kitchens acted the same way for poor families, since such kitchens improved not only these families' access to food but also their social support. These social relationships acted as a buffer between stress and health and gave a sense of coherence while offering an avenue for good nutrition for the whole family. These kinds of projects highlight the social function of meals.

The Growing Problem of Poverty and Food Insecurity

After the second World War in North America, it was believed that the benefits of the consumer society would bring a better life for everyone. Education and work were available for men and women. Parents were looking at a promising future for themselves, and even at a better one for their children. But the economy slowed down at the end of the seventies, and governments had to restraint their implication in social services. Today, material and social deprivation at the individual and geographical level, related with food insecurity, is a source of nutritional and health inequalities in populations.

Being Poor in a Rich Country: The Impact of Material Deprivation

Even in rich countries, nutritional problems at the population level are still a source of concern. First, food access is not equal for everybody. An increasing number of people—including a growing number of families with young children—are not able to buy the food they need or to eat adequately every day, or they are anxious about these issues (Wilson and Tsoa 2001). This phenomenon, called food insecurity[2] or food poverty (Dubois et al. 2000b; Robertson et al. 1999), was evidenced by the rapid expansion in the 1990s of charities such as food banks and collective kitchens (Wilson and Tsoa 2001). Only recently have surveys attempted to measure food insecurity (with or without hunger) at the population level.

The main factor responsible for food insecurity is poverty. Canada, the country classified by the United Nations as the best place to live in the world in 1999 (on the Human Development Index), has been criticized for its high level of poverty (it ranked tenth on a poverty index for developed countries) and especially for the high proportion of children living in poor families (Comité consultatif fédéral 1999a). In Canada in 2001, 15.6% of all children (birth to eighteen years) lived in a low-income family, and children living in single-parent families are more likely to live in poverty than children living in two-parent families (Institut Canadien d'Information sur la Santé 2004). In large Canadian cities, recent research has shown up to 25% of preschoolers to be poor (McIntyre et al. 2000; Jutras and Castonguay 1999). The proportion of children and youth living in low-income Canadian families has increased since the beginning of the 1980s. One-seventh of all children were living in poverty in 1982, one-fifth in 1990, and one-quarter in 1995 (Comité consultatif fédéral 1999a). The Canadian Association of Food Banks has confirmed that their clientele doubled between 1989 and 1998 and that more and more children were among them (Wilson and Tsoa 2001). In 1998, 42% of the clients of the food banks were children and adolescents (younger than eighteen years), whereas they represented only 25% of the population (Comité consultatif fédéral 1999a). Even if the trends seem to have been moderating lately, concern has now turned to the depth of poverty, which has increased between 1989 and 1996 (Campagne 2000).

In its document *Health for All in the 21st Century*, the WHO European Office found increasing poverty in European countries in the late 1990s—a problem that was raising the risk of poor health and lower nutritional status (Organisation Mondiale de la Santé 1999). In the past ten years, social and economic changes in countries such as Finland, Sweden, and Denmark also have caused the emergence of unexpected pockets of poverty (Roos and Prättällä 1999). The Finland Ministry of Health and Social Affairs (1996) mentioned reports of certain people who were hungry in that country, even if there were no data at that time.

In Canada, income inequalities stayed relatively stable between 1985 and 1995 due to the government redistribution of money to the people in need (e.g., poor families) (Comité consultatif fédéral 1999b). Nevertheless, a difference of $4,800 in income has been observed between families with frequent hunger and families with occasional hunger (McIntyre et al. 2001). The cost of a nutritive-value food basket—that is, the basic food needed for a family—has been evaluated at $13 per person per week, for a total of $6,885 for a family of four over a year in Canada (Ross et al. 2000). A pilot project called the Self-sufficiency Project, aimed at increasing parental income and employment, observed a positive difference on food expenditure after thirty-six months and a 5.5% decrease in the number of families using food banks or being unable to afford food (35% in the program versus 41% in the control group) (Morris and Michalopoulos 2000).

In 1998 and 1999, more than 10% of Canadian families experienced food insecurity, and a fifth of those families went to charitable agencies to get food. Thirty-five percent of Canadians living in low-income families, 14% of those living in middle-income families, 33% of single-mother families, and more than 25% of aboriginal people living off-reserve in Canada reported some aspects of food insecurity (Che and Chen 2001).

In Canada, food insecurity is inversely associated with age. Children (younger than eighteen) are five times more likely to experience food insecurity than are elderly people. Education and poverty are also tightly associated with food insecurity. But even if poor people are generally less educated, educating people alone would not be sufficient to prevent food insecurity. In Canada, 15% of the mothers experiencing hunger had completed high school, and 60% had at least some post-secondary school (McIntyre et al. 2001). Nevertheless, being poor and undereducated increase the probability of experiencing food insecurity at one moment or another in life.

The last Social and Health Survey in Québec, conducted in 1998, indicated that 8% of families and 22% of single-parent families had experienced some degree of food insecurity (Dubois et al. 2000b). In the United States in 1995, food insecurity (with or without hunger) affected 12% of all households and 41% of the poor households (i.e., those with incomes less than or equal to 130% of poverty level) with children younger than eighteen (USDHHS 2000). In 1999, 3.8% of American children lived in households experiencing food insecurity with hunger, as did 11.8% of children living in households with incomes below the federal poverty level (Federal Interagency Forum on Child and Family Statistics 2000).

Food Insecurity's Impact on Diet, Health, and Social Functioning

It is important to document poverty and food insecurity in a country because they impair the quality of the diet and, consequently, the health of a growing number of individuals. Even if people are rarely dying from hunger in developed countries, food insecurity has consequences throughout many people's lives. In Canada, hungry families did not report good to excellent health for their children as often as did other families (70% versus 88%) (McIntyre et al. 2001). We found that Québec's food-insecure families were twice as likely as the rest of the population to report that their food habits and their health were fair or poor (Dubois et al. 2000b). In the United States in 1994 through 1996, only 19% of the children aged two to five living below the poverty line had a good diet, compared with 28% of the children above the poverty line (Federal Interagency Forum on Child and Family Statistics 2000).

Food insecurity affects parents and children differently. When food is missing at home, parents skip meals so that their children can eat (McIntyre et al. 2001). Even if children are not directly experiencing hunger, however, they may suffer from the stress that food insecurity imposes on their parents. Hungry mothers are more likely to suffer from chronic health conditions and activity limitations (McIntyre et al. 2001; Rouffignat et al. 2001). We did a study of food-insecure mothers with children younger than eighteen living in the province of Québec in 1998. It showed that 21% of the mothers reported having fair or poor health, and 37% said they felt depressed or anxious. When the family experienced a high level of food insecurity, 35% of the mothers reported fair or poor health and 54% reported depression and anxiety (Rouffignat et al. 2001).

For children, being hungry increases hyperactivity, school absenteeism, and tardiness, and it decreases psychological functioning, independent of maternal education and family income (Olson 1999; Murphy et al. 1998). In the United States, 8% of low-income children younger than five years were growth retarded in 1997 (USDHHS 2000). Between 1988 and 1994, 12% of one- to two-year-olds from poor families and 5% of the three- to four-year-olds were iron deficient (USDHHS 2000). In 1996, 29% of low-income pregnant women in their third trimester were anemic (USDHHS 2000). In Australia, Dixon (1999) found that children younger than five living in poverty were less likely to be breastfed and more likely to show suboptimal growth, in comparison with nonpoor children. From five to nine years of age, they were more likely to suffer from suboptimal growth, obesity, and poor nutrition, and between ten to fourteen they were more prone to show elevated cardiovascular risk factors. Public health programs have proven beneficial for low-income preschoolers deficient in iron due to food insecurity (Yip et al. 1992; Rose et al. 1998).

The first cycle (1994–1996) of the National Longitudinal Survey of Children and Youth (NLSCY) found that 1.2% of Canadian families with children aged two to eleven experienced hunger (McIntyre et al. 2001). Food insecurity was directly related to family income (fig. 6.4).

Our analysis of NLSCY data indicates that the proportion of two- to eleven-year-olds in excellent health was lower for children who had experienced hunger at one time or another since their birth than for those who had not. Moreover, the general health status of children living in food-insecure households may have been deteriorating over the years, as illustrated in figures 6.5 and 6.6.

Food-insecurity problems among children may continue across the lifespan. A study we conducted with poor families receiving food from Québec charities in 1999 and 2000 (Rouffignat et al. 2001) found that 54% of the surveyed families had been living in food insecurity for more than two years, as had 67% of the respondents who had experienced food insecurity during childhood. Hence, food insecurity is transmitted from one generation to the other, probably due to the

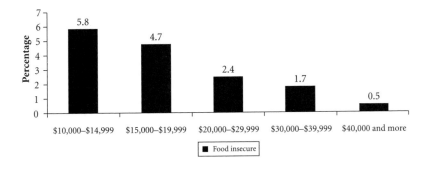

Figure 6.4. Proportion (%) of Canadian children having ever experienced hunger, by family income; *P* ≤.001

Source: Data are from the National Longitudinal Survey of Children and Youth, 1996–1997.

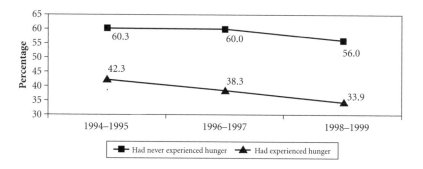

Figure 6.5. Proportion (%) of Canadian children in excellent health who experienced hunger or not, by year of survey; *P* ≤.001

Source: Data are from the National Longitudinal Survey of Children and Youth, 1994–1995, 1996–1997, 1998–1999.

lower level of education and greater poverty among people who experienced food insecurity in their childhood, in comparison with food-secure people who did not have that experience. In the Québec survey, we also measured the depth of food insecurity by the number of dimensions related to the food insecurity experienced by each family. Families experiencing deeper food insecurity reported more negative impacts on the quality of their diet and on physical and mental health, as well as more consultations with health professionals, greater use of health care, and greater general use of community and government services. Along with poverty, social isolation has proven to be a main factor in the depth of food insecurity (Dubois et al. 2000b; Rouffignat et al. 2001), especially for some families. McIntyre, Walsh, and Connor (2001), for example, found that when children were going

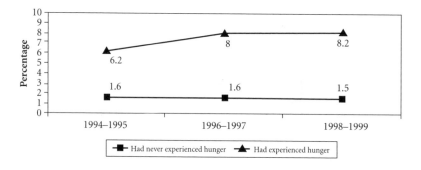

Figure 6.6. Proportion (%) of Canadian children in fair or poor health who experienced hunger or not, by year of survey; *P* ≤.001

Source: Data are from the National Longitudinal Survey of Children and Youth, 1994–1995, 1996–1997, 1998–1999.

hungry, single-parent families and poorer households were more likely to go to a food bank (a signal of social isolation) than to ask relatives for assistance.

Geographic Distribution of Food Insecurity

Nutritional inequalities are geographically distributed in rich countries. Food-insecure households are concentrated in deprived living areas, putting a burden not only on health services and community resources but also on schools, since the children affected by hunger or by stressful home environments may not be able to give their full attention to their teachers. Evidence of these patterns has been gathered from different living areas. For instance, in the province of Québec in 1998, 8% of the households experienced food insecurity, but 12% did in Montreal, the province's largest city. For the whole province, we performed a mapping of material and social deprivation,[3] calculated at the level of enumeration sectors. It shows that social and material deprivation areas are both related to the proportion of food insecure households living in these areas (figure 6.7). In the worst areas, 25% of the households experienced food insecurity, whereas almost none did in the province

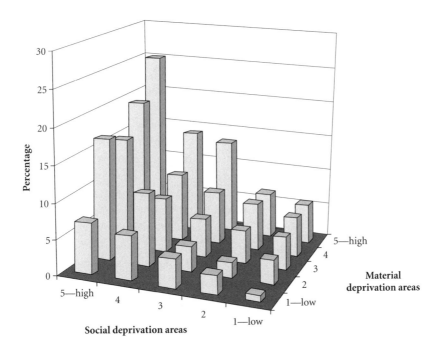

Figure 6.7. Proportion of food insecure families in the province of Québec (Canada) in 1998, by social and material deprivation living areas (in quintiles)

Sources: Data are from the Québec Health and Social Survey, 1998, Institut de la Statistique du Québec; social and material deprivation scale by Pampalon and Raymond 2000.

more affluent areas. Thus, food-insecure families seeking health services and community resources are concentrated in specific areas in the province.

Living areas have also been associated with food insecurity in New Zealand, where 4% of the population fifteen and older reported using food grants or food banks sometimes or often. The figure was the highest for women living in deprived areas, where 31% suffered from a lack of food, 44% had to reduce the variety of food, 29% were stressed about a lack of money for food, and 27% could not afford to eat properly every day (New Zealand Ministry of Health 1999). The relation between living area deprivation and food insecurity may be due to regional variation in food costs. In the United Kingdom, the problem of food insecurity has been attributed in part to the higher price of food in deprived neighborhoods and rural areas, where a nutritive diet can be up to 60% more expensive than in urban supermarkets (U.K. Department of Health 1999b). In a population health perspective, it would be important to adjust the amount of social welfare given to families to the regional variation in food cost.

Food and Nutrition Policy in the Context of Globalization

Nutrition policy can play a central role in the reduction of nutrition and health inequalities in and between countries (Illsley 1990; Acheson et al. 1998). A multisectoral approach is important in a population health perspective; and with regard to nutrition, such an approach should include health, agriculture, education, industry, environment, and finance (Milio 1990).

In view of globalization, nutrition policy that affects many countries requires attention. Food standards, food labeling, and nutrition recommendations must be harmonized for food products to go freely from one country to another. Such processes of standardization are already under way in Europe and in America. We believe that a monitoring system capable of measuring the trends in nutritional inequalities at the population level would be important to ensure that these processes of standardization will not impair the nutritional health of some nations. As nutrition policies may impact other countries, such policies should not be developed in silos. It is also important that they be evaluated during their implementation by experts from outside a given country and adjusted to that country's ever-changing social needs (James 1997).

Food and Nutrition Policy in Different Nations

Because nutrition so strongly affects the development of chronic diseases and their associated costs, most industrialized countries have made the improvement of nutrition part of their global health strategies (Glanz 1997). Different countries have developed food and nutrition policies concerning different aspects of food quality and nutrition for the health of their populations. For instance, in the U.K. document *Reducing Health Inequalities: An Action Report* (1999a), the recommendations for nutrition include nutrition education school programs; study of agriculture policies' impact on health and health inequalities; policies to improve food availability and affordable diet; policies to improve health and nutrition of women of childbearing age and their children, with priority given to eliminate food poverty and reduce obesity; and policies to increase breastfeeding. In the United States, the nutrition policy strategy contends that healthy food choices, nutrition security, safe food and water, and promotion of breastfeeding are important elements for improving nutrition in the population. Nutrition monitoring and human nutrition research, as well as nutrition-sensitive food production, economic policy, and agriculture research, are complements to these priorities (USDA 1996).

In Finland, the 73% decrease in death by cardiovascular disease over the past twenty-five years has been attributed mainly to the modification of eating habits, following the implementation of a coherent food and nutrition policy (Organisation Mondiale de la Santé 1999). This nutrition policy has included intersector administrative activities (e.g., health, agriculture, education) in a collaborative effort to develop uniform objectives for public nutrition (Finland Ministry of Health and Social Affairs 1996). For Puska (2000) the Finnish experience between 1972 and 1997 illustrated the fact that population rates of cardiovascular diseases can be substantially influenced by changes in people's dietary habits.

Food Safety, Novel Foods, and Genetically Modified Foods: New Threats for a Global Economy?

The threat of food- or water-related illnesses is of particular concern to some social groups. For example, more than 30 million people in United States are likely to be particularly susceptible to foodborne diseases, since they are either very young or they have a compromised immune system (USDHHS 2000). A relationship between socioeconomic status and risk of experiencing foodborne illnesses also has been found. In the United Kingdom, one report indicated that hospital admissions for gastrointestinal infections increased with increasing socioeconomic deprivation (USDHHS 2000). Due to worldwide exchanges, controlling products and diseases related to those has become increasingly difficult, and new regulations have been needed (Organisation Mondiale de la Santé 1999). Countries have needed to establish permanent surveillance of contaminants, toxic materials, pesticides, drugs for animals, agrochemicals, and antibiotics for animals used on their territories. Foodborne illnesses could be more of a problem in the years to come (USDHHS 2000), particularly in light of new types of pathogens, the increasing drug resistance of existing pathogens, new lifestyles, and globalization (Danish Ministry of Health 1999; USDHHS 2000; Organisation Mondiale de la Santé 1999; Tamblyn 2000). Some pathogens may travel rapidly from one country to another, increasing preoccupation for food safety at the population level. The recent mad cow disease crisis raises the public and governmental preoccupation for public health related with food safety. Even if such crisis in Canada in 2004 had no direct consequences on the health of individuals, it nevertheless affected the economy of the food and agriculture Canadian industry. Eventually, the price of food may be affected by such situations, and the access to some type of food (e.g., meat) for some groups of the population may become more difficult.

Adding to these concerns has been the recent development of novel foods, including genetically modified foods. The use of biotechnology in the food industry is not new, but new biotechnologies allow the manipulation of plants and animals in unprecedented ways, including genetic manipulation. It is now possible, for example, to transfer a gene from a plant into an animal, and vice versa (Goodyear-Smith 2001). Such developments raise ethical issues and public health concerns about the potential toxicity and unknown impact of these products on the health of populations (WHO 2002, Meningaud et al. 2001). In Europe, food producers must indicate on food labels that a food's content is genetically modified—a requirement that does not exist in North America. Few systematic studies have been done on the impact of novel foods on population health (Pusztai 2002). The development of food from biotechnology may also increase nutritional inequalities in and between populations. For example, laboratories developing genetically modified foods aimed at preventing cardiovascular diseases or cancer—a step that is good for health—will likely sell these high-tech foods at a higher price than traditional foods. A part of the population from lower socioeconomic groups may then not be able to have access to these benefits, whereas the more economically advantaged groups will have. Moreover, in developing countries, when novel foods replace traditional foods, populations become more dependent of international conglomerates and less self-sufficient.

Developing Countries in the Path of Developed Countries: For Better or for Worse

The importance of nutrition for population health became evident in the nutrition transition that preceded the epidemiological transition in developing countries in the 1980s (Popkin et al. 1993; Gonzalez Biosca et al. 1992; Kohlmeier 1991; Sri Kantha 1990). Developing countries have been gaining in chronic diseases what they have been losing in deficiency diseases, due in part to nutrition (Illsley 1990). The twentieth-century health trends of developed countries can help us anticipate what might happen in developing countries in the years to come. Average life expectancy improved from forty-five to seventy-five years in Western countries over a century (Bunker et al. 1994), but it is predicted that developing countries will not gain as many years in life expectancy, due in part to their rapid evolution from subsistence societies to market societies (WHO 1991). For example, in China, the population has become better nourished as the total caloric intake has increased by almost 20% since the 1940s, and life expectancy has almost doubled in the same period, due in part to better nutrition and fewer infectious diseases (Sri Kantha 1990). But infectious diseases and undernutrition have continued to be sources of concern in rural Chinese areas, and obesity and fat consumption have been increasing the prevalence of cardiovascular diseases and cancer in the cities, in line with rapid social transformation and the rise of family income (Popkin et al. 1993). New pockets of poverty have also been appearing in urban areas, thus leading to greater food insecurity (Popkin et al. 1993).

Transformations such as those just described have been occurring within short periods in developing countries (Popkin et al. 1993). Societies in rapid processes of urbanization have had rapid increases in obesity. For instance, in some Central and South American countries, obesity has almost reached levels seen in the United States (Pan American Health Organization 1994). As the WHO has noted, developing countries must try to avoid problems of abundant societies and continue to eat more vegetable products than animal products (WHO 2003). In other countries experiencing rapid transformation, such as the Central European countries, observation of the evolution of food patterns has suggested the likelihood of the eventual development of chronic diseases (Kohlmeier 1991).

Conclusion

The literature and data presented in this text indicates that social inequalities create nutritional inequalities even in rich countries where a huge variety of high quality food is available. These inequalities are all over the social stratum, a better diet being related with a better social position. Nevertheless, materially (poor individuals and families) and socially (isolated people) deprived groups living in rich countries are exposed to the worse nutritional situation, which is especially harmful for children's health, development, school achievement, and later social status. Globally, some nutritional indicators at the population level show that the situation may not be improving in the years to come for all aspects related to food and nutrition. It may be the case with food poisoning and the risk related with the development of food biotechnology. It is also the case with the rapid rise of obesity in developed and developing countries. Living in a globalized world means that foods have no boundaries—the good and the bad ones—transporting with them the risk associated not only with foodborne diseases but also, in the longer term, with chronic diseases.

Nutrition remains an important determinant of population health in both developed and developing countries. Since the current production of food worldwide is sufficient to feed all humans on earth, abundance at the world level is already a reality. But it is estimated that in developing countries, 147.5 million children will still suffer from stunting in 2005, and nearly 800 million people were undernourished in 1999–2001 (United Nations Standing Committee on Nutrition [UNSCN] 2004). Societies must remain vigilant in terms of food safety—through laws, regulations, and education—to lower the risk of contamination, while also promoting diets that reduce chronic disease. At the Millennium Summit of the United Nations in 2000, 189 countries committed themselves to the goal of reducing global undernutrition by half by 2015, and each country agreed to develop a nutrition plan for action to reach this target (UNSCN 2004). In some parts of the world however, such as sub-Saharan Africa, child malnutrition, household food insecurity, and poverty are all moving in the wrong direction (UNSCN 2004).

In the years to come, the marketing strategy of the food industry, coupled with the development of novel foods, will create new areas requiring government intervention to challenge the global food industry and protect the health of populations. To ensure that these interventions will be well adapted to social transformations and will not induce more nutritional and related health inequalities, it is important for government to gather high-quality nutrition data that will permit international comparisons and longitudinal analyses of socioeconomic disparities in food access.

New technologies could help nations produce more healthy foods at a lower cost, but these foods must be redistributed equitably and in respect of traditional food. The real challenge remains the reduction of nutritional inequalities within and between countries.

Notes

1. Body Mass Index (BMI) is calculated by weight in kilograms divided by height in meters squared.

2. Food insecurity exists "whenever the availability of nutritionally adequate and safe foods or the ability to acquire acceptable foods in socially acceptable ways is limited or uncertain." Food security is "assured access at all times to enough food for an active and healthy life" (Che and Chen 2001).

3. This index has been developed by Pampalon and Raymond (2000) for the province of Québec. Material deprivation includes the proportion of persons without a secondary school diploma, the mean personal income, and the level of activity in the enumeration sector; social deprivation includes the proportion of one-person households; separated, divorced, or widowed people; and single-parent families in the enumeration sector (from the Canadian census data 1996).

References

Acheson, D., D. Barker, J. Chambers, H. Graham, M. Marmot, and M. Whitehead. 1998. *Independent Inquiry into Inequalities in Health Report*. London: Stationery Office.

Adler, N. E., T. Boyce, M. A. Chesbey, S. Cohen, S. Folkman, R. L. Kahn, and L. Syme. 1994. Socioeconomic status and health. The challenge in the gradient. *American Psychologist* 49 (1):15–24.

Alberman, E. 1991. Are our babies becoming bigger? *Journal of Research in Social Medicine* 84:257–260.

Anand, R. S., and P. P. Basiotis. 1998. Is total fat consumption really decreasing? *Family Economics and Nutrition Reviews* 11:58–60.

Anand, R. S., P. P. Basiotos, and B. W. Klein. 1999. Profile of overweight children. *Nutrition/ Insights* 13:1–2.

Australian Institute of Health and Welfare. 2000. *Australia's Health 2000. The Seventh Biennial Health Report of the Australian Institute of Health and Welfare.* Canberra: AIHW.

Bal, D. G., and S. B. Forester. 1993. Dietary strategies for cancer prevention. *Cancer* 72 (3 suppl.): 1005–1010.

Barker, M., S. Robinson, C. Osmond, and D. J. P. Barker. 1997. Birth weight and body fat distribution in adolescent girls. *Archives of Disease in Childhood* 77:381–383.

Barker, M. E., S. I. McClean, J. J. Strain, and K. A. Thompson. 1992. Dietary behaviour and health in Northern Ireland: An exploration of biochemical and haematological associations. *Journal of Epidemiology and Community Health* 46:151–156.

Barzi, F., M. Woodward, R. M. Marfisi, L. Tavazzi, F. Valagussa, R. Maechioli, and GISSI-Preventione Investigators. 2003. Mediterranean diet and all-cause mortality after myocardial infarction: Results from the GISSI-Preventione trial. *European Journal of Clinical Nutrition* 57:604–611.

Bolton-Smith, C., W. C. S. Smith, M. Woodward, and H. Tunstall-Pedoe. 1991. Nutrient intakes of different social-class groups: Results from the Scottish Heart Health Study (SHHS). *British Journal of Nutrition* 65:321–335.

Bourdieu, P. 1979. *La distinction. Critique sociale du jugement.* Paris: Les éditions de minuit.

Bourn, J. 1996. *Health of the Nation, a progress report.* London. National Audit Office.

Bowman, S. A., M. Lino, S. A. Gerrior, and P. P. Basiotis. 1998. The Healthy Eating Index, 1994–1996. *Family Economics and Nutrition Review* 11 (3):2–14.

Brown, J. L., and L. P. Sherman. 1995. Policy implications for new scientific knowledge. *Journal of Nutrition* 125:2281S–2284S.

Bunker, J. P., H. S. Frazier, and F. Mosteller. 1994. Improving health: Measuring effects of medical care. *The Milbank Memorial Fund Quarterly* 71:225–258.

Buss, D. H. 1999. MAFF programme of research in support of dietary surveys. *Nutrition and Food Science* 1:5–11.

Campagne [a Canadian coalition]. 2000. *La pauvreté des enfants au Canada.* Toronto: Thistle Printing.

Caraher, M., and D. Dixon 1996. *Buying, Eating and Cooking Food: A Review of the National Data Set on Food Attitudes, Skills and Behavioural Change.* London, Health Education Council.

Carr-Hill, R. 1990. The measurement of inequities in health: Lessons from the British experience. *Social Science and Medicine. Special issue: Health Inequities in Europe* 31:393–404.

Centers for Disease Control and Prevention (CDC). 2004. Trends in intake of energy and macronutrients—United States, 1971–2000. *Morbidity and Mortality Weekly Report* 53:80–82.

Che, J., and J. Chen. 2001. Food insecurity in Canadian households. *Health Reports* 12(4):11–22.

Choquet, M., and S. Ledoux. 1994. *Adolescents. Enquête nationale.* Paris: INSERM.

Comité consultatif fédéral, provincial, territorial sur la santé de la population. Groupe de travail sur le développement sain des enfants. 1999a. *Investir dans le développement durant la petite enfance: la contribution du secteur de la santé.* Ottawa. Santé Canada.

Comité consultatif fédéral, provincial, territorial sur la santé de la population. 1999b. *Pour un avenir en santé. Deuxième rapport sur la santé de la population canadienne.* Ottawa. Santé Canada.

Committee on Medical Aspects of Food Policy. 1994. *Nutritional Aspects of Cardiovascular Disease.* Report of the Cardiovascular Review Group. Report on Health and Social Subjects no. 46. London: Stationery Office.

Crawford, P. 1988. The nutrition connection: Why doesn't the public know? *American Journal of Public Health* 78:1147–1148.

Crost, M., and M. Kaminski. 1998. L'allaitement maternel à la maternité en France en 1995. Enquête Nationale Périnatale, *Archives de Pediatrie* 5:1316–1326.

Danish Ministry of Health. 1999. *The Danish Government Programme on Public Health and Health Promotion 1999–2008. An Action Oriented Programme for Healthier Settings in Everyday Life.* Copenhagen: Danish Ministry of Health.

De Lorgeril, M., P. Salen, J. L. Martin, I. Monjaud, J. Delaye, and N. Mamelle. 1999. Mediterranean diet, traditional risk factors, and the rate of cardiovascular complications after myocardial infarction. Final report of the Lyon Diet Heart Study. *Circulation* 99:779–785.

Dewey, K. G., M. J. Heinig, L. A. Nommsen, J. M. Peerson, and B. Lönnerdal. 1992. Growth of breast-fed and formula-fed infants from 0 to 18 months: The Darling Study. *Pediatrics* 89:1035–1041.

Dixon, J. 1999. *A National R & D Collaboration on Health and Socioeconomic Status for Australia. First Discussion Paper.* Canberra: National Center for Epidemiology and Population Health.

Doan, R. M. 1989. Class and family structure: A study of child nutritional status in four urban settlements in Amman, Jordan. *Dissertation Abstracts International.* 49 (10):3174A.

Drummond, S., T. Kirk, and A. Looy. 1996. Are dietary recommendations for dietary fat reduction achievable? *International Journal of Food Sciences and Nutrition* 47:221–226.

Dubois, L. 1996. L'aliment: Futur miracle de la bio-technologie? Numéro thématique sous la direction de Marc Renaud et Louise Bouchard: Technologies médicales et changements de valeurs. *Sociologie et sociétés* 28 (2):45–57.

Dubois, L., B. Bédard, M. Girard, and É. Beauchesne. 2000a. L'alimentation. Dans: *Étude longitudinale du développement des enfants du Québec (ÉLDEQ 1998–2002) Volet 1: les nourrissons de 5 mois,* vol. 1, no. 5. Québec: Institut de la statistique du Québec.

Dubois, L., B. Bédard, M. Girard, L. Bertrand, and A. M. Hamelin. 2000b. Alimentation: Perceptions, pratiques et insécurité alimentaire, In *Enquête sociale et de santé 1998.* Québec: Institut de la statistique du Québec.

Dubois, L., and M. Girard. 2001. Social position and nutrition: A gradient relationship in Canada and the USA. *European Journal of Clinical Nutrition* 55:366–373.

Dubois, L., and M. Girard. 2003. Social inequalities in infant feeding during the first year of life. The Longitudinal Study of Child Development in Quebec (LSCDQ 1998–2002). *Public Health Nutrition* 6 (8):773–778.

Dubois, L., J. Labrecque, M. Girard, R. Grignon, and N. Damestoy. 1999. Déterminants des difficultés reliées à l'alimentation dans un groupe de personnes âgées non-institutionnalisées du Québec. *L'année Gérontologique, Nutrition et vieillissement* (supplément): 21–52.

Dunkin, A. J. M., A. E. Johnson, J. M. Lilley, K. Morgan, R. J. Neale, R. M. Page, and R. L. Silburn. 1998. Gender and living alone as determinants of fruit and vegetable consumption among the elderly living at home in urban Nottingham. *Appetite* 30:39–51.

Egan, M. C. 1994. Public health nutrition: A historical perspective. *Journal of the American Dietetic Association* 94:298–304.

Fall, C. H. D., D. J. P. Barker, C. Osmond, P. D. Winter, P. M. S. Clark, and L. N. Hales. 1992. Relation of infant feeding to adult serum cholesterol and death from ischemic heart disease. *British Medical Journal* 304:801–805.

Farchi, G., F. Fidanza, P. Grossi, A. Lancia, S. Mariotti, and A. Menotti. 1995. Relationship between eating patterns meeting recommendations and subsequent mortality in 20 years. *European Journal of Clinical Nutrition* 49:408–417.

Farchi, G., F. Fidanza, S. Mariotti, and A. Menotti. 1994. Is diet an independent risk factor for mortality? Twenty year mortality in the Italian rural cohorts of the Seven Countries Study. *European Journal of Clinical Nutrition* 48:19–29.

Federal Interagency Forum on Child and Family Statistics. 2000. *America's Children: Key National Indicators of Well-being.* Washington, DC: Government Printing Office.

Finland Ministry of Health and Social Affairs. 1996. *Public Health Report Finland.* Helsinki: Finland Ministry of Health and Social Affairs.

Flandrin, J. L., and M. Montanari, eds. 1996. *Histoire de l'alimentation.* Paris: Ed Fayard.

Fogel, R. W. 1994. Economic growth, population theory and physiology: The bearing of long-term processes on the making of economic policy. Working paper no. 4638, Cambridge: National Bureau of Economic Research.

Ford, E. S., I. B. Ahluwalia, and D. A. Galuska. 2000. Social relationships and cardiovascular disease risk factors: Finding from the Third National Health and Nutrition Examination Survey. *Preventive Medicine* 30:83–92.

Fortes, C., F. Forastiere, S. Farchi, S. Mallone, T. Trequattrinni, F. Anatra, G. Schmid, and C. A. Perucci. 2003. The protective effect of the Mediterranean diet on lung cancer. *Nutrition and Cancer* 46:30–37.

Frankel, S., D. J. Gunnell, T. J. Peters, M. Maynard, and G. Davey-Smith. 1998. *British Medical Journal* 316:499–504.

Gallo, A. M. 1996. Building strong bones in childhood and adolescence: Reducing the risk of fractures in later life. *Pediatric Nursing* 22:369–374.

Glanz, K. 1997. Behavioral research contributions and needs in cancer prevention and control: Dietary change. *Preventive Medicine* 26:S43–S55.

Godlee, F. 1996. The food industry fights for salt. But delaying salt reduction has public health and commercial costs. *British Medical Journal* 312:1239–1240.

Gonzalez Biosca, D., S. Mizushima, M. Sawamura, Y. Nara, and Y. Yamori. 1992. The effect of nutritional prevention of cardiovascular disease on longevity. *Nutrition Reviews* 50: 407–412.

Goodyear-Smith, F. 2001. Health and safety issues pertaining to genetically modified foods. *Australian and New Zealand Journal of Public Health.* 25:371–375.

Guérard, F. 1996. L'hygiène publique au Québec de 1887 à 1939: Centralisation, normalisation et médicalisation. *Recherches Sociographiques* XXXVII (2):203–227.

Guidotti, T. L. 1997. Why are some people healthy and others not? A critique of the population-health model. *Annals RCRSC* 30:203–206.

Gunnell, D. J., S. Frankel, K. Nanchahal, F. E. M. Braddon, and G. Davey-Smith. 1996. Lifecourse exposure and later disease: A follow-up study based on a survey of family diet and health in pre-war Britain (1937–1939). *Public Health* 110:85–94.

Gunnell, D. J., S. Frankel, K. Nanchahal, T. J. Peters, and G. Davey-Smith. 1998. Childhood obesity and adult cardiovascular mortality: A 57-y. follow-up study based on the Boyd Orr Cohort. *American Journal of Clinical Nutrition* 67:1111–1118.

Guo, S. S., A. F. Roche, W. C. Chumlea, J. D. Gardner, and R. M. Siervogel. 1994. The predictive value of childhood body mass index values for overweight at age 35 years. *American Journal of Clinical Nutrition* 59:810–819.

Hamlin, C. 1995. Public health then and now. Could you starve to death in England in 1839? The Chadwick-Farr controversy and the loss of the "social" in public health. *American Journal of Public Health* 85:856–866.

Hamm, P., R. B. Shekelle, and J. Stamler. 1989. Large fluctuations in body weight during young adulthood and twenty-five-year risk of coronary death in men. *American Journal of Epidemiology* 129:312–318.

Harris, B. 1997. Growing taller, living longer? *Ageing and Society* 17:513–532.

Hautvast, J. G. A. J. 1997. Adequate nutrition in pregnancy does matter. *European Journal of Obstetrics and Gynecology and Reproductive Biology* 75:33–55.

Helsing, E. 1993. Trends in fat consumption in Europe and their influence on the Mediterranean diet. *European Journal of Clinical Nutrition* 47 (suppl. 1):S4–S12.

Heude, B., L. Lafay, J. M. Borys, N. Thibult, A. Lommez, M. Romon, P. Ducimetiere, and M. A. Charles. 2003. Time trend in height, weight, and obesity prevalence in school children from Northern France, 1992–2000. *Diabetes and Metabolism* 29:235–240.

House, J. S., K. R. Landis, and D. Umberson. 1988. Social relationships and health. *Science* 241:540–545.

Huijbregts, P., E. Feskens, L. Räsänen, F. Fidanza, A. Nissinen, A. Menotti, and D. Kromhout. 1997. Dietary patterns and 20 year mortality in elderly men in Finland, Italy, and the Netherlands: Longitudinal cohort study. *British Medical Journal* 315:13–17.

Hulshof, K. F. A. M., M. R. H. Löwik, F. J. Kok, M. Wedel, M. A. M. Brants, R. J. J. Hermus, and F. ten Hoor. 1991. Diet and other life-style factors in high and low socioeconomic groups (Dutch Nutrition Surveillance System). *European Journal of Clinical Nutrition* 45: 441–450.

Hurt, E. 2002. International guidelines and experiences on health claims in Europe, *Asia Pacific Journal of Clinical Nutrition* 11:S90–S93.

Illsley, R. 1990. Comparative review of sources, methodology and knowledge. *Social Science and Medicine. Special issue: Health Inequities in Europe.* 31:229–236.

Institut Canadien d'Information sur la Santé. 2004. *Amèliorer la santé des Canadiens.* Initative sur la Santé de la population canadienne.

International Obesity Task Force. 2001. *Obesity in Europe.* London. European Association for the Study of Obesity.

Irish Department of Health and Children. 2000. *The national health promotion strategy 2000–2005.* Dublin.

James, W. P. T. 1997. Summary and conclusions: Comparative national nutrition policies in Europe: An international expert conference for the World Health Organization. *Nutrition Reviews* 55:S74–S76.

Johansen, H., R. Semenciw, H. Morrison, Y. Mao, P. Verdier, M. E. Smith, and D. T. Wigle. 1987. Important risk factors for death in adults: A 10-year follow-up of the Nutrition Canada survey cohort. *Canadian Medical Association Journal* 136:823–828.

Jutras, S., and G. Castonguay. 1999. *La contribution des facteurs de l'environnement physique au développement des enfants vivant en milieu défavorisé.* Montréal, Laboratoire de recherche en écologie humaine et sociale. Université du Québec à Montréal.

Katz, D. L., R. L. Brunner, T. St-Jeor Sachiko, B. Scott, J. F. Jekel, and K. D. Brownell. 1998. *American Journal of Health Promotion* 12:382–390.

Kennedy, E., and J. Goldberg. 1995. What are American children eating? Implications for public policy. *Nutrition Reviews* 53:111–126.

Kessler, D. A. 1995. The evolution of a national nutrition policy. *Nutrition Policy Annual Reviews* 15:xiii–xxvi.

Keys, A., A. Menotti, M. Karvonen, C. Aravanis, H. Blackburn, R. Buzina, B. S. Djordjevic, A. S. Dontas, F. Fidanza, M. H. Keys, D. Kromhout, S. Nedelkkovic, S. Punsar, F. Seccareccia, and H. Toshima. 1986. The diet and 15-year death rate in the Seven Countries Study. *American Journal of Epidemiology* 124:903–915.

Kohlmeier, L. 1991. Food patterns and health problems: Central Europe. *Annals of Nutrition and Metabolism* 35 (suppl. 1):22–31.

Kubzansky, L. D., L. F. Berkman, T. A. Glass, and T. E. Seeman. 1998. Is educational attainment associated with shared determinants of health in elderly? Findings from the MacArthur Studies of Successful Aging. *Psychosomatic Medicine* 60:578–585.

Kushi, L. H., R. A. Lew, F. J. Stare, C. R. Ellison, M. el Lozy, G. Bourke, L. Daly, I. Graham, N. Hickey, R. Mulcahy, and J. Kevaney. 1985. Diet and 20-year mortality from coronary heart disease. The Ireland-Boston Diet-Heart Study. *New England Journal of Medicine* 312:811–818.

Launer, L. J., T. Harris, C. Rumpel, and J. Madans. 1994. Body mass index, weight change, and risk of mobility disability in middle-age women and older women. The epidemiological follow-up study of NHANES I. *Journal of the American Medical Association* 271:1093–1098.

Lawson, M. 1995. Iron in infancy and childhood. Iron nutritional and physiological significance. *Report of the British Nutrition Foundation Task Force.* London: Chapman and Hall. 93–105.

Levenstein, H. 1988. *Revolution at the Table. The Transformation of the American Diet.* New York: Oxford University Press.

Levenstein, H. 1993. *Paradox of Plenty. A Social History of Eating in Modern America.* New York: Oxford University Press.

Levenstein, H. 1996. Diététique contre gastronomie: Traditions culinaires, sainteté et santé dans les modèles de vie des américains. In *Histoire de l'alimentation,* ed. J. L. Flandrin and M. Montarani. Paris: Éditions Fayard.

Lino, M., P. P. Basiotis, R. S. Anand, and J. N. Variyam. 1998a. The diet quality of Americans. Strong links with nutrition knowledge. *Nutrition/Insights* 7:1–2.

Lino, M., S. A. Gerrior, P. P. Basiotis, and R. S. Anand. 1998b. Report card on the diet quality of children. *Nutrition/Insights* 9:1–2.

Little, J. C., D. R. Perry, and S. L. Volpe. 2002. Effect of nutrition supplement education on nutrition supplement knowledge among high school students from a low-income community. *Journal of Community Health* 27:433–450.

Lobstein, T., L. Baur, and R. Uauy. 2004. Obesity in children and young people: A crisis in public health. *Obesity Reviews* 5 (suppl. 1):4–85.

Lorant, V., and R. Tonglet. 2000. Obesity: Trend in inequality. *Journal of Epidemiology and Community Health* 54:637–638.

Lozoff, B., G. M. Brittenham, and A. W. Wolf. 1991. Long-term developmental outcome of children with iron deficiency. *New England Journal of Medicine* 325:687–694.

Mackenbach, J. P. 1993. The contribution of medical care to mortality decline: McKeown revisited. In *Prosperity, Health and Well-being.* Toronto: L'Institut Canadien de Recherches Avancées.

Marquart, L., K. L. Wiemer, J. M. Jones, and B. Jacob. 2003. Whole grains health claims in the USA and other efforts to increase whole-grain consumption. *Proceedings of the Nutrition Society* 62:151–160.

Martinez, J. A., J. M. Hearney, A. Kafatos, S. Paquet, and M. A. Martinez-Gonzales. 1999. Variables independently associated with self-reported obesity in the European Union. *Public Health Nutrition* 2 (1a):125–133.

McCreary Centre Society. 1993. *Adolescent Health Survey.* Province of British Columbia, Vancouver.

McIntosh, W. A. 1996. *Sociologies of Food and Nutrition.* New York: Plenum Press.

McIntyre, L., S. K. Connor, and J. Warren. 2000. Child hunger in Canada: Results of the 1994 National Longitudinal Survey of Children and Youth. *Canadian Medical Association Journal* 163:961–965.

McIntyre, L., G. Walsh, and S. K. Connor. 2001. *A Follow-up Study of Child Hunger in Canada.* Hull. Développement des Ressources Humaines Canada.

McKeown, T. 1988. *The Origins of Human Disease.* Oxford: Basil Blackwell.

Meningaud, J. P., G. Moutel, and C. Herve. 2001. Ethical acceptability, health policy and foods biotechnology bades foods: Is there a third way between the precaution principle and overly enthusiastic dissemination of CMO? *Medicine and Law* 20 (1):133–141.

Milio, N. 1990. *Nutrition Policy in Food-rich Countries. A Strategic Analysis.* Baltimore: John Hopkins University Press.

Milio, N. 1991. Toward healthy longevity. Lessons in food and nutrition policy development from Finland and Norway. *Scandinavian Journal of Social Medicine* 19:209–217.

Milio, N. 1998. European food and nutrition policies in action. Finland's food and nutrition policy: Progress, problems, and recommendations. WHO Regional Publications. *European Series* 73:63–75.

Millar, J. S. 1998. *A Report on the Health of British Columbians: Provincial Health Officer's Annual Report. 1997. The Health and Well-being of British Columbia's Children.* Victoria: Ministry of Health and Ministry Responsible for Seniors.

Morris, P., and C. Michalopoulos. 2000. *The Self-sufficiency Project at 36 Months: Effect on Children of a Program that Increased Parental Employment and Income.* Ottawa: Human Resources Development Canada (HRDC).

Morrison, H. I., D. Schaubel, M. Desmeules, and D. T. Wigle. 1996. Serum folate and risk of fatal coronary heart disease. *Journal of the American Medical Association* 275:1893–1896.

Morton, J. F., and J. F. Guthrie. 1998. Changes in children's total fat intakes and their food group sources of fat, 1989–91 versus 1994–95: Implications for diet quality. *Family Economics and Nutrition Review* 11 (3):44–57.

Murphy, J. M., C. A. Wehler, M. E. Pagano, M. Little, R. E. Kleinman, and M. S. Jellinek. 1998. Relationship between hunger and psychosocial functioning in low-income American children. *Journal of the American Academy of Child and Adolescent Psychiatry* 37: 163–170.

Must, A. 1996. Morbidity and mortality associated with elevated body weight in children and adolescents. *American Journal of Clinical Nutrition* 63 (suppl.):445S–447S.

Nestle, M. 2002. *Food Politics.* Berkeley: University of California Press.

New Zealand Ministry of Health. 1999. *NZ Food: NZ People. Key Results of the 1997 National Nutrition Survey.* Wellington: New Zealand Ministry of Health.

New Zealand Ministry of Health. 2000. *Social Inequalities in Health, New Zealand 1999: A Summary.* Wellington: New Zealand Ministry of Health.

North, K., P. Emmett, and the Alspac Study Team. 2000. Multivariate analysis of diet among three-year-old children and associations with socio-demographic characteristics. *European Journal of Clinical Nutrition* 54:73–80.

Norum, K. R., L. Johansson, G. Botten, G.-E. A. Bjorneboe, and A. Oshaug. 1997. Nutrition and food policy in Norway: Effects on reduction of coronary heart disease. *Nutrition Reviews* 55:S32–S39.

Nube, M., J. P. Vanderbroucke, C. van der Heide-Wessel, and R. M. van der Heide. 1987. Scoring of prudent dietary habits and its relation to 25-year survival. *Journal of the American Dietetic Association* 87:171–175.

Olson, C. M. 1999. Nutrition and health outcomes associated with food insecurity and hunger. *Journal of Nutrition* 129 (2S suppl.):521S–524S.

Organisation Mondiale de la Santé. 1999. *Santé 21. La politique-cadre de la santé pour tous pour la région européenne de l'OMS.* Copenhagen: Organisation Mondiale de la Santé.

Oski, F. A. 1993. Infant nutrition, physical growth, breastfeeding and general nutrition. *Current Opinion in Pediatrics* 5:385–388.

Pampalon, R., and G. Raymond. 2000. Un indice de défavorisation pour la planification de la santé et du bien-être au Québec. *Maladies chroniques au Canada.* 21:113–122.

Panagiotakos, D. B., C. H. Pitsavos, C. Chrysohoouu, J. Skoumas, L. Papadimitriou, C. Stefanadis, and P. K. Toutouzas. 2003. Status and management of hypertension in Greece: Role of the adoption of a Mediterranean diet: The Attica Study. *Journal of Hypertension* 21:1483–1489.

Pan American Health Organization. 1994. Nutritional situation in the Americas. *Epidemiological Bulletin* 15 (3):1–6.

Pande, M., C. Unwin, and L. L. Haheim. 1997. Factor associated with the duration of breastfeeding: Analysis of the primary and secondary responders to a self-completed questionnaire. *Acta Paediatrica* 86:173–177.

Parmenter, K, J. Waller, and J. Wardle. 2000. Demographic variation in nutrition knowledge in England. *Health Education Research* 15:163–174.

Parsons, T. J., C. Power, S. Logan, and C. D. Summerbell. 1999. Childhood predictors of adult obesity: A systematic review. *International Journal of Obesity* 23 (suppl 8):S1–S107.

Pérusse, L., Y. C. Chagnon, and C. Bouchard. 1998. Etiology of massive obesity: Role of genetic factors. *World Journal of Surgery* 22:907–912.

Plancoulaine, S., M. A. Charles, L. Lafay, M. Tauber, N. Thibult, J. M. Borys, E. Eschwège, and the Fleurbaix-Laventie Ville Santé Study Group. 2000. Infant feeding patterns are related to blood cholesterol concentration in prepubertal children aged 5–11 y: The Fleurbaix-Laventie Ville Santé Study. *European Journal of Clinical Nutrition* 54:114–149.

Popkin, B. M., G. Keyou, Z. Fengying, X. Guo, M. Haijiang, and N. Zohoori. 1993. The nutrition transition in China: A cross-sectional analysis. *European Journal of Clinical Nutrition* 47:333–346.

Poulain, J. P. 1998. Les jeunes séniors et leur alimentation. *Cahiers de l'OCHA. Observatoire CIDIL de l'harmonie alimentaire,* no. 9.

Power, C., J. K. Lake, and T. J. Cole. 1997. Measurement and long-term health risks of child and adolescent fatness. *International Journal of Obesity* 21:507–526.

Power, C., O. Manor, and J. Fox. 1991. *Health and Class, The Early Years.* London: Chapman and Hall.

Prättälä, R., M.-A. Berg, and P. Puska. 1991. Diminishing or increasing contrasts? Social class variation in Finnish food consumption patterns, 1979–1990. *European Journal of Clinical Nutrition* 46:279–287.

Puska, P. 2000. Nutrition and mortality: The Finnish experience. *Acta Cardiologica* 55:213–220.

Pusztai, A. 2002. Can science give us the tools for recognizing possible health risks of GM foods? *Nutrition and Health* 16: 73–84.

Ravelli, A. C. J., J. H. P. van der Meulen, R. P. J. Michels, C. Osmond, D. J. P. Barker, C. N. Hales, and O. P. Bleker. 1998. Glucose tolerance in adults after prenatal exposure to famine. *Lancet* 351:173–177.

Robertson, A., E. Brunner, and A. Sheiham. 1999. Food is a political issue. In *Social Determinants of Health,* ed. M. Marmot and R. G. Wilkinson. Oxford: Oxford University Press.

Robertson, A., C. Torado, T. Lobstein, M. Jermini, C. Knai, J. H. Jensen, A. Ferro-Luzzi, and W. P. James. 2004. Food and health in Europe: A new basis for action. *WHO Regional Publications. European Series* (96):1–385.

Roos, E., E. Lahelma, M. Virtanen, R. Prättälä, and P. Pietinen. 1998. Gender, socioeconomic status and family status as determinants of food behaviour. *Social Science and Medicine* 46:1519–1529.

Roos, G., and R. Prättällä. 1999. *Disparities in Food Habits. Review of Research in 15 European Countries.* Helsinki: National Public Health Institute.

Rose, D., J. P. Habitch, and B. Devaney. 1998. Household participation in the food stamp and WIC programs increases the nutrient intakes of preschool children. *Journal of Nutrition* 128:548–555.

Rosengren, A., H. Wedel, and L. Wilhelmsen. 1999. Body weight and weight gain during adult life in men in relation to coronary heart disease and mortality. *European Heart Journal* 20:269–277.

Ross, D. P., K. Scott, and P. Smith. 2000. Données de base sur la pauvreté au Canada. *Conseil de développement social* no. 558.

Rouffignat, J., L. Dubois, J. Panet-Raymond, P. Lamontagne, S. Cameron, and M. Girard. 2001. *De la sécurité alimentaire au développement social. Les effets des pratiques alternatives dans les régions du Québec. 1999–2000.* Rapport de recherche. Québec. Conseil Québécois de la Recherche Sociale et Ministère de la Santé et des Services sociaux du Québec.

Ryan, A. S. 1997. The resurgence of breast-feeding in the United States. *Pediatrics* 99:1–5.

Sanders-Phillips, K. 1994. Correlates of healthy eating habits in low income black women and Latinas. *Preventive Medicine* 23:781–787.

Schneider, D. 2000. International trends in adolescent nutrition. *Social Science and Medicine* 51:955–967.

Scottish Office Department of Health. 1998. *Working Together for a Healthier Scotland. A Consultation Document.* London: Stationery Office.

Scrimshaw, N. S. 1995. The new paradigm of public health nutrition. *American Journal of Public Health* 85:622–624.

Semenciw, R. M., H. I. Morrison, Y. Mao, H. Johansen, J. W. Davies, and D. T. Wigle. 1988. Major risk factors for cardiovascular disease mortality in adults: Results from the Nutrition Canada survey cohort. *International Journal of Epidemiology* 17:317–324.

Shi, L. 1998. Sociodemographic characteristics and individual health behaviors. *Southern Medical Journal* 91:933–941.

Silfverdal, S. A., L. Bodin, S. Hugosson, Ö. Garpenholt, B. Werner, B. Esbjörner Em Lindquist, and P. Olcès. 1997. Protective effect of breastfeeding on invasive *Haemophilus influenzae* infection: A case–control study in Swedish preschool children. *International Journal of Epidemiology* 26:443–450.

Smith, A. M., and K. I. Baghurst. 1992. Public health implications of dietary differences between social status and occupational category groups. *Journal of Epidemiology and Community Health* 46:409–416.

Société canadienne de pédiatrie, les diététistes du Canada, and Santé Canada. 1998. *La nutrition du nourrisson né à terme et en santé.* Ottawa: Ministre des travaux publics et services gouvernementaux Canada.

Sri Kantha, S. 1990. Nutrition and health in China. *Progress in Food and Nutrition Science* 14:93–137.

Stephen, A. M., and G. M. Sieber. 1994. Trends in individual fat consumption in the UK 1900–1985. *British Journal of Nutrition* 71:775–788.

Strandhagen, E., P. O. Hansson, I. Bosaeus, B. Isaksson, and H. Eriksson. 2000. High fruit intake may reduce mortality among middle-aged and elderly men. The study of men born in 1913. *European Journal of Clinical Nutrition* 54:337–341.

Szreter, S. 1986. The importance of social intervention in Britain's mortality decline c. 1850–1914: A re-interpretation of the role of public health. *Society for the History of Medicine* 1(1):1–37.

Tamblyn, S. E. 2000. The frustration of fighting foodborne disease. *Canadian Medical Association Journal* 162:1429–1430.

Tanner, J. M. 1992. Growth as a measure of the nutritional and hygienic status of a population. *Hormone Research* 38 (suppl. 1):106–115.

Tarlov, A. R. 1996. Social determinants of health. The sociobiological transition. In *Health and Social Organization*, ed. D. Blane, E. Brunner, R. Wilkinson, 71–93. London: Routledge.

Trichopoulou, A., T. Costacou, C. Bamia, and D. Trochopoulos. 2003. Adherence to a Mediterranean diet and survival in a Greek population. *New England Journal of Medicine* 348:2599–2608.

U.K. Department of Health. 1999a. *Reducing Health Inequalities: An Action Report. Our Healthier Nation.* London: Stationery Office.

U.K. Department of Health. 1999b. *Saving Lives: Our Healthier Nation.* London: Stationery Office.

United Nations Standing Committee on Nutrition. 2004. *Fifth Report on the World Nutrition Situation. Nutrition for Improved Development Outcomes.* New York: United Nations.

U.S. Department of Agriculture. 1996. *Nutrition Action Themes for the United States. A Report in Response to the International Conference on Nutrition.* Washington, DC: Center for Nutrition Policy and Promotion.

U.S. Department of Health and Human Services. 2000. *Healthy People 2010. Understanding and Improving Health.* Washington, DC: Author.

U.S. Food and Drug Administration and National Institutes of Health. 2000. *Healthy People 2010. Objectives for Improving Health. Nutrition and Overweight.* Washington, DC: U.S. Government Printing Office.

Vaz de Almeida, M. D., P. Graça, C. Alfonso, A. D'Amicis, R. Lappalainen, and S. Damkjair. 1999. Physical activity levels and body weight in a nationally representative sample in the European Union. *Public Health Nutrition* 2 (1a):105–113.

Wahlqvist, M. L., A. Kouris-Blazos, and B. H. Hsa-Hage. 1997. Ageing, food, culture and health. *Southeast Asian Journal of Tropical Medicine and Public Health* 28 (suppl. 2):100–112.

Walter, T. 1993. Impact of iron deficiency on cognition in infancy and childhood. *European Journal of Clinical Nutrition* 47:307–316.

Warwick, C. 2004. Gastrointestinal disorders: Are health care professionals missing zoonotic causes? *Journal of the Royal Society of Health* 124:137–142.

Watt, R. G., J. Dykes, and A. Sheiham. 2001. Socio-economic determinants of selected dietary indicators in British pre-school children. *Public Health Nutrition* 4:1229–1233.

Williams, P. L., S. H. Innis, and A. M. P. Vogel. 1996. Breastfeeding and weaning practices in Vancouver. *Canadian Journal of Public Health* 87:231–236.

Wilson, B., and E. Tsao. 2001. *HungerCount 2001: Food Bank Lines in Insecure Times.* Toronto: Canadian Association of Food Banks.

Woo, J., S. S. F. Leung, S. C. Ho, A. Sham, T. H. Lam, and E. D. Janus. 1999. Influence of educational level and marital status on dietary intake, obesity, and other cardiovascular risk factors in a Hong Kong Chinese population. *European Journal of Clinical Nutrition* 53:461–467.

World Health Organization. 2001. *Report of the Expert Consultation on the Optimal Duration of Exclusive Breastfeeding*. Geneva: Department of Nutrition for Health and Development.

World Health Organization. 2002. *WHO Global Strategy for Food Safety: Safer Food for Better Health*. Geneva: Department of Nutrition for Health and Development.

World Health Organization. 2003. *Diet, Nutrition and the Prevention of Chronic Diseases. Report of a Joint WHO/FAO Expert Consultation*. Geneva: WHO Technical Report Series 916.

World Health Organization Study Group on Diet, Nutrition and Prevention of Noncommunicable Disease. 1991. Diet, nutrition and the prevention of chronic diseases. *Nutrition Reviews* 49:291–301.

Yang, E. J., H. K. Chung, W. Y. Kim, J. M. Kerver, and W. O. Song. 2003. Carbohydrate intake is associated with diet quality and risk factors for cardiovascular disease in U.S. adults: NHANES III. *Journal of the American College of Nutrition* 22 (1):71–79.

Yip, R., I. Parvanta, K. Scanlon, E. W. Borland, C. M. Russell, and F. L. Trowbridge. 1992. Pediatric nutrition surveillance system—United States, 1980–1991. *Morbidity and Mortality Weekly Report, CDC Surveillance System* 41:1–24.

Yoneyama, K., H. Nagata, and H. Asano. 1994. Growth of Japanese breast-fed and bottle-fed infants from birth to 20 months. *Annals of Human Biology* 21:597–608.

Yoshinaga, M., A. Shimago, C. Koriyama, Y. Nomura, K. Miyata, J. Hashiguchi, and K. Arima. 2004. Rapid increase in the prevalence of obesity in elementary school children. *International Journal of Obesity and Related Metabolic Disorders* 28:494–499.

Zizza, C. 1997. The nutrient content of the Italian food supply, 1961–1992. *European Journal of Clinical Nutrition* 51:259–265.

Chapter 7

Work and Health: New Evidence and Enhanced Understandings

Cam Mustard, John N. Lavis, and Aleck Ostry

Since the beginning of the industrial revolution, the nature of work has been continuously transformed. Scientific discoveries have led to the replacement of human labor with technology and have spawned entirely new modes of work. The productivity gains associated with technological innovation have driven economic growth in the developed economies, and the rising living standards following from this growth have led to safer, cleaner work environments and declining average weekly hours of work.

Throughout this long-term transformation of the nature of work, labor market participation has remained a defining experience for most people. Between the ages of twenty-two and sixty-five, we spend about 40% of our waking hours at work. Earning income in the labor market is the principal distributive mechanism in the modern state, the mechanism by which the material resources of an economy are distributed among its citizens. Jahoda (1981) has called these material returns to labor market participation the "manifest meaning" of work. However, Jahoda and other scholars of the sociology of work (Orth-Gomer and Weiss 1994) have also noted the significance of the latent meanings of work. Participation in employment may offer opportunities for personal growth and development, and it can engage the individual in shared goals and pursuits. An individual's work role (often categorized as his or her occupation or career) is a defining characteristic of social status and helps identify a person's place in the social hierarchy. Work environments are also social communities that may provide rich and rewarding or restricted and harmful social and psychological experiences for the individual.

A large majority of workers in the industrialized countries have reported being very satisfied with their work experience (*Economist* 2004). Although there are important differences across the economies of the member states of the Organization for Economic Cooperation and Development (OECD), people in those countries have typically ranked work experiences as among the most rewarding of

173

their roles and activities (Statistics Canada 1999). But for some people, work is detrimental to health and well-being. It can expose individuals to harmful physical environments, restrict their personal development and sense of worth, and fail to provide for the household's economic security.

In this chapter we focus on how labor market experiences affect workers' health. An integrated framework for thinking about how work may influence health is presented, with a specific focus on the cumulative effects of labor market experiences over the work career. We then briefly review the evidence documenting the biological consequences of adverse work experiences. Next, we describe significant changes in the structure and organization of work over the past two decades that have implications for the health of working-age adults. Finally, some potential implications of these labor market changes for public and private sector labor market policies and practices are outlined.

Characteristics of Labor Market Experiences That Affect Health

Work experiences have pervasive consequences for the health of populations in developed economies. Though annual rates of temporarily disabling occupational morbidity in North America have declined significantly over the past quarter-century, they remain as high as 40 per 1,000 worker-years (Courtney and Webster 1999). Compensable occupational disease and illness account for approximately 3% of the total population burden of disability (Leigh et al. 1996; Murray and Lopez 1996). Evidence has accumulated rapidly over the past decade that these established causes of work-attributable morbidity represent only the tip of the iceberg of health consequences of work. We now know that common diseases such as coronary heart disease, mental illness, and degenerative musculoskeletal disease may be initiated or accelerated by chronically adverse work experiences (Marmot and Feeney 1996). It is difficult to document precisely the contribution of work experiences to the onset and progression of such disorders, due to a long latency and multiple causes (Frank and Maetzel 2000). However, the emerging research evidence, distilled from robust longitudinal observational studies, has increasingly indicated that processes embedded in the experience of work are important causes of the pervasive occupational gradient in life expectancy—where workers in low-skill and low-wage occupations have higher mortality than workers in high-skilled, high wage occupations—observed in all developed economies (Sorlie and Rogot 1990; Siegrist and Marmot 2004; Kunst et al. 1998). Prospective studies of young adults entering the labor market have now documented the health effects of adverse labor market experiences (Wadsworth et al. 1999; Morrell et al. 1997, Graetz 1993; Matthews et al. 1998; Power and Hertzman 1997; Blane et al. 1996). In healthy working adults followed up over time, work environment characteristics (e.g., the range of control over how to respond to the demands of work) have been shown to explain, separately and strongly, the emergence of occupational morbidity gradients. This remains true even after adjustment for behavioral risk factors such as smoking or diet (Hemingway and Marmot 1999; Bosma et al. 1997; Mustard et al. 2003; Borg et al. 2000).

What are the characteristics of work environments and labor market experiences that have potential direct or interactive effects on health? Work roles and work environments are varied and diverse, as are the motivations, attachments, and values of individuals with regard to their work roles. Microlevel social relations are shaped by coworkers and immediate supervisors. The tasks and expectations of work are shaped by features of firm-level organizational culture, as well as by the industrial sector in which the firm or work organization is integrated. Legal and regulatory policies shape the practices and policies of labor markets. The phase of the macroeconomic business cycle or the stage of national economic development also plays a role in shaping work environments and labor market experiences.

A Conceptual Framework Encompassing the Availability and Nature of Work

We propose a framework developed by one of us (Lavis) that conceptually integrates experiences related to the availability of work to the nature of work, since such a framework provides a means of organizing the micro- and macrolevel influences noted above. This framework weaves together currently fragmented perspectives that look separately at the relationships between unemployment and health, job insecurity and health, overwork and health, job characteristics and health, employment grade and health, or work organization and health. The absence of an integrating conceptual framework for examining these specific labor market experiences and health relationships has fragmented research. It has also limited public and private sector policy actors' appreciation of the range of labor market experiences that affect health. In the absence of this understanding, employers and government alike have been unable to articulate the tradeoffs between policies that affect the economic outcomes of labor market experiences and policies that affect the health consequences of these experiences (Lavis 1997).

Aspects of the Two Main Dimensions of Labor Market Experiences

There are six important experiences within the dimension of the availability of work. Three of these experiences represent underwork: discouraged workers who have withdrawn from the labor market, unemployed workers (people actively seeking work), and conditions of underemployment (which can be defined in terms of both hours of work and skill utilization). The fourth experience represents employment circumstances in which an individual endures consistent fear of underwork. The remaining two types of experiences within the domain of the availability of work are being fully employed and being overemployed or overworked.

The dimension of the nature of work is represented by three features: job characteristics, job position within the firm or society, and the organizational characteristics of the firm. Job characteristics may be defined using a single attribute, such as the work's repetitive nature or physical demands. Alternatively, job characteristics may be described in more complex terms representing, for example, their mix of effort and reward (Siegrist et al. 1988, 1990; Siegrist 1996) or their sociopsychological profile (Karasek et al. 1981, 1982; Karasek and Theorell 1990). Job position within the firm captures the idea of occupation and the specific roles, authority, and status that arise from a person's occupation. The differences in roles, authority, and status across various occupations give rise to a hierarchy of occupations in most societies, wherein prestige, income, and control over the work environment are distributed unequally (Townsend and Davidson 1982; Lynch and Kaplan 2000). The final feature of this dimension, the organizational characteristics of the firm, has four relevant components: the ways in which work is organized, the way in which workers are paid, the degree of attention to skills upgrading, and the mechanisms of workplace governance (O'Grady 1993). Work organizations are structured around an explicit authority structure in which worker roles are subordinate to management roles that are in turn subordinate to the authority of executive roles. Levels of compensation, status, and prestige are ordered to reflect this hierarchy. In the broad labor market, there is a strong income and status hierarchy across occupations, expressed by skill levels, educational requirements, and professional qualifications.

The risks of exposure to adverse experiences in the labor market often appear to cluster around characteristics of occupation (Johnson and Hall 1995). As an example of the clustering of risks, the chance of experiencing a period of unemployment is higher among low-wage, low-skill occupations than among occupations requiring professional qualifications. Adverse psychosocial work exposures—such as those occurring when employees have limited control over the manner in which work is performed (decision latitude) or face expectations of fast-paced work tasks requiring high concentration (psychological demands)—are also distributed unequally across the occupational hierarchy. In most OECD economies, approximately 20% of workers are engaged in occupations with low decision latitude and high psychological demands (Karasek et al. 1998). However, fully 25% of workers in low-status Canadian occupations experience conditions of low control and high demands, compared with 11% of workers in high-status occupations (Mustard et al. 2003). Similarly, individuals in lower-status occupations more commonly experience limited profit sharing, contingent employment relationships, and highly hierarchical authority structures.

Static versus Dynamic Perspectives on the Dimensions of Labor Market Experiences

These two main dimensions of labor market experience, the availability of work and the nature of work, can be viewed from either a static or a dynamic perspective. Most typically, the relationship between labor market experiences and health has been described from a static perspective, as in the body of research examining the health consequences of unemployment. There is a large body of literature composed of both cross-sectional and prospective study designs that have estimated the acute consequences to individual physical and mental health of (as well as behavioral responses to) the involuntary loss of employment (Gore 1978; Graetz 1993; Iversen et al. 1987; Kasl et al. 1975; Kasl and Cobb 1980; Kasl et al. 1995; Klein-Hesselink and Spruit 1992; Kraut et al. 2000; Lavis 1999; Morrell et al. 1997; Sorlie and Rogot 1990; Wadsworth et al. 1999). The evidence of health effects arising from unemployment is sufficiently substantial to consider the relationship causal (Bradford Hill 1965). This literature has also examined many hypotheses concerning pathways and mechanisms for work-related health effects, ranging from the material consequences of job loss to the disruptions of social ties by which involuntary loss of employment might lead to disturbance in physical and mental health and function (Jahoda 1981; Bartley 1994; Kessler et al. 1987). There is also an emerging body of research focused on the degree to which the health consequences of unemployment are mediated by labor market policies such as the degree and duration of unemployment benefits (Rodriguez 2001).

The perspective of this research is static in that the focus is on a single moment or event in an individual's labor market career—specifically, a discrete spell of unemployment. But the dimensions of the availability of work and the nature of work can also be viewed from a dynamic perspective that takes into account the cumulative history of labor market experiences. Viewed in this way, the cumulative effect of an individual's sequence of occupations and work roles (which might include periods of voluntary and involuntary withdrawal from the labor market) is examined for the relationship to changes in health status. This perspective is most congruent with a view that the health effects of labor market experience are dominated not by single events but rather by the cumulative effects of chronic or repeated experiences. Although there is much less empirical research on the cumulative effects of labor market experiences, important research cohorts are beginning to be used for such investigations (Amick et al. 2001; Manor et al. 2003).

A dynamic perspective has also proven important in the emerging research on the mechanisms through which adverse psychosocial exposures rooted in particular types of work environment and labor market experiences may initiate or accelerate physiological changes to central biological pathways. We turn next to a description of the insights offered by this research.

The Biological Basis of Links between Work Experiences and Health

To have consequences for health, experiences and exposures rooted in work environments must influence biological mechanisms. The biological systems responsible for homeostatic regulation are the central pathways of interest in understanding how experiences arising from the social ordering of society lead to socioeconomic gradients in morbidity and mortality (see chapter 2). All organisms have evolved biological mechanisms that regulate homeostasis in response to turbulence, challenge, or deprivation in the external environment. Classic work by early physiologists established the homeostatic function of the endocrine system in humans, wherein circulating hormones such as catecholamines and corticosteroids act as agents of metabolic self-regulation (Cannon 1928; Selye 1956). In addition to maintaining metabolic and physiological homeostasis, these mechanisms also regulate the acute response to external challenge. In humans, this exquisitely complex set of biological adaptations includes a sensitivity to social cues, social environments, and social stimuli (McEwen and Seeman 1999; Cohen et al. 1997, Sapolsky 1992).

There are three important physiological control systems that are sensitive to perceptions of social environments: the hypothalamic–pituitary–adrenal system (HPA axis), which controls cortisol secretion; the sympatho–adrenal–medullary system (SAM axis), which controls epinephrine and norepinephrine secretion; and the psycho–neuro–immune system (PNI axis), which links central nervous system influences to immune system function and blood clotting factors. A well-replicated body of research has demonstrated the direct responsiveness of these biological regulatory systems to the challenges of social experiences, and in particular to those experiences associated with position in a social hierarchy. This sensitivity of homeostatic regulation to social stimuli is an evolutionary adaptation that has contributed to the fitness of humans as a social species.

Hypotheses about Disease Causation Mechanisms

A mechanism is required, however, that links the adaptive physiological response to challenge to the emergence of states of pathology and disease. There is a family of contemporary hypotheses that propose disease causation mechanisms arising from the chronic arousal of these regulatory axes. Some researchers have hypothesized that chronic exposure to stressors and challenge may over time be translated into modified neuroendocrine function, with later consequences for susceptibility to disease (Brunner 1997; Cohen et al. 1997). Others have linked Selye's (1956) original idea of adrenal exhaustion with a contemporary view of the functional consequences of chronic physiological arousal. For example, the allostatic load hypothesis, developed by McEwen (1998), proposes that organisms pay a price over time for the adaptation to external stressors, the result of chronic overactivity of the neuroendocrine regulatory mechanisms. This wear and tear, viewed as accelerated aging, produces deterioration in functioning of the cardiovascular and immune systems, as well as of cognitive function (McEwen 1998; Seeman et al. 1997).

Documenting the Biological Consequences of Adverse Work Experiences

To establish the biological consequences of adverse work experiences, two classes of evidence are required: (1) documentation that regulatory physiology is responsive to conditions arising from experiences associated with the availability of work or the nature of work and (2) documentation that repeated exposure to adverse work conditions can lead to regulatory dysfunction. In turn, links need to be shown between regulatory dysfunction and altered metabolism, physiology, or immune function associated with the initiation or progression of disease. The availability and coherence of evidence linking specific experiences in the labor market to physiological response and in turn to altered states of metabolism, physiology, or immune function were assessed in a recent systematic review (Lavis et al. 1998). In this review the studies selected were restricted to prospective observational designs where exposure to labor market experiences preceded the measurement of health outcome. Studies identified in this review were concentrated on the assessment of the health effects of unemployment and job insecurity (the availability of work) and job characteristics and job position within the firm (the nature of work). Studies of unemployed individuals have measured serum cortisol, serum cholesterol, blood pressure, and lymphocyte reactivity, yielding evidence of altered regulatory function following unemployment (table 6 in Lavis et al. 1998). Although Lavis and colleagues found no definitive studies linking unemployment to the initiation or progression of disease, a large body of work had consistently found the experience of unemployment to be associated with the risk of death in the period following the unemployment spell (table 10 in Lavis et al. 1998).

In the case of the nature of work, a body of evidence has been established over the past decade showing a strong and consistent association between job characteristics, such as decision latitude, and disease incidence (especially cardiovascular disease), as well as between job position in the firm and disease risk. Lavis and colleagues (1998, table 15), for example, reviewed the relationship between job demands, job control, and physiological measures including blood pressure, serum cholesterol, and prolactin. In examining the role of the nature of work on disease initiation and progression, Brunner (1996) focused on cardiovascular disease and the related cluster of features known as the metabolic syndrome (central adiposity, elevated insulin, high blood pressure, and elevated serum cortisol). The preponderant finding in this general research area has been that individuals chronically exposed to adverse psychosocial working environments have an elevated risk of both cardiovascular disease incidence and cardiovascular disease mortality (Belkic et al. 2004; Bosma et al. 1998; Hemingway and Marmot 1999). Although based on observational research designs, these findings appear robust, in that the studies have generally achieved adequate measurement of potential confounders and the results have not appeared to be due to the distribution of health behaviors in different occupational groups.

Health Effects as Related to Occupational and Social Hierarchies

Jobs characterized by adverse psychosocial conditions are not randomly distributed throughout the occupational hierarchy. High-status occupations, which have professional-level entry criteria and relatively high compensation, are most commonly characterized by high levels of demands and responsibilities. At the same time, there are also high levels of latitude, control, and autonomy in the individual's approach to responding to these demands. In contrast, many low-status occupations, especially those associated with machine-paced production or scheduled performance requirements, are characterized by the unhealthy combination of high demands and limited discretionary autonomy to respond to these demands. Evidence is increasing that this distribution of benign and adverse job characteristics across the occupational hierarchy is among the factors accounting for the distribution of cardiovascular risk factors in working-age populations. These risk factors include SAM axis dysfunction arising from chronic arousal (high blood pressure), lipid metabolism dysfunction associated with atherogenic processes (cholesterol and arterial plaque), and differences in coagulation parameters such as fibrinogin level (Belkic et al. 2000). These cardiovascular disease risk factors are distributed in working-age populations in a gradient corresponding to socioeconomic position, a gradient that closely corresponds to the observed socioeconomic gradient in cardiovascular disease mortality.

In the past decade, research based on longitudinal cohort studies has demonstrated the emergence of this occupational gradient in risk of morbidity among individuals who had no diagnosed disorder at the time of enrollment in the studies. The U.K. National Child Development Study, for instance, yielded data about occupational gradients in health status that had emerged through differential exposure to labor market experiences associated with the availability of work. Through that study, researchers documented that the frequency of spells of unemployment between the ages of twenty and thirty had been strongly related to individuals' subsequent development of mental health disorders and declines in perceived health status (Power et al. 1997).

Several important cohort studies have also documented the emergence of occupational hierarchy-related health status gradients associated with the nature-of-work exposures. In a study of more than 5,000 Danish workers who had reported good health at baseline, differential exposure to adverse job psychosocial characteristics was related to the risk of reporting a decline in perceived health status over a five-year follow-up period (Borg et al. 2000). The results of this study were not accounted for by other potential explanations, such as differences in health behaviors among members of different occupational groups. Similar results have been replicated in cohorts in separate OECD economies (figure 7.1) (Mustard et al. 2003, Martikainen et al. 1999).

Those taking a Darwinian perspective would argue that the observed health status advantage of people ranked highest in a social hierarchy is simply the expression of genetic fitness. Those who are genetically fittest will tend to have the best adapted cognitive, behavioral, and biological responses to their physical and social environments. They will therefore tend to be the most successful in ascending status and rank hierarchies. In short, health produces social status. This perspective is not without some evidentiary basis. Position in the occupational hierarchy is associated not only with adult height (with rank advantage conferred on taller individuals) but also with the average height of parents (a marker of genetic potential) (Power and Hertzman 1997; Marmot et al. 1991; Davey Smith et al. 2000). Children in the 1946 British birth cohort with chronic physical health conditions have been found to be less upwardly mobile than children with good health (Wadsworth 1986, 1997).

However, there is also a growing body of observational and experimental evidence suggesting that social environments can profoundly alter and may frequently

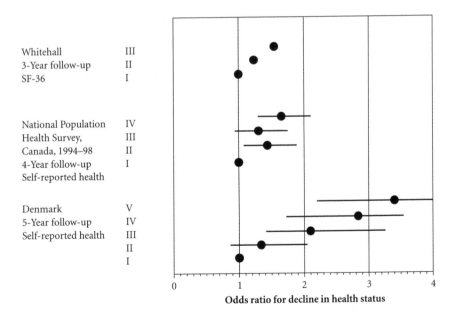

Figure 7.1. Prospective risk of decline in health status by position in occupational hierarchy

dominate biological potential. For example, in an elegant study of the relationship between social status and cardiovascular disease process, small groups of captive female macaque monkeys with established dominance hierarchies were experimentally manipulated by switching animals between groups (Shively and Clarkson 1994). The health consequences of adapting to the new social hierarchy were dramatic. Dominant animals that became subordinate developed a fivefold excess of coronary occlusion compared with animals that remained dominant. Subordinate animals that became dominant following the experimental manipulation had twice the risk of developing atherosclerosis compared with animals that maintained a subordinate position across the experimental manipulation. The implication of this evidence is that insecurity and instability in social environments can affect the health of individuals across a ranking of attained status.

The Transformation of Work

As we noted in this chapter's introduction, the nature of work has been continuously transformed since the beginning of the industrial revolution. New modes of work have emerged following the technological applications of scientific discoveries. Old forms of work have disappeared as machines have replaced human labor. In this section, we focus on two prominent changes in the world of work in the past twenty-five years: (1) the demographic change in the world of work arising from increased female labor force participation and (2) the structural change in the nature and availability of work arising from technological and organizational innovation in contemporary workplaces. We will use these case studies to explore the potential implications for the health of workers and for the design of private and public sector policies. In some of these case studies, there is strong research evidence to guide labor market policy intervention aimed at moderating conditions that are harmful to health. In other areas, the evidence base provides ambivalent guidance on the health consequences of the changing world of work.

Demographic Change: Female Labor Force Participation

One of the most substantial changes in contemporary working life in developed economies has arisen not from technological innovation but from demography. Many women have entered the labor market over the past fifty years. Women have, of course, always worked. In agrarian and early industrial economies, the traditional role for women was to work within the home and to care for children. Beginning with the Second World War, female labor force participation in the United States increased from approximately 10% to more than 70% of working-age women by 1990 (figure 7.2) (Heymann 2000). This dramatic increase in female labor force participation has had effects both on the world of work and on the

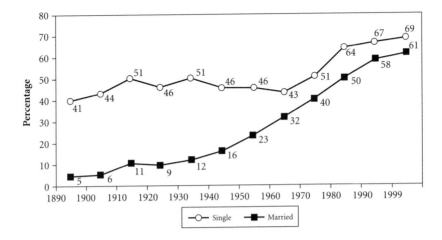

Figure 7.2. Labor force participation rate of single and married women, 1890–1999 (based on data for 1890 to 1970 from U.S. Bureau of the Census, *Historical Statistics of the United States: Colonial Times to 1970,* part 1, series D 49-62, 1890–1970, decennial census [Washington, DC, 1997] for 1999 from U.S. Bureau of Labor Statistics, unpublished tabulations calculated from the Current Population Survey).

Source: Reprinted, by permission of the publisher, from J. Heymann, *The Widening Gap: Why America's Working Families Are in Jeopardy and What Can Be Done about It* (New York: Basic Books, 2000), 213.

raising of children. By the 1990s, for example, more than 70% of U.S. children lived in households in which both parents were in the labor force. Where once women's work provided food, clothing, and other sustaining elements of the household, by the end of this period most families no longer had any adult working at home full-time. They were increasingly dependent on wages and salaries rather than domestic labor for the provision of these essentials.

The increased participation by women in paid work has led to a focus on three potential consequences to their health. The first relates to reproductive health. In the last half-century, fertility has fallen in the developed economies, declining below the replacement rate in some countries. This fertility decline is significantly, but not exclusively, related to female role expectations generally and to labor force participation opportunities specifically. The pattern of declining fertility in these countries has two important features: smaller family size and delayed initiation of childbearing. These changes are generally viewed as beneficial to women's health. Maternal mortality and morbidity associated with reproduction have fallen precipitously in the twentieth century. Although the largest share of this improvement must be attributed to advances in medicine and in the organization and delivery of medical care, these contributions have been made against the backdrop of reduced female exposure to maternity-related life- and health-threatening experiences.

However, the consequences to women's health from rising female participation in the labor force may also be viewed from a less sanguine perspective. As women come to participate in the labor force with the same frequency as men, it is possible that they will adopt male behaviors or have greater exposure to traditionally male work environments. This could lead to women having a higher risk of mortality from heart disease, lung cancer, automobile accidents, and other causes of the excess male mortality in developed economies (Nathanson 1995). There is some evidence for this proposition: Rates of female smoking and rates of female lung cancer mortality have increased during the period of rising social and occupational equality.

Yet rising rates of female labor force participation appear to have had little effect on the rates or causes of female mortality. As women have entered the labor force over the past half-century, the sex differential in life expectancy (which is currently approximately five years in Canada) has been preserved (Vallin 1995). This evidence is not consistent with the hypothesis that greater exposure to work environments adversely affects women's health (Waldron 1991). At the same time, however, it is clear that the pervasively observed male gradient in risk of morbidity and mortality in relation to position in the occupational hierarchy is expressed in women as well (Sorlie and Rogot 1990; Bosma et al. 1997). In most developed economies, women, on average, occupy lower-status positions in the occupational hierarchy (Hall 1989; Mustard et al. 2003; Matthews et al. 1998). There is no substantial evidence that there are profound sex differences in the physiology of stress responses that might confer differential protection on women relative to men in hierarchically ranked work environments. Therefore, given the relatively long latency of expression of chronic disease arising from cumulative exposures to socially cued behaviors and to socially determined environments, it may be premature to conclude that rising rates of female labor force participation have only benign implications for women's health.

Other consequences to women's health arising from increasing labor force participation relate to the potential detrimental effects of multiple role demands. In households with children, women have retained primary responsibility for family caregiving and for domestic labor (Heymann 2000). Working women are more likely than working men to be caring for a child or spouse who is disabled or for an elderly relative. There has been substantial research attention focused on examining the consequences (particularly the psychological ones) for health and well-being of the increased complexity of women's roles. Substantial numbers of women have reported enhanced well-being arising from the opportunity to participate simultaneously in a work role and in the role of primary domestic care-giver (Roxburgh 1996). For some women, role complexity may in fact be protective of health.

Role complexity can be expected to have very different implications for health, depending on the socioeconomic position of women. A secure and demanding occupational role may enhance well-being and health for middle-class mothers in emotionally sustaining dual-parent households. However, in a study of white-collar women holding a university degree, the combination of adverse work environments (characterized by high demands and low control) and large family responsibilities was associated with elevated systolic and diastolic blood pressure (both during working hours and during evenings) (Brisson et al. 1999). Perhaps more importantly, multiple role demands that may enhance a woman's well-being in an economically secure household may overwhelm a single mother in an insecure and low-paid position in the labor market. Much more informative research is needed on the consequences of multiple role demands for women in disadvantaged positions in the socioeconomic hierarchy. Overall, there is very little evidence as yet that the dramatic increase in female labor force participation has brought with it a substantial change in the risk to women's health.

Changes in the Nature of Work

Continuous change in the structure of labor markets and in the organization of work has occurred over the past twenty-five years. A dramatic shift in the sectoral distribution of employment, reminiscent of the equally sharp changes as labor moved from farms to factories in the first quarter of this century (Reich 1996; Rifkin 1996), has been among the most profound changes in developed economies' labor markets over this period. From the 1970s to the early 1990s, manufacturing employment decreased and employment in the service sector has expanded, such that by 1991, 78% of the Group of Seven countries workforce was employed in services (Daniels 1993; Castells and Aoyama 1994).

As well as changes in the sectoral distribution of employment, several related structural trends have occurred within occupations. During the past two decades, an overall upgrading of the skill level required in jobs in the United States (Howell and Wolff 1991), Canada (Myles 1988; Livingstone 1999), and the United Kingdom (Gallie 2000) has occurred. Among British workers asked about their perception of skill requirements from 1981 to 1992, 26.2% reported an increase in the skill requirements of their job (Gallie 2000). The highest proportion of workers reporting increased skill requirements were among the semi- and unskilled manual occupational categories. In the absence of other changes in the nature of work, increases in skill requirements would be expected to be translated into higher earnings and, potentially, into higher job satisfaction. In a substantial paradox emerging from the performance of the labor market over the past two decades, there is compelling evidence that increasing worker productivity has become disconnected from the earnings received by workers (figure 7.3) (Palley 1998).

In addition to increased skill requirements within jobs, there has also been a trend toward increasing entry requirements (a trend known as credential inflation), independent of actual skill requirements, particularly for unskilled jobs (Holzer 1996; Livingstone 1999). For example, in a large study of Ontario workers, Holzer

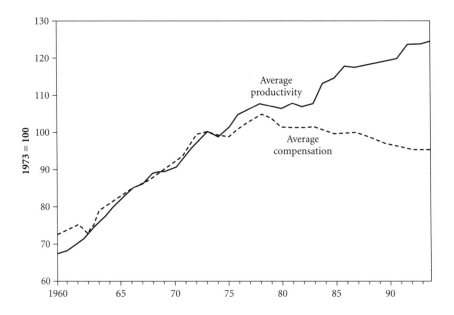

Figure 7.3. Nonsupervisory average productivity and compensation (data provided by Economic Policy Institute, Washington, DC)

Source: Figure reprinted, by permission of the publisher, from T. I. Palley, *Plenty of Nothing: The Downsizing of the American Dream and the Case for Structural Keynesianism* (Princeton, NJ: Princeton University Press, 1998).

(1996) compared the qualifications required for various occupations in the early 1980s and the mid-1990s. He found that the requirement for postsecondary education in unskilled manual and clerical occupations increased by 60% and 96%, respectively, compared with a decrease of 3% for managerial occupations and an increase of 6% for professional jobs. These high relative rates of credential inflation for unskilled workers are one example of the labor market transformations that have altered the availability of work among low-skilled occupations. Another example is a change in the demand for low-skilled labor in regional economies arising from global economic integration. The labor market changes during the last quarter of a century have occurred against a backdrop of historically high unemployment (Hobsbawm 1994). In the United States, annual average unemployment rates from 1973 to the early 1990s generally were at least 2% higher than the rates from 1947 to 1973 (Mishel et al. 1997). In OECD nations, unemployment rates during the 1980s were approximately double those of the 1970s (Navarro 2001).

Persistently high unemployment has also contributed to a pervasive perception of employment insecurity among workers. Between the 1970s and the 1990s, job insecurity (measured on a six-point scale ranging from secure to insecure jobs) increased from 3.5 to 4.5 or 1.5 standard deviations (Karasek et al. 1998). This suggests that weakening norms concerning the employment contract, the declining influence of organized labor in defining the nature of work, and an ascendancy of shareholders' interests in corporate governance have increased employees' exposure to the risk of layoff. Also indicative of employers' increasing authority to define the terms of employment has been the decline in median job tenure (figure 7.4). For example, at least in the United States, throughout the economic expansion of the 1990s, the annual proportion of workers experiencing dislocation increased from 8% to more than 12% of the labor force (Osterman 1999). Although some of this increase in employee insecurity may have been cyclical, there has been an increased turbulence in the labor market even during periods of economic expansion. The risk of dislocation is even higher among lower-paid and lower-quality occupations. The health consequences of job insecurity and the anticipation of job loss are poorly understood but may be substantial (Lavis et al. 1998; McDonough 2000). As noted earlier in this chapter, the perception of insecurity can provoke acute biological responses that are involved in homeostatic regulation.

Another major trend in labor market dynamics over the past quarter-century in Europe, North America, and Australia has been a rise in nontraditional work arrangements such as part-time work, shift work, self-employment, multiple job holding, and casual or temporary work (Quinlan 1998; Quinlan et al. 2001). These new flexible labor arrangements have been evident across many economic sectors.

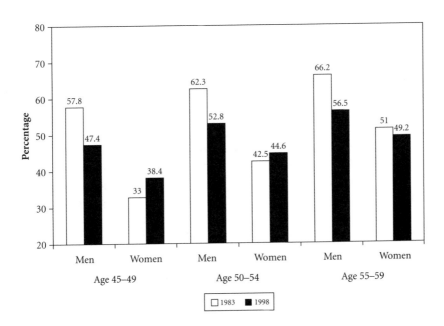

Figure 7.4. Percentage of men and women with ten or more years' tenure, 1983 and 1998

Source: U.S. Bureau of Labor Statistics, "Employee Tenure in 1998," news release, 23 September 1998. Figure cited in P. Osterman, *Securing Prosperity: The American Labor Market, How It Has Been Changed, and What to Do about It* (Princeton, NJ: Princeton University Press, 1999).

The increase in part-time employment has been particularly marked. In 1953 in Canada, 3.8% of the workforce was employed part-time; by 1980, this had risen to 13.5% and by 1993, to 17.3% (Duffy et al. 1997). By 1989, the share of the workforce employed part-time in Sweden was 24%; in the United Kingdom, 22%; and in Japan and the United States, 18% (Livingstone 1999). Increases in part-time employment have gone hand in hand with increases in multiple job holding. During the 1980s in Canada, the number of multiple-job holders increased by 89% among females and 28% among males (Duffy and Pupo 1992).

Although the emergence of nontraditional work arrangements is a visible example of the structural changes occurring in the nature of work in developed economies' labor markets, it is important to note that the proportion of the labor force in employment arrangements that are formally insecure (i.e., limited in the duration of employment) is relatively small. Fewer than 10% of U.S. workers are in contract, on-call, or temporary agency employment (Osterman 1999). There is also good evidence that the growth in these forms of employment, which have been called contingent work, leveled off in the 1990s in the United States (Osterman 1999).

In addition to declines in the security of employment arrangements, important changes in the organization of work within firms in many economic sectors have been occurring. In particular, management hierarchies have flattened in many service and manufacturing industries as employers adopt models of high-performance work organizations (Osterman 1999). Evidence suggests that the prevalence of job strain and work intensity has increased in workplaces in both the United States and some European nations (Landsbergis et al. 1999). European surveys have shown that the proportion of high-strain jobs (i.e., work with high demands, low control, and low support) increased from 25% to 30% between 1991 and 1996 (European Foundation 1997; Bond et al. 1998). From 1990 to 2000, three waves of the European Survey on Working Conditions documented important increases in the pace and intensity of work, especially among white-collar workers (European Foundation 1997). The monitoring of changes over time in the organization of work has produced an uneven portrait, with disquieting evidence of decline in the quality of many occupational roles and in a range of working conditions, while also documenting the development of new organizational practices which have the potential to improve aspects of working life quality (Lowe 2000).

Implications for the Health of the Workforce

The health implications of these labor market changes over the past quarter-century can be summarized in five dimensions. First, work clearly has become safer, both as a result of regulatory actions to reduce exposures to physical and chemical hazards and as a result of the replacement of human labor with machines made possible by advances in technology.

Second, the increase in female labor force participation has not—at least not yet—been associated with women's declining health in the developed economies, relative to the period when women were engaged primarily in nonwage domestic labor. There is little evidence to date that the increased rates of female labor force participation have had adverse effects on the health of working women arising from workplace exposures or from the multiple role demands of working life and domestic life. At the same time, many institutions in society that support the raising of children by families have been slow to adapt to the increase in female labor force participation. Institutional supports for the care of children, including day-care services and the formal education system, may not fully meet the demands of families with two adult labor market participants (Heymann 2000). Over time, these challenges may present cumulative risk to the health and well-being of parents and children.

Third, as global economic integration has altered the demand for labor in regional economies, increased instability in the availability of work in many sectors of the developed economies has increased. Whereas the service sector has expanded, many traditional sectors have contracted. This churning of the labor market has been associated with higher rates of employment dislocation, shorter median work tenure, longer duration of unemployment spells, and the growth of insecure work arrangements in the formal wage economy. Health consequences from an increasingly insecure labor market may arise as a result of insecurity in labor market income and, simultaneously, as a result of the cumulative effects of physiological responses to the perception of insecurity or the experience of job dislocation.

Fourth, labor market changes have altered the nature of work in many firms. With the reduction of demand for low-skilled occupations or with the restructuring of work associated with pressures to increase productivity, evidence has emerged in some sectors of increased intensification of work and an increase in the prevalence of high-strain work environments (Ostry et al. 2000; Woodward et al. 1999). From both a biomechanical and a physiological perspective, an optimal evolution of work environments would see a reduction, rather than an increase, in these potentially adverse exposures.

Finally, the reduction in demand for low-skill occupations has led to a stagnation of market income among those workers, contributing to a widening of earned income inequality in the developed economies. There are reasons to be concerned that the proportion of workers whose labor market income is below a minimally adequate level is increasing, rather than decreasing. For example, the real value of the U.S. minimum wage declined from 117% of the three-person family poverty threshold in 1968 to 80% of the threshold in 1998 (Pollin and Luce 1998). The health effects of poverty are well documented. It is a paradox that a sustained period of economic growth over the past twenty-five years has produced an increase in the numbers of people whose labor market income is below a minimum level of adequacy. The greatest risk of exposure to adverse working experiences has always been associated with lower-status occupations, and the evidence summarized here indicates that both the availability of work and the nature of work have deteriorated over the past two decades among persons in low-status occupations. The magnitude of these changes in the nature and availability of work is sufficiently large to be concerned about the short-term and especially the long-term consequences to the health of working-age populations.

To this point in the chapter, we have presented two bodies of evidence: (1) the basis for concluding that there is a causal relationship between labor market experiences and health (and the associated biological pathways) and (2) a description of some current trends in the labor market that may be magnifying the risks to health of labor force participation. There are many contradictions in this composite portrait. For example, the rise in female labor force participation has not produced strong evidence for harmful consequences to the health of women. Similarly, the long period of economic growth experienced over the past 25 years has, paradoxically, been associated with a deterioration in some dimensions of the availability of work and the nature of work. Understanding these contradictory and paradoxical patterns does not easily lead to conclusive policy guidance. In the final section of this chapter, we will consider some of the possible policy implications arising from these two bodies of evidence.

Implications for Labor Market Policies

Several policy implications arise from an appreciation of the health effects of labor market experiences, and these illustrate some of the opportunities for applying a health lens to the examination of public policy alternatives in the labor market arena. The potential health consequences of changes in the labor market and in the nature of work are likely to be much more extensive than would be implied in the traditional view of the health effects of work. This traditional view is concerned with acute occupational injury and a specific group of diseases arising from chemical or physical occupational exposures. The perspective on the health effects of work articulated here views adverse work experiences as cumulative exposures that can initiate or accelerate chronic disease processes ranging from cardiovascular disorders to degenerative musculoskeletal conditions. Potential adverse work exposures are differentially distributed in relation to workers' relative positions in the occupational hierarchy, with workers in higher-status occupations being more protected from such exposures.

Although most of these labor market exposures are amenable to policy intervention, policy making appears to have become increasingly neglectful of work's health effects, as economic objectives and the interests of shareholders and executives have come increasingly to dominate policy formulation (as noted earlier).

Ideally, labor market policy would find an equitable balance among the interests of corporations, workers, and society at large, and the health effects of labor market experiences would be an important part of the policy-making calculus. At the very least, one might hope to find the health consequences of labor market experiences informing policy choices "at the margin." Established to pursue economic objectives, industrial policy has been informed at the margin by societal interests concerning the environmental consequences of different policy options.

The policy options discussed in this section explore extensions or elaborations of active labor market policies that use regulatory and fiscal instruments to influence the behaviors of employers and workers making choices about conditions in the labor market. We view the proposition that a society must choose between active labor market policies and robust economic growth to be a false policy contrast (it is, in essence, a subset of a much broader and long-standing debate about whether increased economic efficiency must come at the price of equity). Despite the confidence with which neoclassical economic theory predicts that active labor market policies will inhibit job creation and economic growth, no convincing empirical evidence of such effects has been found (Blank 1994; Abraham and Houseman 1994; Newmark and Wascher 2000; Arjona et al. 2001; Lindert 2004). The discussion of potential policy actions that follows is informed by the assumption that active labor market policies and robust institutional structures in the labor market need not inhibit economic growth.

We focus our comments in three areas: (1) policies addressing the intersection of work and family, (2) policies designed to increase the profile and range of health implications considered by firms in the design of work, and (3) broader income distribution (or redistribution) policies and the extent to which they take into account the health effects of income inequality.

Family-supportive Labor Market Policies

Over the past two decades, employers and public policy makers, responding to the growth in female labor market participation, have increasingly focused on employment policies that affect the functioning of families. Public-sector policies that have emerged include day-care or child-care funding programs, maternity leave rights, and maternity wage replacement insurance. Private-sector policies have included family leave provisions, the provision of subsidized day care, and the extension of eligibility for sick leave so that workers can care for children and other family members. It is important to note that public and private sector policies have emerged in response to different objectives. Family-supportive public programs, either universal or targeted to lower-income households, have the objective of establishing common entitlement within similar groups in the labor force. Private-sector policies are structured to advance the competitive advantage of individual firms, and they focus on attracting and retaining scarce labor talent. It is not surprising, then, that the generosity of private-sector family-supportive leave policies or benefit packages is directly related to occupational status, with individuals in higher-status occupations having access to more generous benefits (Heymann 2000).

This inequality in the availability of family-supportive employment benefits has unrecognized consequences for the health of children and parents and for parental labor market participation. Families with limited work-leave options cannot provide the same response to the caregiving needs of sick children or disabled family members as families with more generous benefits. In contemporary labor market circumstances in the developed economies, where two-income households are the norm, most working adults cannot meet all the care needs of children and adults in their families. The voluntary initiatives of employers have not been sufficient to equitably address these needs.

Active labor market policies motivated by the dual objectives of improving equity and mitigating the potential harmful consequences to health would focus on several dimensions. Consideration would be given to the regulation of minimum working conditions for families, including rights to unpaid leave and flexibility in work arrangements that are not tied to place of employment or job classification. Minimum working conditions for families would also include the universal right to income insurance in circumstances requiring work leave for family caregiving responsibilities. Finally, minimum working conditions for families would be based on the principle that all working households derive adequate income from work. These principles have begun to receive policy attention through the use of instruments such as the National Child Benefit Supplement in Canada and the Earned Income Credit in the United States. These policies are designed to achieve the simultaneous ends of enhancing income in low-income households with children, presenting neutral consequences for employer costs, and encouraging labor force participation.

Policies to Influence Work Environments

In the industrial economies, health-related interventions in work environments have been almost exclusively concerned with the regulation of physically hazardous materials and processes. Occupational health protection efforts have produced immeasurably safer, cleaner, and healthier work environments. Workers' compensation systems in many developed economies have also used fiscal incentives to influence firm-level practices concerning the prevention and rehabilitation of compensable occupational illnesses and injury. There is strong evidence that these incentive-based policies are effective instruments for influencing firm behavior (Hyatt 1998).

With the exception of the experience in Scandinavian countries, however, governments and employers have given very little concerted attention to the control of workers' exposure to adverse work environment characteristics related to the nature of work or to labor market conditions related to the availability of work. There are perhaps three principal explanations for this general absence of policy commitment. First, the scientific evidence for the causal attribution of chronic cardiovascular, musculoskeletal, and mental health disorders to psychosocial work conditions and to labor market experiences related to the availability of work has emerged clearly only in the past decade (Hemingway and Marmot 1999). Furthermore, the evidence that the disorders in question are inherently multifactorial and, therefore, only partially attributable to work experiences has complicated policy decision making (Frank and Maetzel 2000). Second, the implications of this evidence for modifications to work processes and work organization impinge directly on the principle—strongly held by employers—that firms should retain considerable autonomy in dictating work processes and environments. Regulatory constraints on this autonomy have been aggressively contested in most jurisdictions (*Washington Business Journal* 2000). Third, government regulation of labor market practices concerning the rights and duties of employers and workers, hours of work, and employment insurance and pension systems have not traditionally incorporated a prominent health-impact perspective.

This history notwithstanding, clear opportunities exist to improve the present and future health of working-age populations through improvements in work environments. As an example, Theorell has recently estimated that 7% of cardiovascular disease in males aged forty-five to sixty-four may be attributable to cumulative exposure to high-strain working conditions (Theorell 1999). This attributable fraction is equivalent in magnitude to that of elevated serum lipids or hypertension. If the contribution of other working conditions, such as the physiological arousal associated with shift work, is considered, the work-related etiologic component of cardiovascular disease can be understood to be even greater.

Active labor market policies focused on modifying work environments might productively focus on three areas: (1) research and monitoring, (2) regulatory actions, and (3) economic incentives for the employer. First, ongoing research efforts are needed to continue to clarify the magnitude of health effects associated with working conditions and labor market experiences. In addition, it will be necessary to monitor adverse labor market experiences, at the level both of the population/workforce level and of work organizations (Smulders et al. 1996; Lavis et al. 2001). Second, regulatory intervention, with a focus on reform and innovation in the institutional structure of the labor market, may be needed to redress the significant shift over the past quarter-century toward greater employer, versus worker, authority determining the nature of work (e.g., the quality of working conditions and employment security). There is accumulating evidence, for example, that mandatory joint labor-management mechanisms can effectively improve both the health and productivity of the work environment (Theorell 1999; Kompier and Cooper 1999; O'Grady 2000). The growth of nonstandard employment and the decline in union membership (particularly in the private sector) can be expected to weaken the effectiveness of joint management-management mechanisms. In this context, policy actions designed to strengthen joint governance authority in firms and across economic sectors would contribute to halting the deterioration in working conditions that have implications for the health of the workforce.

Regulation will also continue to be important in defining limits to the biomechanical and psychosocial intensity of work. Policy initiatives are not keeping pace with research evidence that has clarified the long-term health effects of cumulative exposure to adverse psychosocial work environments.

Policy initiatives also need to address the structuring of reward and deterrence incentives to signal desirable employment practices to firms. In this area, policy makers may draw lessons from the workers' compensation system practices regarding insurance premiums, which are now broadly applied in North America and Europe. These practices provide premium reductions to firms with low injury rates and charge higher premiums to firms with high injury rates. It may be useful to consider extending such firm-level incentives to other payroll tax instruments. For example, firms with high rates of employment dislocation over time could be charged premium supplements on employment insurance premiums that recognize the short-term health care costs associated with unemployment (Betcherman 1995; Kraut et al. 2000). On a longer time horizon, a similar mechanism could be explored to set differential firm premiums in universal pension programs and health insurance programs to anticipate higher or lower rates of work disability arising from firm-level work organization practices.

Income Distribution Policies

One interpretation of changes in labor market demand over the past twenty years proposes that there has been a decline in low-skill employment and a strong increase in demand for high-skill workers. Although there has been controversy concerning the degree to which differentials in the wage returns to education have accompanied this structural change in the demand for labor, it is increasingly clear that wage differentials between low-skill and high-skill occupations have increased (Picot 1998; Betcherman 1995; Gottschalk and Smeeding 1997). At the population level, this dynamic will produce wider inequalities in earned income.

Within the OECD economies, income redistribution policies express a range of social welfare objectives. In Canada, for example, employment insurance and health insurance both have redistributive consequences. The employment insurance program is financed by workers and employers, and the benefits flow disproportionately to workers in occupations and geographic regions with high rates of unemployment. The Canadian universal health care insurance programs are also redistributive, with program financing drawn in part from progressive income taxes and with health care benefits flowing disproportionately to lower-income households. There are also several tax credit programs focused on low-income households with children that have the effect of transferring income, through the tax system, from high-income to low-income households. In Canada, for example, the National Child Benefit Supplement has contributed to the reduction of the number of low-income families with children from 20.4% in 1996 to 17.2% in 1999. None of these redistribution policies, however, has the explicit objective of addressing the inequality in earned income produced by labor market dynamics.

Conclusion

In the industrial economies, people rank work experiences as being among the most rewarding aspects of their lives. However, when labor market experiences expose workers to adverse psychosocial work environments, there is compelling evidence that a significant fraction of these individuals will be subjected to stressors that initiate or accelerate chronic degenerative disease processes. These adverse psychosocial work environments are not distributed randomly: Persons in lower-status occupations will experience a greater cumulative burden of physiological challenge arising from unstable and insecure work environments.

This chapter has argued that over the past twenty years the prevalence of job insecurity has increased and the quality of the nature of work has deteriorated in the developed economies, despite strong economic growth. This deterioration in the quality of work and in the availability of work has been concentrated in lower-status positions in the occupational hierarchy.

Active labor market policies can address these changes, and there is ample evidence of effective instruments available to the state to mitigate the adverse health consequences of the contemporary labor market. Optimal labor market policy would find an appropriate balance amongst the interests of corporations, workers, and society at large, and the health effects of labor market experiences should be an important part of the policy-making calculus. However, policies appear to have become increasingly neglectful of worker health effects. The evidence presented in this chapter argues for more accounting of the health consequences of labor market experiences in informing policy choices that influence the experience of workers in the labor market.

Acknowledgments

We acknowledge the very helpful comments provided by Peggy McDonough, Patricia Baird, Ben Amick, Alison Earle, and Jody Heymann, which have greatly improved the clarity of this chapter.

References

Abraham, K., and S. Houseman. 1994. Does employment protection inhibit labor market flexibility? Lessons from Germany, France and Belgium. In *Social Protection vs Economic Flexibility*, ed. R. Blank. Chicago: University of Chicago Press.

Amick, B., P. McDonough, H. Chang, W. H. Rogers, C. Pieper, and G. Duncan. 2001. The relationship between all-cause mortality and working life course psychosocial and physical exposures in the United States labor market from 1968–1992. *Psychosomatic Medicine Journal* 64: 370–381.

Arjona, R., M. Ladaique, and M. Pearson. 2001. *Growth, Inequality and Social Protection*. Paris: Social Policy Division, OECD.

Bartley, M. 1994. Unemployment and ill-health: Understanding the relationship. *Journal of Epidemiology and Community Health* 48:333–337.

Belkic, K., P. Landsbergis, P. Schnall, and D. Baker. 2004. Is job strain a major source of cardiovascular disease risk? *Scandinavian Journal of Work, Environment and Health* 30: 85–128.

Belkic, K., J. Schwartz, P. Schnall. 2000. Evidence for mediating econeurocardiologic mechanisms. In *The Workplace and Cardiovascular Disease. Occupational Medicine: State of the Art Reviews in Occupational Medicine*, ed. P. Schnall, K. Belkic, P. Landisbergis, and D. Maker. Vol. 15, No. 1. Philadelphia: Hanley & Belfus.

Betcherman, G. 1995. Inside the black box: Human resource management and the labour market. In *Good Jobs, Bad Jobs, No Jobs: Tough Choices for Canadian Labour Law*, ed. R. J. Adams, G. Betcherman, and B. Bilson. Toronto: CD Howe Institute.

Blane, D., C. Power, and M. Bartley. 1996. Illness behaviour and the measurement of class differentials in morbidity. *Journal of the Royal Statistical Society A* 59:77–92.

Blank, R. 1994. Does a larger social safety net mean less economic flexibility? In *Working Under Different Rules*, ed. R. Freeman. New York: Sage.

Bond, T. J., E. Galinsky, and J. E. Swanberg. 1998. *The 1997 National Study of the Changing Workforce*. New York: Families and Work Institute.

Borg, V., T. S. Kristensen, and H. Burr. 2000. Work environment and changes in self-rated health: A five year follow-up study. *Stress Medicine* 16:37–47.

Bosma, H., M. Marmot, H. Hemingway, A. Nicholson, E. Brunner, and S. A. Stansfeld. 1997. Low job control and risk of coronary heart disease in Whitehall II (prospective cohort) Study. *British Medical Journal* 314:558–565.

Bosma, H., R. Peter, J. Siegrist, and M. Marmot. 1998. Two alternative job stress models and the risk of coronary heart disease. *American Journal of Public Health* 88:68–74.

Bradford Hill, A. 1965. The environment and disease: Association or causation? *Proceedings of the Royal Society of Medicine* 58:295–300.

Brisson, C., N. Laflamme, J. Moisan, A. Milot, B. Masse, and M. Vezina. 1999. Effect of family responsibilities and job strain on ambulatory blood pressure among white-collar women. *Psychosomatic Medicine* 61:205–213.

Brunner, E. 1996. The social and biological basis of cardiovascular disease in office workers. In *Health and Social Organization*, ed. D. Blane, E. Brunner, and R. Wilkinson. London: Routledge.

———. 1997. Stress and the biology of inequality. *British Medical Journal* 314:1472–1476.

Cannon, W. B. 1928. The mechanisms of emotional disturbance of bodily functions. *New England Journal of Medicine* 198:877–884.

Castells, M., and Y. Aoyama. 1994. Paths towards the informational society: Employment structure in G-7 countries, 1920–90. *International Labour Review* 133 (1):6–33.

Cohen, S., W. J. Doyle, D. P. Skoner, B. S. Rabin, and J. M. Gwaltney Jr. 1997. Social ties and susceptibility to the common cold. *Journal of the American Medical Association* 277: 1940–1944.

Courtney, T. K., and B. S. Webster. 1999. Disabling occupational morbidity in the United States: An alternative way of seeing the Bureau of Labor Statistics' data. *Journal of Occupational and Environmental Medicine* 41:60–69.

Daniels, P. W. 1993. *Service Industries in the World Economy.* Oxford: Blackwell.

Davey Smith, G., C. Hart, M. Upton, D. Hole, C. Gillis, G. Watt, and V. Hawthorne. 2000. Height and risk of death among men and women: Aetiological implications of associations with cardiorespiratory disease and cancer mortality. *Journal of Epidemiology and Community Health* 54:97–103.

Duffy, A., D. Glenday, and N. Pupo. 1997. *Good Jobs, Bad Jobs, No Jobs: The Transformation of Work in the 21st Century.* Toronto: Harcourt Brace.

Duffy, A., and N. Pupo. 1992. *Part-time Paradox: Connecting Gender, Work and Family.* Toronto: McClelland & Stewart.

Economist. 2004, May 6. Emerging market indicators. 355:108.

European Foundation. 1997. *Time Constraints and Autonomy at Work in the European Union.* Dublin: European Foundation for the Improvement of Living and Working Conditions.

Frank, J., and A. Maetzel. 2000. Determining occupational disorder: Can this camel carry more straw? In *Injury and the New World of Work,* ed. T. Sullivan. Vancouver: University of British Columbia Press.

Gallie, D. 2000. The polarization of the labor market and exclusion of vulnerable groups. In *Health Effects of the New Labor Market,* ed. K. Isaksson, C. Hogstedt, C. Ericksson, and T. Theorell. New York: Plenum Publishers.

Gore, S. 1978. The effect of social support in moderating the health consequences of unemployment. *Journal of Health and Social Behavior* 19:157–165.

Gottschalk, P., and T. M. Smeeding. 1997. Cross-national comparisons of earnings and income inequality. *Journal of Economic Literature* 35:633–687.

Graetz, B. 1993. Health consequences of employment and unemployment: Longitudinal evidence for young men and women. *Social Science and Medicine* 36:715–724.

Hall, E. M. 1989. Gender, work control, and stress: A theoretical discussion and an empirical test. *International Journal of Health Services* 19:725–745.

Hemingway, H., and M. Marmot. 1999. Psychosocial factors in the aetiology and prognosis of coronary heart disease. Systematic review of prospective cohort studies. *British Medical Journal* 318:1460–1467.

Heymann, J. 2000. *The Widening Gap: Why America's Working Families Are in Jeopardy and What Can Be Done about It.* New York: Basic Books.

Hobsbawm, E. A. 1994. *Age of Extremes: The Short Twentieth Century, 1914–1991.* London: Abacus.

Holzer, H. J. 1996. *What Employers Want: Job Prospects for Less-educated Workers.* New York: Russell Sage Foundation.

Howell, H. J., and E. N. Wolff. 1991. Trends in the growth and distribution of skills in the U.S. workplace, 1960–1985. *Industrial and Labor Relations Review* 44:486–502.

Hyatt, D. 1998. *Evidence on the Efficacy of Experience Rating in British Columbia.* Royal Commission on Workers' Compensation in British Columbia.

Iversen, L., O. Andersen, P. K. Andersen, K. Christoffersen, and N. Keiding. 1987. Unemployment and mortality in Denmark 1970–1980. *British Medical Journal* 295:879–884.

Jahoda, M. 1981. Work, employment and unemployment: Values, theories and approaches to social research. *American Psychologist* 36 (2):184–191.

Johnson, J. V., and E. M. Hall. 1995. Class, work, and health. In *Society and Health,* ed. B. C. Amick, S. Levine, A. R. Tarlov, and D. Chapman Walsh. New York: Oxford University Press.

Karasek, R., D. Baker, F. Marxer, A. Ahlbom, and T. Theorell. 1981. Job decision latitude, job demands, and cardiovascular disease: A prospective study of Swedish men. *American Journal of Public Health* 71:694–705.

Karasek, R., C. Brisson, N. Kawakami, I. Houtman, P. Bongers, and B. Amick. 1998. The Job Content Questionnaire (JCQ): An instrument for internationally comparative assessments of psychosocial job characteristics. *Journal of Occupational Health Psychology* 3:322–355.

Karasek, R. A., and T. Theorell. 1990. *Healthy Work.* New York: Basic Books.

Karasek, R. A., T. Theorell, J. Schwartz, C. Pieper, and L. Alfredsson. 1982. Job, psychological factors and coronary heart disease: Swedish prospective findings and U.S. prevalence findings using a new occupational inference method. *Advances in Cardiology* 29:62–67.

Kasl, S. V., and S. Cobb. 1980. The experience of losing a job: Some effects on cardiovascular functioning. *Psychotherapy and Psychosomatics* 34:88–109.

Kasl, S. V., S. Gore, and S. Cobb. 1975. The experience of losing a job: Reported changes in health, symptoms and illness behavior. *Psychosomatic Medicine* 37:106–122.

Kasl, S. V., E. Rodriguez, and K. E. Lasch. 1995. The impact of unemployment on health and well-being. In *Adversity, Stress and Psychopathology*, ed. B. P. Dohrenwend. Washington, DC: American Psychiatric Press.

Kessler, R. C., J. B. Turner, and J. S. House. 1987. Intervening processes in the relationship between unemployment and health. *Psychological Medicine* 17:949–961.

Klein-Hesselink, D. J., and I. P. Spruit. 1992. The contribution of unemployment to socioeconomic health differences. *International Journal of Epidemiology* 21:329–337.

Kompier, M., and C. Cooper. 1999. *Preventing Stress, Improving Productivity: European Case Studies in the Workplace.* London: Routledge.

Kraut, A., C. A. Mustard, R. Walld, and R. Tate. 2000. Unemployment and health care utilization. In *Health Effects of the New Labour Market*, ed. K. Isaksson, C. Hogstedt, C. Eriksson, and T. Theorell. London: Plenum Press.

Kunst, A. E., F. Groenhof, J. P. Mackenbach, and E. W. Health. 1998. Occupational class and cause specific mortality in middle aged men in eleven European countries: Comparison of population based studies. *British Medical Journal* 316:1636–1642.

Landsbergis, P., J. Cahill, and P. Schnall. 1999. The impact of lean production and related new systems of work organization on worker health. *Journal of Occupational Health Psychology* 4:108–130.

Lavis, J. N. 1997. The links between labour-market experiences and health: Towards a research framework. Toronto: Institute for Work & Health Working Paper 62.

———. 1999. Unemployment and mortality in the United States, 1968–1992. Toronto: Institute for Work & Health Working Paper 63.

Lavis, J. N., C. A. Mustard, J. I. Payne, and M. S. R. Farrant. 1998. Employment, working conditions and health: Towards a set of population-level indicators. Toronto: Institute for Work & Health Working Paper 99.

———. 2001. Work-related population health indicators. *Canadian Journal of Public Health* 92:72–78.

Leigh, J., P. Macaskill, C. Corvalan, E. Kuosma, and J. Mandryk. 1996. *Global Burden of Disease and Injury Due to Occupational Factors.* WHO/EHG/96.20, 1–56. Geneva: Office of Global and Integrated Environmental Health, World Health Organization.

Lindert, P. 2004. *Growing Public: Social Spending and Economic Growth Since the Eighteenth Century.* Cambridge: Cambridge University Press.

Livingstone, D. 1999. *The Education–Jobs Gap: Underemployment or Economic Democracy.* Toronto: Garamond Press.

Lowe, G. 2000. *The Quality of Work.* Toronto: Oxford University Press.

Lynch, J., and G. Kaplan. 2000. Socioeconomic position. In *Social Epidemiology,* ed. L. Berkman and I. Kawachi. New York: Oxford University Press.

Mackenbach, J. P., A. E. Kunst, A. Cavelaars, F. Groenhof, J. Geurts, and the European Union Working Group on Socioeconomic inequalities in Health. 1997. Socioeconomic inequalities in morbidity and mortality in western Europe. *Lancet* 349:1655–1659.

Manor, O., S. Matthews, and C. Power. 2003. Health selection: the role of inter- and intra-generational mobility on social inequalities in health. *Social Science and Medicine* 57:2217–2227.

Marmot, M. G., G. Davey Smith, S. Stansfeld, C. Patel, F. North, J. Head, I. White, E. Brunner, and A. Fenney. 1991. Health inequalities among British civil servants: The Whitehall II Study. *Lancet* 337:1387–1393.

Marmot, M., and A. Feeney. 1996. Work and health: Implications for individuals and society. In *Health and Social Organization,* ed. D. Blane, E. Brunner, and R. Wilkinson. London: Routledge.

Martikainen, P., S. Stansfeld, H. Hemingway, and M. Marmot. 1999. Determinants of socioeconomic differences in change in physical and mental functioning. *Social Science and Medicine* 49:499–507.

Matthews, S., C. Hertzman, A. Ostry, and C. Power. 1998. Gender, work roles and psychosocial work characteristics as determinants of health. *Social Science and Medicine* 46:1417–1424.

McDonough, P. 2000. Job insecurity and health. *International Journal of Health Services* 30:453–476.

McEwen, B. S. 1998. Protective and damaging effects of stress mediators. *New England Journal of Medicine* 338:171–179.

McEwen, B. S., and T. Seeman. 1999. Protective and damaging effects of mediators of stress. Elaborating and testing the concepts of allostasis and allostatic load. *Annals of the New York Academy of Sciences* 896:30–47.

Mishel, L., J. Bernstein, and J. Schmitt. 1997. *The State of Working America: 1996–1997.* Armonk: M. E. Sharpe.

Morrell, S., R. Taylor, S. Quine, C. Kerr, and J. Western. 1997. A cohort study of unemployment as a cause of psychological disturbance in Australian youth. *Social Science and Medicine* 38:1553–1564.

Murray, C. J. L., and A. D. Lopez, eds. 1996. *The Global Burden of Disease.* Cambridge, MA: Harvard University Press, on behalf of the World Health Organization.

Mustard, C. A., M. Vermeulen, and J. N. Lavis. 2003. Is occupational class a determinant of decline in perceived health status? *Social Science and Medicine* 57:2291–2303.

Myles, J. 1988. The expanding middle: Some Canadian evidence on the deskilling debate. *Canadian Review of Sociology and Anthropology* 25:335–364.

Nathanson, C. A. 1995. Mortality and the position of women in developed countries. In *Adult Mortality in Developed Countries: From Description to Explanation,* ed. A. Lopez, G. Caselli, and T. Valkonen. Oxford: Clarendon Press.

Navarro, V. 2001. *The Political Economy of Social Inequalities: Consequences for Health and Quality of Life.* New York: Baywood.

Newmark, D., and W. Wascher. 2000. Minimum wages and employment: A case study of the fast food industry in New Jersey and Pennsylvania. *American Economic Review* 90:1362–1396.

O'Grady, J. 1993. *Direct and Indirect Evidence in the Extent of Changes in Work Organization in Canada*. Toronto: Premier's Council on Economic Renewal.

———. 2000. Joint health and safety committees: Finding the balance. In *Injury and the New World of Work*, ed. T. Sullivan. Vancouver: University of British Columbia Press.

Orth-Gomer, K., and S. Weiss. 1994. *Behavioral and Psychological Aspects of Prevention: First International Teaching Seminar in Behavioral Medicine*. Stress Research Reports no. 245. Stockholm: Karolinska Institute.

Osterman, P. 1999. *Securing Prosperity: The American Labor Market, How It Has Been Changed, and What to Do about It*. Princeton, NJ: Princeton University Press.

Ostry, A., S. Marion, L. Green, P. Demers, K. Teschke, R. Hershler, S. Kelly, and C. Hertzman. 2000. Downsizing and industrial restructuring in relation to changes in psychosocial conditions of work in British Columbia. *Scandinavian Journal of Work, Environment and Health* 26:273–278.

Palley, T. I. 1998. *Plenty of Nothing*. Princeton, NJ: Princeton University Press.

Picot, G. 1998. What is happening to earnings inequality and youth wages in the 1990s? *Canadian Economic Observer* 3 (September):1–18.

Pollin, R., and S. Luce. 1998. *The Living Wage: Building a Fair Economy*. New York: New Press.

Power, C., and C. Hertzman. 1997. Social and biological pathways linking early life and adult disease. *British Medical Bulletin* 53:210–221.

Power, C., C. Hertzman, S. Matthews, and O. Manor. 1997. Social differences in health: Life-cycle effects between ages 23 and 33 in the 1958 British birth cohort. *American Journal of Public Health* 87:1499–1503.

Quinlan, M. 1998. Labour market restructuring in industrialised societies: An overview. *Economic and Labour Relations Review* 9 (1):1–30.

Quinlan, M., C. Mayhew, and P. Bohle. 2001. The global expansion of precarious employment, work disorganization, and consequences for occupational health: A review of recent research. *International Journal of Health Services* 31:335–414.

Reich, R. 1996. *The Work of Nations*. New York: Vintage Books.

Rifkin, J. 1996. *The End of Work: The Decline of the Global Labor Force and the Dawn of the Post-market Era*. New York: Putnam.

Rodriguez, E. 2001. Keeping the unemployed healthy: The effect of means-tested and entitlement benefits in Britain, Germany, and the United States. *American Journal of Public Health* 91:1403–1411.

Roxburgh, S. 1996. Gender differences in work and well-being: Effects of exposure and vulnerability. *Journal of Health and Social Behavior* 37 (September):265–277.

Sapolsky, R. M. 1992. *Stress, the Aging Brain and the Mechanisms of Neuron Death*. Cambridge, MA: MIT Press.

Seeman, T. E., B. H. Singer, J. W. Rowe, R. I. Horwitz, and B. S. McEwen. 1997. Price of adaptation-allostatic load and its health consequences. *Archives of Internal Medicine* 157:2259–2267.

Selye, H. 1956. *The Stress of Life*. New York: McGraw-Hill.

Shively, C. A., and T. B. Clarkson. 1994. Social status and coronary artery atherosclerosis in female monkeys. *Arteriosclerosis and Thrombosis* 14:721–726.

Siegrist, J. 1996. Adverse health effects of high-effort/low-reward conditions. *Journal of Occupational Health Psychology* 1:27–41.

Siegrist, J., and M. Marmot. 2004. Health inequalities and the psychosocial environment-two scientific challenges. *Social Science Medicine* 58:1463–1473.

Siegrist, J., H. Matschinger, P. Cremer, and D. Seidel. 1988. Atherogenic risk in men suffering from occupational stress. *Atherosclerosis* 69:211–218.

Siegrist, J., R. Peter, A. Junge, P. Cremer, and D. Seidel. 1990. Low status control, high effort at work and ischemic heart disease: Prospective evidence from blue-collar men. *Social Science Medicine* 31:1127–1134.

Smulders, P. G. W., M. A. J. Kompier, and P. Paoli. 1996. The work environment in the twelve EU-countries: Differences and similarities. *Human Relations* 49:1291–1313.

Sorlie, P. D., and E. Rogot. 1990. Mortality by employment status in the National Longitudinal Mortality Study. *American Journal of Epidemiology* 132:983–992.

Statistics Canada. 1999. Overview of the time use of Canadians in 1998. Ottawa: General Social Survey Cycle 12. Catalogue 12F0080XIE.

Theorell, T. 1999. How to deal with stress in organizations? A health perspective on theory and practice. *Scandinavian Journal of Work, Environment and Health* 25:616–624.

Townsend, P., and N. Davidson. 1982. *Inequalities in health: The Black Report.* Harmondsworth, UK: Penguin.

Vallin, J. 1995. Can sex differentials in mortality be explained by socio-economic mortality differentials? In *Adult Mortality in Developed Countries: From Description to Explanation,* ed. A. Lopez, G. Caselli, and T. Valkonen. Oxford: Clarendon Press.

Wadsworth, M. E. J. 1986. Serious illness in childhood and its association with later-life achievement. In *Class and Health: Research and Longitudinal Data,* ed. R. G. Wilkinson. London: Tavistock.

———. 1997. Health inequalities in the life course perspective. *Social Science Medicine* 44:859–869.

Wadsworth, M. E. J., S. M. Montgomery, and M. J. Bartley. 1999. The persisting effect of unemployment on health and social well-being in men early in working life. *Social Science and Medicine* 48:1491–1499.

Waldron, I. 1991. Effects of labor force participation on sex differences in mortality and morbidity. In *Women, Work, and Health: Stress and Opportunities,* ed. M. Frankenhaeuser, U. Lundberg, and M. Chesney. New York: Plenum Press.

Washington Business Journal. 2000. Business groups sue to stop OSHA's ergonomic rule. November 17, 2000.

Woodward, C., H. Shannon, C. Cunningham, J. McIntosh, B. Lendrum, D. Rosenbloom, J. Brown. 1999. The impact of re-engineering and other cost reduction strategies on the staff of a large teaching hospital. *Medical Care* 37:556–569.

Chapter 8

Income Inequality as a Determinant of Health

Nancy Ross, Michael Wolfson, George A.
Kaplan, James R. Dunn, John Lynch, and
Claudia Sanmartin

In all wealthy economies, the least well off tend to have relatively poorer health, despite the facts that they are typically living well above subsistence levels and that their income levels are higher than those of their counterparts in much poorer countries. There is also evidence to suggest, furthermore, that the income gap within a country, the degree of income inequality, is also associated with overall measures of health status, such as life expectancy and mortality. Health, it turns out, may be compromised by social and economic contexts that produce wider differences in life opportunities between those on the bottom and those on the top.

Is it possible that income inequality is a determinant of population health? If so, then we would expect to find that places that deliberately even out individuals' life chances produce better overall health for their inhabitants. This better health could be achieved both by the provision of very tangible, material things for the less well off and, perhaps, by the reduction in the perception of inequality that may itself cause adverse health outcomes. This latter mechanism may operate through feelings of inferiority and shame; the associated biochemical physiologic responses, generated by being lower on the social ladder, may contribute to poor health over the course of one's life. It is thought that the combination of lacking enough material resources for health and feeling inferior may be sufficient to produce aggregated measures of population health that are lower than might be possible in the presence of policies that reduce income inequality. It is on such observations and possibilities that we focus in this chapter.

In this chapter we first review research evidence on the relationship between income and health at the individual level, highlighting some studies that have followed individuals through time to demonstrate the direction of the relationship. This is a fundamental starting point since the individual relationship between income and health likely underlies any analysis examining the connection between income inequality, a characteristic of groups of individuals, and health. In other words, individual incomes matter a great deal for health, a fact that is important to bear in mind despite the emphasis here on the relationship between income *inequality* and health.

The groups of individuals that have been studied to assess the relationship between income inequality and health are all place based—be they countries, states or provinces, cities, counties, or census tracts. A particularly intriguing series of analyses draws on a compelling natural experiment that compares jurisdictions within Canada and the United States. As noted later, Canadian provinces and cities are very different from their American counterparts, both on measures of income inequality and population health; in fact, these differences are so compelling that they cannot be ignored or dismissed. Along the way, we examine a variety of other research findings, particularly the work that demonstrates social hierarchies' deleterious effects on health. The chapter concludes with a series of hypotheses about why health outcomes in Canada and the United States are so different.

Wealthier Is Healthier for Individuals

There is now overwhelming evidence that for *individuals*, higher socioeconomic position (SEP) is associated with better health. This relationship at the individual level is found for most disease groups, as well as across places and through time, regardless of how SEP is measured. Wilkins and colleagues (2002) completed a comprehensive analysis of overall life expectancy and mortality rates for multiple causes of death by neighborhood income level (intended as a proxy for individual SEP) for Canada between 1971 and 1996. With the important exceptions of prostate cancer and breast cancer—for which mortality is positively related to neighborhood income—virtually all other causes of death are inversely related to neighborhood income level. Whether one measures life expectancy at birth or probability of survival until age seventy-five, the outcomes become increasingly favorable as one moves from the poorest to the richest neighborhood incomes (fig. 8.1). Figure 8.1 makes abundantly evident the fact that the relationship between SEP and health at the individual level involves more than poverty. Every step up the SEP ladder is generally associated with an increment in health and a reduction in mortality. In other words, there is an individual-level gradient.

Many earlier epidemiological studies examining the SEP–health relationship tended to focus on the effects of poverty on health. Despite the many exceptions to this tendency (e.g., Berkman and Syme 1979), this seemed to make sense because it was reasoned that health was threatened by absolute material deprivation. So,

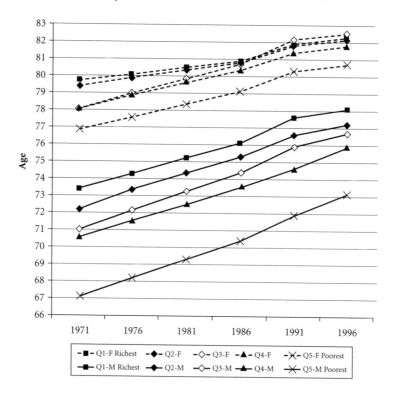

Figure 8.1. Relationship between income and life expectancy for men and women, 1971–1996, by neighborhood income quintile

Source: Wilkins et al. 2002.

above some threshold level of income or social status, it was argued, we should not expect to see improvements in health. All one needed to achieve good health was to have sufficient income to meet basic needs for food, shelter, and protection. But as indicated in figure 8.1 (which is consistent with a wide range of other evidence discussed later), this way of thinking about the problem of socioeconomic differences in health status, is oversimplified.

British Civil Servants, Baboons, and Social Hierarchies

In our effort here to journey from the individual-level relationship between SEP and health to the societal-level relationship between income inequality and the health of populations, it is worthwhile to take a slight detour to examine some subpopulation research that suggests that social hierarchies, both human and animal, may damage health. A widely known epidemiological study of male British civil servants showed that each higher occupational grade in the British civil service provided ever more protection against a wide range of damaging health behaviors, diseases, and death (Marmot et al. 1978; Rose and Marmot 1981; Marmot et al. 1984). As the authors noted, these results could not be attributable to poverty. None of the participants was impoverished per se, yet there was a clear gradient—incremental and sizeable health benefits every step up in the occupational hierarchy—within the British civil service.

Models developed in occupational health research provide at least a glimpse of what might underlie some of the enduring (van Rossum et al., 2000) employment status and health gradients in this cohort of workers. Since 1981, one of the leading ways of thinking about how work environments are associated with poor health is through Karasek and colleagues' "demand-control" model. The idea here is that jobs characterized by low decision latitude (the worker doesn't have the opportunity to use skills or influence the pace or direction or their work) and high psychological demands (the worker doesn't have enough time to complete the tasks and there may be conflicting demands) are linked to ongoing occupational stress, psychological strain, and then eventually poor health (Karasek et al. 1981; see Levi et al. 2000 for a review of the models). These kinds of low-control and high-demand jobs are characteristic of those in lower occupational grades and provide us with one way of thinking about why hierarchies in the work environment might be detrimental to health for those on the bottom. Indeed, much of the inverse social gradient in heart disease first identified back in the initial studies of British civil servants was later attributable to low control at work (Marmot et al. 1997). Low control at work was even more important than smoking status toward the explanation of why there was such an elevated in risk of developing heart disease for those in the lowest occupational grades compared with those in the highest.

Some potentially interesting parallels have also been seen in research on non-human primates, although the health effects of societal rank seem to be context- and species-dependent for nonhuman primates but generally not for humans. In his book *Why Zebras Don't Get Ulcers,* the neuroscientist Sapolsky (1998, 307–308) ended his chapter "The View from the Bottom" with the following:

> Do low-ranking monkeys have a disproportionate share of disease, more stress-related disease? And the answer was, "Well it's actually not that simple." It depends on the sort of society that animal lives in, its personal experience of that society, its coping skills, its personality, the availability of social support. Change some of those variables and the rank-health gradient can shift in the exact opposite direction. . . . Do poor humans have a disproportionate share of disease? And the answer was, "Yes, yes, over and over." Regardless of gender or age or race. In societies with universal health care and those without.

What do we make of the (nonhuman) primate–human differences in the health effects of social rank? Sapolsky conjectured that the key to understanding these differences is to be found in the fundamental shift for humans from a hunter–gatherer social organization to one where agriculture made social stratification, and in turn, hierarchies, possible. Yet the influence of advanced market economies (which are inherently hierarchical) on the health of human populations has generally been favorable if viewed on sufficiently broad temporal and spatial scales. Omran's (1971, 1983) model of epidemiological transition links health outcomes at the population scale to the social and economic development of nations. According to this model, as nations move from subsistence to postindustrial economies, mortality typically declines (along with fertility rates), and the major causes of death and disability shift from parasitic and deficiency diseases to chronic diseases such as heart disease and cancer. Despite this, with few exceptions, even though the major causes of death have shifted for the wealthiest nations, those on the bottom rungs even in those nations tend to suffer more frequently from the diseases of the day.

Success in the British civil service and on the savannah seemingly gives one a health edge over colleagues and troop mates lower in the hierarchy, even if (in the case of the human hierarchy), those lower-ranked colleagues are not "in poverty." Could this relative health edge be somehow due to a preexisting health "endowment" that allows the healthier among us to reach the top? In other words, is some sort of selection effect allowing the healthiest to get ahead while dooming the sick to spiral downward? This possibility was raised in the August 1980 United Kingdom Department of Health and Social Security (DHSS) publication, *Report of the Working Group on Inequalities in Health,* also known as the Black Report (after Sir Douglas Black, the group's chairman and the president of the Royal College of Physicians at the time). This report raised the public consciousness in Britain about the degree to which poor health was unequally distributed throughout British society even after the establishment of the National Health Service in 1948 (see DHSS 1980, plus Gray 1982 for a good summary of the report). One explanation offered for the consistent relationship between social class and health status in the United Kingdom was that a selection effect was operating—namely, that poor health precedes and results in both poor labor market success and higher mortality, or in other words, that illness causes socioeconomic disadvantage, rather than the other way around.

More recently, cumulative evidence generated from the analysis of powerful longitudinal datasets—ones that follow individuals in general populations over time—has clearly pointed to the conclusion that in most cases socioeconomic position is predictive of poor health, rather than the reverse. The most persuasive studies have involved prospective analyses of large, representative cohorts (e.g., Rogot et al. 1988; Wolfson et al. 1993). Wolfson and colleagues looked at the relationship between past earnings and mortality for more than half a million male Canada Pension Plan contributors and retirees. Figure 8.2 shows the relationship between mortality between the ages of 65 and 70 and each individual's average level of

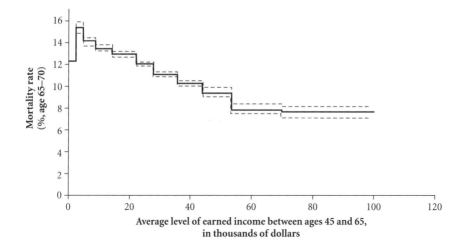

Figure 8.2. Career earnings and death for 500,000 Canadian men

earned income between ages 45 and 65. The graph shows a clear gradient. It must be emphasized that this is not just at a point in time; these are longitudinal data, so they show the connection between markers of socioeconomic status as early as age 45 and mortality experienced decades later, after age 65. The causality, for most cases, must run from socioeconomic status to mortality, and not the other way around.[1] Moreover, the magnitude of this gradient in terms of the public health impact is substantial. If the 80% of men with the lowest earnings were somehow able to achieve the survival rates of the top 20%, the increase in life expectancy would be roughly the same as if cancer as a cause of death were eliminated for this cohort of men.

To summarize the main points so far, there is a relationship between individual-level income, or SEP more broadly, and individual health. This relationship is not just about the difference in health states between the poor and the rich: In terms of health outcomes, being middle class is better than being poor, and being rich is better still. Also, the balance of evidence from follow-up studies has suggested that the individual relationship is causal—although health will certainly affect socioeconomic position for some individuals, the predominant direction of causality is from socioeconomic position to health.

From Individuals to Populations

Although many causal pathways for this SEP gradient have been discussed, and the connections are certainly multifactorial, there is no consensus on the relative importance of various mechanisms (Evans et al. 1994; Macintyre 1997), or of the appropriate analytical strategies to evaluate their relative causal contributions

(Lynch et al. 2000). During the last two decades, while many researchers (e.g., Brunner 1997; Wilson et al. 1993) turned their attention to the bloodstream (e.g., to uncover biological mechanisms), other researchers (e.g., Kaplan 1995; Diez-Roux et al. 2001) focused on the health effects attributable to the broader character of social organization or the social milieu in which individuals live. While Rose (1985) noted, almost two decades ago, that that understanding of the biological mediators of socioeconomic factors helps us understand how social inequality affects health at the cellular level, it does not shed light on the question of why such socioeconomic exposures are differentially distributed across populations.

At the population level, the best-known social gradient is the relationship observed among countries between life expectancy or mortality rates, on the one hand, and gross domestic product (GDP) per capita or other measures of economic standing on the other. Higher levels of GDP per capita are strongly associated with greater longevity, for example, as shown in figure 8.3, reproduced from the 1993 World Development Report.

These data also show a general tendency for the relationship to have drifted upward over time: The same level of GDP per capita has become associated with greater life expectancy. As a result, GDP per capita is commonly regarded as a correlate of health status (e.g., World Bank 1999).

As for individuals, the country-level story is not simply about deprivation. The greater the GDP, in general, the longer the population lives, even at levels of GDP well above widespread poverty. But the relationships in figure 8.3 are all curvilinear, so that the beneficial association of GDP per capita with life expectancy tails off in moving from very poor to very wealthy countries. More wealth does not seem to buy a country significantly more health at the top end of the distribution. This weakened relationship among higher-income countries has been noted by Wilkinson (1992, 1994, 1996) and others before him (e.g., Preston 1975; Rodgers 1979). Wilkinson in particular has argued that above some threshold level of affluence, differences in national life expectancy and mortality are much more strongly associated with income disparities than with average income (i.e., GDP per capita), and that average level of income becomes relatively unimportant. In his best-known study, using mortality and income data from nine Organization for Economic Cooperation and Development (OECD)[2] nations for the late 1970s and early 1980s, life expectancy at birth was clearly associated with the share of disposable income held by the least well-off 70% of the population (Wilkinson 1992). Controlling for average national incomes did not affect this association. This finding became known as the big idea—namely, that the winner in the "Health Olympics" (Bezruchka 2001) would be the country that not only generated wealth for its citizens but also spread it around equitably.

However, Wilkinson's results have generated considerable debate. One concern about his empirical claims is that for OECD countries, the relationship between inequality and mortality appears to vary with the sample of countries included

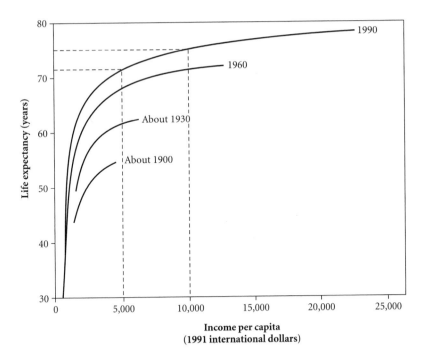

Figure 8.3. Income per capita versus life expectancy

Source: Adapted from World Bank Report, *World Development Report 1993: Investing in Health* (New York: Oxford University Press, 1993), p. 34.

(Lynch et al. 2001, 2004) and the particular choice of measure of inequality, such as share of income accruing to the bottom 70% rather than some other proportion of the population (Judge 1995). Indeed, a recent analysis of sixteen wealthy countries (including the nine examined by Wilkinson) using updated income data, could not reproduce the relationship between income inequality and life expectancy found earlier by Wilkinson. In fact, the earlier results may have reflected the sample of countries available at that time (Lynch et al. 2001). This recent work examining countries included in the most recent wave of the Luxembourg Income Study showed that there was no universal association between income inequality and life expectancy or age-specific all-cause mortality. However, greater income inequality was generally associated with poorer child health outcomes in the Lynch and associates (2001) study.

In general, analyses based on international comparisons have not provided persuasive evidence one way or the other (Lynch et al. 2004). Results have been shown to depend on the specific choice of countries and measures of income inequality. Moreover, the underlying data on national income distributions are not nearly as comparable as the data on mortality. Finally, there is a methodological question about whether to weight the data points by population size (i.e., to give the more populous nations more emphasis in the regression or correlation analyses). This has important implications for the interpretation of the findings, given that the United States often seems to stand out because of its characteristic large population, high GDP per capita, relatively high income inequality, but only middling life expectancy by OECD standards.

But perhaps the most important point to be made here is that there are many historical and cultural contingencies that can intervene in the relationship between income inequality and population health (Lynch et al. 2001; 2004). Every nation has its own population health story with chapters of social, economic, and political history that are undeniably influential in any given year's summary measure of population health.

That said, income distribution seems to be naggingly important—more equitable distributions seem to be a hallmark of at least some of the most successful societies in the world—and, coupled with other social, economic, and cultural factors, is likely an important determinant of health. Certainly there are relatively compelling arguments as to why income inequality might be detrimental to health, whereas one finds no equally compelling rationales for a health-enhancing effect from income inequality.

The Economic Inequality Gradient—What Is the Evidence?

Whereas the international results continue to be a subject of academic disagreement and debate, on empirical or statistical grounds (e.g., choice of inequality measure, choice of countries to include), the same cannot be said for results from recent analyses of states and cities within the United States. Comparisons of mortality and income inequality have shown a very clear association (Kaplan 1996; Kennedy et al. 1996; Lynch et al. 1998), with states and cities characterized by greater income inequality having worse population health. This relationship has proven far stronger than the association between mortality and average state income.

Yet this association, too, has been the subject of recent critiques. The main issue has been not the data comparability or choice of jurisdictions, but rather the possibility that the results are a product of investigating the relationship using an ecological study design (i.e., one where places, and not individuals, are the unit of analysis). The claim is that the individual-level relationship between income and mortality is sufficient to produce a place-level correlation between income inequality and mortality if there are disproportionate numbers of poor living in high-inequality places. In other words, the place-level relationship is a "statistical artefact" (Gravelle 1998; Judge 1995). Certainly, the concern is legitimate at a theoretical level. Indeed, earlier authors (Orcott-Duleep 1995; Lynch and Kaplan 1997) used exactly the same argument as Gravelle to speculate on why we should expect population group–level associations between income inequality and mortality.

Whatever the logical merits of the argument, however, its relevance must turn on its empirical importance. And careful empirical work has established that the "statistical artefact effect" has only marginal significance (Wolfson et al. 1999). The artifact critique is tied to the fact that the individual-level relationship between income and mortality is nonlinear. For example, figure 8.4 shows a clear, statistically very significant, and nonlinear relationship between the risk of dying and household income. This relationship was estimated from data on household income and other demographic characteristics from the U.S. Census Bureau's Current Population Survey matched to the National Death Index, providing about 7.6 *million* person-years of mortality exposure from ten years of follow-up. (The "population density" curve on the same graph shows how many individuals there were at each income level. It shows the characteristic shape where more than half of the population have incomes below the mean, because of the long upper tail of the distribution.)

Figure 8.5 illustrates Gravelle's critique in a very simple case involving two societies, A and B, each with two members. Society A is highly unequal, with member a1 having very low income, whereas the other member, a2, has very high income. In contrast, incomes of b1 and b2 in society B are much closer together, hence more equally distributed. (By design, both societies have the same average income, to prevent the intrusion of other statistical distractions.) We assume, however, that no matter what the distribution of income is in a society, at the individual level, the same relationship between the risk of dying and income applies, shown by the downward-sloping curve, with a shape similar to that observed for the United States in figure 8.4 and Canada in figure 8.2. And from the research underlying figure 8.2, plus the regression analysis underlying the curve in figure 8.4, but going

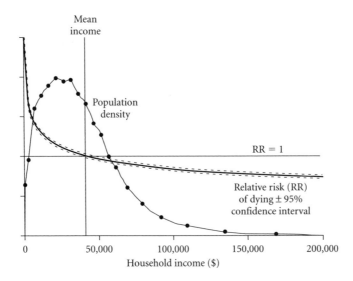

Figure 8.4. Relative risk of dying and population distribution for U.S. individuals by household income ($)

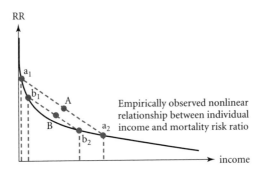

Figure 8.5. Hypothetical pair of societies

beyond it, we assume that the relationship is 100% causal. (A more realistic as-sumption is that it is largely causal, but that for some individuals, unobserved poor health at or before the starting period of the data leads both to lower incomes and higher risks of dying—i.e., there are some selection effects, but these are not the major part of the explanation.)

The larger dots at A and B along this relative risk curve are simply the average mortality risks of the two societies. Clearly, the dot for A is above that for B, so that the more unequal society A would be observed to have the higher mortality rate. The important point is that this aggregate observation would have nothing at all to do with income inequality per se. Rather, it would simply be the result of the *curvilinear* relationship between income and mortality operating at the indi-vidual level.

Wolfson and associates (1999) provided an empirical assessment of this claim by working through the implications of Gravelle's critique *as if* it were 100% true. They calculated hypothetical mortality rates for each state if the U.S. relative risk curve shown in figure 8.4 were the sole source of mortality differences between states. Data from the U.S. Census Bureau were employed to generate analogues for each state/age/sex/income group using the curve in figure 8.4. The weighted average was computed for each state based on that state's income distribution. The results of these hypothetical calculations for two demographic subgroups are shown in figures 8.6a and 8.6b (unfilled circles) and are compared to the actual mortality rates (filled circles).

The dashed lines show a simple linear regression for the hypothetical mortality rates, whereas the solid line is a fit to the actual data. There is a clear slope to the dashed line, so that Gravelle (as well as earlier authors) is certainly correct: Income inequality combined with a curvilinear relationship at the individual level between income and mortality risk can indeed account for an observed relationship at the aggregate level (in this case, states) between inequality and mortality. However, it is very clear from these graphs that the slope of the dashed line is nowhere near

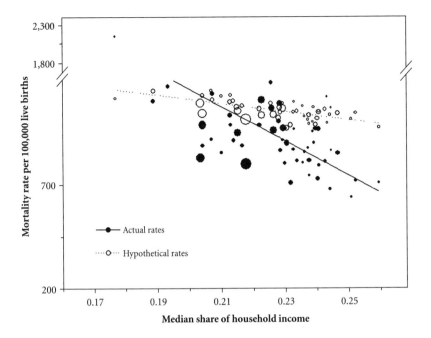

Figure 8.6a. Scatter plot of hypothetical and actual mortality rates for infants by income inequality (as measured by median share of household income)

as steep as the slope of the observed relationship. Therefore, something must be going on beyond any statistical artifact in this relationship among U.S. states.

This finding is more than a response to Gravelle's concerns. It also raises questions about earlier interpretations of the inequality–mortality association by Preston (1975), Rodgers (1979), Orcott-Duleep (1995), Wagstaff and van Doorslaer (2000), and Mellor and Milyo (1999). All of these authors observed (or rediscovered) that a curvilinear individual-level relationship between income and health would result, mechanically, in an observed correlation between income inequality and mortality rates at the population level. However, as shown in figures 8.6a and b, the situation in the United States goes well beyond this—there is something about the social milieu or social context of economically unequal places, beyond individual characteristics, that profoundly influences health, at least among U.S. states, and as will be shown below, likely among U.S. metro areas. Moreover, whatever factor is at work in the United States, as will be shown below, is apparently not at work in Canada.

Something Other Than Inequality at Play?

The second line of critique of the relationship between inequality and population health at the city/state level is that there are other characteristics of places that

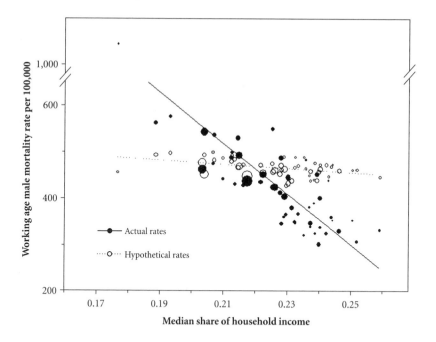

Figure 8.6b. Scatter plot of hypothetical and actual mortality rates for working-age males by income inequality (as measured by median share of household income)

might account for the relationship between income inequality and mortality. For example, Deaton and Lubotsky (2003) have suggested that including a race variable, operationalized as the proportion of an area's (state's or metropolitan area's) population that is black, in multivariate regression analyses, renders income inequality insignificant in its effect on mortality. In other words, according to these authors, results showing an effect running from income inequality to mortality are the simple result of an omitted factor (i.e., a missing measure) with race being the actual explanatory variable but "lurking" in the background and, because it is highly correlated with income inequality, forcing income inequality to be observed as significant for state- or city-level variations in mortality.

However, this explanation does not accord with the data. Figure 8.7 shows the relationship between income inequality and mortality among U.S. urban areas, after taking account of the "percentage black" indicator. Urban areas have been grouped into quartiles ranked by percentage black. The diagram does show (not surprisingly, given higher black mortality rates in general) (Rogers et al. 2000) that cities with larger proportions of blacks do have higher working-age mortality rates. But within each of the four graphs, there is a clear and statistically significant relationship between income inequality and mortality.

Moreover, the Deaton and Lubotsky hypothesis bestows upon the statistical construct—"percentage black"—intrinsic meaning that fails to address or capture the

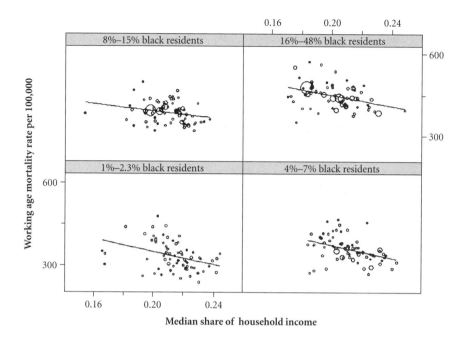

Figure 8.7. The relationship between income inequality (as measured by median share of household income) and mortality for U.S metropolitan areas, 1991, by proportion of black residents

essence of the fundamental fact that states and cities with relatively high proportions of black residents have higher mortality rates—for both blacks *and* whites. As figure 8.7 makes clear, there is more going on here than simply the effects of population mixtures with a larger fraction predisposed to a higher mortality rate. It may be, for example, that the percentage black is a marker or proxy for unmeasured characteristics of U.S. urban places, such as the provision of local public goods or the extent of spatially concentrated affluence and poverty (rather than more heterogeneous neighborhoods) that are really the driving force for the observed relationship between income inequality and mortality. A recent study by Subramanian and Kawachi (2003) has, furthermore, provided strong empirical evidence against the idea that race can explain the effects of income inequality on health. Although these authors found that race is associated with poor self-rated health at the individual level, they found no association between poor self-rated health and the proportion of black residents in U.S. states.

Multilevel Studies—The "Gold Standard"?

If we could design the perfect study to determine whether income inequality affects population health, what would we do? Clearly, it would be imperative to employ a study design that could accommodate the possibility that health is a function of both individual characteristics and features of the environment, physical as well as social. Advances in statistics now allow for the specification of models that simultaneously account for effects at both the individual level and at the social contextual level (e.g., Fiscella and Franks 1997; Kennedy et al. 1998; Daly et al. 1998; Mellor and Milyo 1999; Lochner at al. 2001; LeClere and Soobader 2000; Subramanian et al. 2001). This makes it possible to tease out the independent effects on health of societal-level inequality while controlling for individual characteristics such as income.

The results of these studies have been mixed (for reviews, see Wagstaff and van Doorslaer 2000; Lynch et al. 2004), perhaps due to variations in the studies' sample sizes and the variety of geographic scales at which income inequality has been measured. One concern with studies showing no effects (e.g., Mellor and Milyo 1999) is that the researchers drew stronger negative conclusions than their results would support. Because of the extensive data demands of these multilevel analyses, rather large sample sizes are required, so the absence of a statistically significant result (as in the work of Mellor and Milyo 1999) may be the consequence of insufficient statistical power rather than the absence of the hypothesized relationship in the underlying population.

In one of these studies, Subramanian, Kawachi, and Kennedy (2001) did find an independent effect of state-level inequality on individual mortality. Furthermore, preliminary results from another multilevel analysis, with a sample of more than half a million individuals followed for between five and ten years, showed that a statistically significant effect of state-level income inequality was observed, though only among working-age men. This relationship remained intact after adjustment for individual-level factors such as age, race, education, income (explicitly taking account of the curvilinear relationship), and employment status. (Backlund et al. n.d.). This finding is consistent with Wolfson and colleagues' (1999) results, as previously described, and suggests that the curvilinear association between income and health cannot fully explain observed associations between income inequality and health at the population level.

It would be premature to suggest that this debate has been settled. Additional work using multilevel techniques is very important and needs to be continued. More definitive results, however, await sufficiently large datasets to provide adequate statistical power, as well as an appropriate range of (spatially defined) communities or social contexts, as along with further conceptual consideration of the interpretation of results from such multilevel analyses (Kaplan and Lynch 2001; Diez-Rouz 1998). For example, these types of studies almost always assume that the direction of causal effect is from the community or the neighborhood to the individual. In reality, it is quite likely that the relationship is subtler and works in both directions, where individuals both shape and are shaped by the communities in which they live. It is quite unlikely that any amount of mathematical modeling is going to completely capture such subtle and complex pathways linking individuals and their social milieux.

Moreover, there are some conceptual issues that no sample size will help settle. For example, there are tensions in the broader multilevel literature as to what exactly distinguishes a contextual effect from an individual effect. Is individual income truly an individual-level characteristic, or is it more accurately tied to the range of possible incomes available to an individual in a given place at a particular time? Strictly speaking, if individual income were purely an individual property, individuals would be completely free to choose their incomes. Misspecification of multilevel models (i.e., omitting appropriate contextual-level or individual-level variables) will lead to false conclusions about the true source of any health effect. Diez-Roux (1998, p. 220) has summed up the problem nicely:

> Obviously, if it affects health, "context" must somehow "get into the body," and it ultimately operates through individual-level processes; thus if one were to include enough individual-level variables in the regression models, the group-level effect would disappear. However, this does not imply that individual-level variables, rather than group-level variables, are the "true" cause of the outcome.

There are two further important points to be made here about the nature of multilevel models, and they pertain to the handling of time and space. First, to the extent that unequal social environments do compromise the health of individuals inhabiting them, these effects almost certainly act over quite a long period of time, manifesting in the slow onset of multifactorial chronic diseases, rather than resulting in sudden death. Although place-based mortality rates embody some of this effect, study designs would be improved by incorporating time and broadening outcomes beyond mortality to things like heart disease incidence, mental health, and health-related behaviors. Second, the question of the appropriate spatial unit of analysis for the investigation of the effects of social inequality has not received adequate attention. The choice of geographic scale for studies of social contextual effects is a difficult one and is often dictated by data availability. Understanding the net effects of social influences while taking account of individual-level effects requires enough individuals within the community while also having enough communities to ensure that there is some community-level variance to analyze.

The added difficulty of contextual studies examining the effects of income inequality is that small geographic areas like neighborhoods or census tracts tend to be fairly homogeneous and therefore equal, even though they may be located in a broader region or metropolitan area that is quite unequal. For example, in their multilevel study of income inequality and self-reported health status for white working-age male respondents to the U.S. National Health Interview Survey, Soobader and LeClere (1999) found that income inequality exerted an independent influence on health at the county level but that the effect was greatly reduced at the census tract level. The appropriate geographic scale at which to measure income inequality in terms of its meaning for individuals remains an open question requiring both theoretical and empirical attention.

A "Natural Experiment"—Comparing Canada and the United States

None of these ongoing methodological issues and conceptual controversies calls into question the income inequality–mortality gradient in the United States, especially at the level of metropolitan areas. The existence of this gradient appears now to be uncontested—which makes it all the more remarkable that comparable analyses on Canadian data have *not* produced this relationship (Ross et al. 2000a). Initially, in typical Canadian fashion, this was viewed as the "Canada paradox" (rather than a "U.S. paradox"). But, more recent analyses of 528 cities in five industrialized countries demonstrated that both Canada and the United States have company (fig. 8.8). The relationship is found among cities in the United States and Great Britain (with the British finding corroborated by Weich, Lewis, and Jenkins [2002]) but not among those in Canada, Australia, or Sweden (Ross et al. 2005).

Interestingly, there is a strong statistical relationship between income inequality and working-age mortality across the pooled group of 528 cities. In other words,

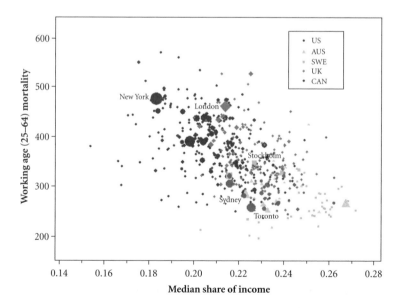

Figure 8.8. Working-age mortality by median share of income—Canadian, U.S., Australian, Swedish, and British cities

income inequality accounts fairly effectively for the pattern of urban working-age mortality in these five industrialized countries. But, despite the overall relationship among the pooled group, the null within-country results for Australia, Canada, and Sweden, the similar results from recently released studies based in Denmark (Osler et al. 2002) and Japan (Shibuya et al. 2002), and questions about the quality of the evidence underlying the 1992 Wilkinson results, leave only the United States (states and metropolitan areas) and Great Britain showing a clear within-country relationship between income inequality and mortality. The United States and Great Britain were the two most unequal countries in the five-country analysis. If anything, this suggests that something about a country's overall stance with regard to income inequality—citizens' tolerance for obvious disparities; the emphasis placed on redistribution in kind through government programs such as education, health care, and housing; and the generally accepted "stories" in popular culture about the sources and legitimacy of social inequalities—may underlie the different patterns observed within a country across its subpopulations defined by states and provinces or by metropolitan areas.

We can safely say that Canada no longer seems paradoxical in this arena and that the United States has at least a little company. The international comparisons seem to suggest that there are mechanisms mitigating the potentially health-damaging effects of U.S.- or British-style income inequality.

A strong and nonartifactual relationship between income inequality and mortality is certainly possible, and evident in the United States as shown by figures 8.6a and b above. At the same time, such a relationship is clearly not universal, as just shown in figure 8.8. The most compelling counterexample, in terms of the excellent international comparability of the data and general similarity of cultures, is Canada, but this is reinforced by recent analyses (with similarly rigorous attention to data comparability) showing that Australia and Sweden are similar to Canada. The different results from different countries—and particularly the fact that a gradient is found in the two most unequal countries and not in the other three—clearly suggests that other country-specific factors influence whether or not income inequality is associated with health. To delve into what these factors might be, we focus next on some ideas about why Canada and the United States differ so starkly on the income inequality-population health gradient.

"Natural Experiment," Unnatural Differences?

The existence of an association between income inequality and mortality in the United States and Great Britain but not in Canada, Australia, or Sweden has prompted several new lines of research, as well as challenges to the results. The first major empirical challenge was that the original association was artifactual. As noted earlier, this explanation, although theoretically possible, is empirically insufficient to account for the strength of the observed association in the United

States. Another possible counterargument is that the U.S. result is virtually all due to racial distributions. Again, as noted earlier, this argument does not withstand scrutiny and would not, in any case, explain the British results.

Yet another challenge is that the Canadian data do not have the same range of inequality to reveal an association, even if it were there. This concern is easily addressed. If we consider only that subset of U.S. cities with income inequality in the same low range as that of the Canadian cities, a significant negative slope remains for the U.S. metropolitan areas (fig. 8.9) (Ross et al. 2000b). The evidence therefore suggests real differences in this relationship between Canada and the United States.

The fact that there is evidence of a relationship, at the state and metropolitan area level, between the distribution of income and mortality in the United States but not in Canada leads us, at the very least, to the conclusion that there is no necessary innate and inviolable relationship between income inequality and health. Of course, the fact that we observe an association in the United States but not in Canada leaves wide open the question of whether, in the United States, income inequality leads to (i.e., causes) higher mortality. It may be that income and its distribution is a marker for a complex set of other more deeply rooted factors relating to the differing extent and character of social inequality in the two countries (Lynch et al. 2001).

For example, some aspects of basic social values, such as trust in government or tolerance of inequality, may lie behind the differences between Canada and the

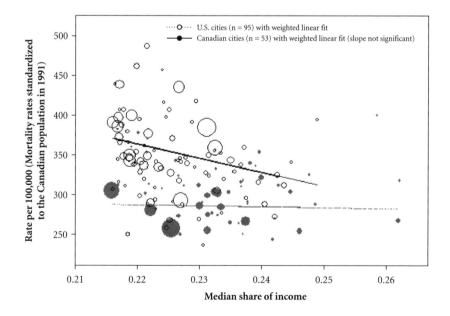

Figure 8.9. Comparison of Canadian and U.S. metropolitan areas on the income inequality–mortality relationship over the Canadian range of income inequality

United States, both in levels of income inequality and in levels of mortality. Of course, widespread trust in government is, itself, the result of social decisions, such as investments in employment insurance or in education and other social supports for children. Thus, trust in government can be viewed as a marker for a history of material and structural social investments, laws, and public policies that are transparently intended to improve the life chances of most of the population. In fact, Lynch and colleagues (2001) have shown that the countries with the highest levels of overall trust are the Nordic social democratic welfare states. It is in these countries where such social investments have been at the core of public policy for decades and in some places for more than a century (Kautto et al. 2001).

Another possibility is that characteristics of the labor market are at the root of the relationship, and these are masked, to some extent, in the Canadian data relative to the U.S. data. For example, the nature of hierarchical organization in the workplace could affect workers' decision latitude or effort-reward imbalances (Levi et al. 2000), which are, in turn, reflected in the distribution of income from working. In the United States, household income after transfer payments but before taxes may be a better marker for labor market income, whereas in Canada, with its more progressive income tax structure and more substantial transfer system, household income after transfer payments may be too blurred a mix of transfers and employment income to show a relationship between income inequality and health. In other words, one could argue that all of the health-damaging action is in labor market inequality, and other studies were not able to see this for Canada, at least not in the initial pretax, posttransfer income inequality and mortality study (Ross et al. 2000a). There remains the possibility that inequalities generated in the labor market are health compromising, even though the bottom-line income for many Canadians' households is supplemented with transfers. Income earned through a well-paid job may be more important for health (for some of the reasons discussed at the outset of the chapter) than income received but not earned.

The Earnings Gap and Mortality

A recent analysis of different concepts of income inequality and working-age mortality among U.S. and Canadian metropolitan areas sheds some light on the effect of labor market inequality on the health of Canadians. The study considered the population health correlates of inequality generated from three different income concepts: (1) earned income inequality for the subset of households reporting at least $1,000, intended to capture inequality among those households with non-trivial attachments to the labor force; (2) earned income inequality for all households, including the unemployed (i.e., households reporting zero or negative earnings); and (3) total income (the traditional posttransfer, pretax measure that was used in the original study and seen in fig. 8.8) for all households. In the United States, the association between income inequality and working-age mortality is clearly not a function of the income concept examined. That is, health-compromising inequality exists in the labor force, among both high and low earn-ers (fig. 8.10a), as well as among those with and without jobs (fig. 8.10b). In Canada, however, the only evident relationship between income inequality and mortality at the metropolitan-area level is found when we consider inequality in labor market income including the unemployed (fig. 8.10b).

In essence then, metropolitan-scale mortality in Canada *is* related to inequalities in income generated by labor market exclusion. In the United States, in contrast, whether or not labor market exclusion is considered appears to make no difference. This may reflect the nature of the U.S. labor market, where there is less distinc-tion—at least in terms of mortality risk—between being employed in a low-wage job at the bottom of the earnings distribution and being unemployed (Sanmartin et al. 2003).

On balance, the income inequality–mortality relationship at the metropolitan scale is very consistent in the United States but much less so in Canada. This finding points to some underlying factors that could account not only for the persistence across measures and concepts of income inequality of the observed U.S. relationship but also for the relatively scant evidence of the same relationship in Canada.

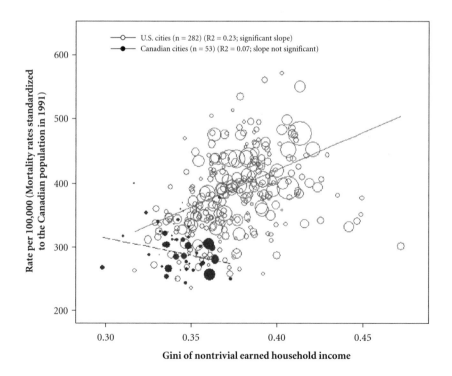

Figure 8.10a. Relationship between working-age mortality and Gini coefficient for nontrivial earnings (> = \$1,000)

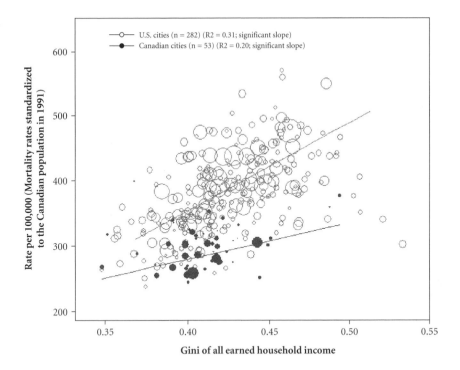

Figure 8.10b. Relationship between working-age mortality and Gini coefficient for all earned household income (including those households reporting zero earnings)

There are three main hypotheses. One intuitively appealing possibility is that Canada has a universal health care system that eliminates financial access barriers to health-repairing care for those at the lower end of the income spectrum, whereas in the United States access to health care is significantly constrained at the lower end of the income spectrum, with approximately 38 million Americans without health insurance in 2001 (Fronstin 2001).

A second possibility is that there are basic differences not only in taxation, transfers, and social policy but also in primary market income inequality—that is, the distribution of incomes generated by the market, particularly from work but also from investments. It may be that the driving factor is labor market inequality, which in turn is important not so much because it plays an obvious role in providing purchasing power but because it may be a marker for the distribution of decision latitude or effort–reward imbalance in the population—factors already known to be important individual-level determinants of health. In turn, the smaller tax and transfer systems (per capita) in the United States mean that labor income inequality, which is higher in the United States to begin with (see the following discussion), is also more strongly reflected in measured household income inequality than in Canada.

A third possibility is that something about the character of the places people live, beyond access to health care and income distribution patterns, is the key influence. In particular, we conjecture that U.S. cities have much more spatially concentrated areas of affluence and poverty than Canadian cities, with associated differential patterns of public goods and urban amenities, and that these could be the key factors underlying the dramatic difference between Canada and the United States on the income inequality-mortality relationship. In what follows, we address each of these possible explanations.

UNIVERSAL HEALTH CARE

The most obvious difference between Canada and the United States is the accessibility of health care. Canada has universal coverage for a wide range of health care services, whereas the United States has a substantial population with limited and precarious coverage. Where this might matter most is in the area of primary care. Looking cross-nationally, there are suggestive relationships between inequality and characteristics of primary health care systems. Health indicators such as birth outcomes, life expectancy, and mortality tend to be more favorable in more egalitarian countries with strong primary care like Canada, Sweden, and The Netherlands and less favorable in more unequal countries with weaker primary care infrastructures such as the United States (Starfield 2000). At the state level in the United States, income inequality (measured by the Gini coefficient[3]) is strongly inversely correlated with primary care (measured by the ratio of primary care physicians to population). Thus, it would appear that in the United States, at least, that unequal places are marked by relatively poorer access to primary care and this lack of access may be one of the mechanisms through which income inequality influences health (Shi and Starfield 2000; Shi et al. 1999). However, there is far more to health than health care (Evans et al. 1994), and health care does not prevent the onset of disease or the occurrence of accidents or homicide. Therefore, although universal availability of primary care in Canada may be important, it is unlikely to be a predominant factor.

Publicly provided health insurance also has benefits beyond the direct effect of removing financial barriers in accessing health care services. It means that those with lower incomes are under less financial pressure to pay for health care and therefore effectively have more disposable income. Disposable incomes in the lower and lower–middle ranges of the income spectrum in Canada are almost certainly higher than in the United States not only directly as a result of lower out-of-pocket spending on health care (both insurance premiums and direct costs like copayments) but also, likely, indirectly because the employer-paid portions of health care benefits are smaller in Canada. Canada's universal health insurance coverage, furthermore, is a source of personal security and eliminates a potential major source of stress that many in the United States experience. Even for insured people in the United States, this coverage is so often tied to employment that it is also often an impediment to labor force mobility. This fact will tend to lock more workers in the United States than in Canada into jobs they detest, with all the resulting personal stress associated with low job satisfaction.

COMPARATIVE TRENDS IN INCOME INEQUALITY IN CANADA AND THE
UNITED STATES

The second main possible determinant of the difference in the relationship between mortality and income inequality in Canada and the United States is the character of the two countries' distributions of income. Unfortunately, comparable data on the inequality–mortality relationship for Canada and the United States have been produced only for 1990 through 1991, and the 2000 through 2001 censuses have yet to be fully analyzed. But some speculation is possible using survey data[4] that allow national-level patterns of income inequality to be reliably compared.

As shown by Wolfson and Murphy (1998), family income inequality remained almost constant from 1974 to 1997 in Canada. (In fact, both the bottom and the top quintiles increased their income shares, so that in the conventional sense, no unambiguous trend in inequality can be detected.) In contrast, inequality increased substantially over this period in the United States.

Table 8.1 shows the trends in family total income inequality for Canada and the United States, based on the data used by Wolfson and Murphy (1998). A series of indicators is reported. The first row shows the same median share (i.e., the share of income accruing to the bottom half of the income spectrum) as used in the Canada-U.S. income inequality-mortality comparisons shown earlier. Q1 to Q4 are the shares of income accruing to the first four quintiles of the population (0–20%, 20–40%, 40–60%, and 60–80%), D9 is the share for the ninth decile (80–90%), and V19 and V20 are the income shares for the nineteenth and twentieth "vingtiles" (90–95% and 95–100%). Finally, the Gini coefficient is a widely used overall

Table 8.1. Family total income inequality in Canada and the United States. Trends in two summary measures (median share, Gini) and in quantile shares

Summary measure or share	Canada			United States		
	1974	1985	1997	1974	1985	1997
Median Share	22.9	22.8	22.3	21.9	21.1	19.6
Q1 (first quartile)	4.0	4.7	4.7	4.6	3.7	3.5
Q2 (second quartile)	10.9	10.5	10.2	10.1	9.9	9.1
Q3 (third quartile)	17.7	17.1	16.4	16.4	16.7	15.7
Q4 (fourth quartile)	24.9	24.9	24.5	24.8	24.8	24.4
D9 (ninth decile)	16.3	16.7	16.8	17.1	16.9	17.5
V19 (nineteenth vingtile)	10.1	10.4	10.6	10.7	10.7	11.3
V20 (twentieth vingtile)	16.2	15.8	16.7	16.5	17.1	18.4
Gini	0.388	0.387	0.396	0.414	0.414	0.439

measure of inequality. The specific years were chosen to span a wide time interval, while being at similar points in the business cycle. The second interval, from 1985 to 1997, includes the 1990 to 1991 period of the Canada and U.S. censuses that form the basis for the comparative Canada-U.S. data on inequality in relation to mortality shown above.

The first row indicates that inequality started out higher in the United States in 1974 (i.e., a smaller median share) and was rising on both sides of the border, but by a much greater extent in the United States (2.3 percentage points decline in the United States versus a 0.6 percentage point decline in Canada). This effect is echoed in the Gini coefficients, which show a small increase in Canada and a much larger increase in the United States. Per the quintile, decile, and vingtile shares (to look more closely at the income distributions in the two countries), the share of the bottom quintile in Canada actually increased, while the bottom 60% in the United States saw a declining share of the income pie.[5] At the top of the income spectrum, in contrast, income shares generally rose—and by considerably more in the United States than in Canada. Thus, not only did Canada have lower levels of income inequality than the United States, as already indicated in figure 8.8, but also inequality was trending differently, with the United States experiencing a much more substantial increase.

These comparative trends raise a number of questions. In particular, could the higher levels of inequality in the United States, compared with Canadian levels, in 1990 and 1991 be the main factor accounting for the different relationship between income inequality and mortality between the two countries, or is the lack of a relationship in Canada due to the lack of a dramatic *trend* toward increasing inequality in Canada, compared with that seen in the United States? Answers to this question must await publication and analysis of the 2000 through 2001 round of population censuses in the two countries and other more recent data.

URBAN STRUCTURE

A third major possible explanation for the differences between Canada and the United States regarding the income inequality-mortality relationship is the two countries' urban structures. Although there are clear similarities in terms of the appearance of the overall built environment (i.e., city skylines tend to taller in the city core) and the presence of highways (Yeates 1998), Canadian and American cities do differ in many important respects (Goldberg and Mercer 1986). In their systematic review of Canadian and U.S. metropolitan areas on urban form (population change, transportation, housing, and local government fragmentation) and urban processes (economic restructuring, immigration, and inequality), Mercer and England (2000) concluded that the distinctiveness of Canadian cities, when viewed in a North American context, is best summarized by their essentially "public" nature. In contrast, the "private" city is one where social problems are dealt with on an individual basis.

More fundamentally, the same level of income inequality in a Canadian and a U.S. city may be associated with very different levels of spatial segregation on the basis of income, and there is some limited preliminary evidence to suggest that this type of segregation is linked to mortality in U.S., but not Canadian, cities (Waitzman and Smith 1998; Ross et al. 2002). The general sense is that communities in Canadian cities are more economically heterogeneous, with more diversity in housing stock (Mercer and England 2000). In turn, spatial economic segregation may be associated in the United States, more than in Canada, with inequalities in the availability of local public goods. In addition, any discussion of U.S. residential segregation warrants at least a passing comment on the interplay between race and class and their coeffects on segregation (Farley et al. 1978). There is clearly no Canadian counterpart to Massey and Denton's (1988b) characterization of some U.S. cities as being "hypersegregated," nor is there a Canadian counterpart to the inner-city decline experienced most profoundly by the industrial manufacturing cities of the U.S. Northeast and Midwest. Jargowsky (1996) demonstrated a rapid increase in economic segregation and a rise in the concentration of poverty and affluence in American cities during the 1980s. The most recent findings from analyses of the 2000 U.S. census show, however, a dramatic decline in both the number of high-poverty neighborhoods and the size of the population living in high-poverty neighborhoods in the United States (Jargowsky 2003). This overall trend masks considerable variation in the geography of the decline of concentrated poverty with older suburban areas just outside of the center of many U.S. cities showing only very slight declines in the numbers of and population residing in low-income neighborhoods and cities like Washington, D.C., and Los Angeles actually showing a large increase in the concentration of poverty. So although the overall decline in the concentration of poverty over a very short period in the United States is impressive, Jargowsky (2003) warns that the outlook for older "inner ring" suburbs in the United States is worrisome. In terms of the Canadian story, economic segregation increased in many large Canadian cities throughout the first half of the 1990s (Ross et al. 2004).

Socioeconomic segregation in the United States is layered on top of often regressive metropolitan governance and fiscal structures (Jargowsky 1996, 1997; Orfield 1997). In many U.S. cities, a large proportion of the funds used to deliver public services is generated from local property taxes. However, this kind of funding makes the fiscal capacity of a municipality vulnerable to property values and the incomes of those who live there. This heightened vulnerability, in turn, affects the quantity, quality, and price of public services that are offered. The situation is further exacerbated by incentives for municipal fragmentation[6] and economic flight. Both of these strategies are employed by higher-income communities to get higher-quality public services at a lower cost, and they are often enabled by the exclusionary zoning policies (e.g., minimum lot sizes, no zoning for multiple-family units) of affluent municipalities. Ultimately, these factors create a considerable patchwork of inequitable services and public goods across an urban landscape (Jargowsky 1997; Orfield 1998; Altshuler 1999). The result is that U.S. municipal governance structures may act synergistically with a complex matrix of other social investments to amplify the health effects of pure income inequalities alone. In contrast, in Canada, municipal structures, combined with provincial government roles—for example, in funding education, roads, and welfare—often serve to attenuate such differences.

Therefore, income inequality at the metropolitan level in the United States is often associated with spatial economic segregation, and this in turn translates into inequalities in the availability of public goods and, possibly, an incapacity to produce public goods at all. More fundamentally, these factors relating to spatial economic segregation are also associated with systematic underinvestment across wide ranges of human, physical, social, and health infrastructures. They not only influence the private resources available to individuals but also shape the nature of public infrastructure, education, health services, transportation, environmental controls, availability of food, quality of housing, and occupational health regulations that form the material basis of contemporary life. In the United States, higher income inequality is significantly associated with many aspects of infrastructure, unemployment, health insurance, social welfare, work disability, educational and medical expenditure, and even library books per capita (Kaplan et al. 1996; Lynch et al. 2000).

The precise mechanisms linking many of these public goods to population health are not well understood. Local public goods can influence the cumulative stresses of everyday life by providing collective resources (e.g., parks, recreation, transportation) for coping with the demands of life (Kaplan 1996). Public goods such as high-quality schools, libraries, community recreational and sports centers, and other educational services can substantially improve the life chances (and the health chances) of those (especially the young) near them and who cannot afford to purchase them privately (Kohen et al. 1999). Universal high-quality elementary and secondary education, available regardless of income in Canada, is an important factor in reducing disparities in life chances across the social spectrum. In terms of effective income, high-quality publicly available education functions in a manner very similar to the health care system.

Income inequality also plays out on the urban landscape by sorting similar individuals into similar neighborhoods. Social isolation deprives residents, particularly those in poorer neighborhoods, of resources and the kind of social contacts and role models needed to get ahead in modern society (Wilson 1987). However, such sorting or economic segregation is likely much more pronounced in the United States than in Canada, and these differences probably have existed for decades. A common feature of economically segregated U.S. cities is a large contiguous area, in either the inner city or the nearby suburbs, characterized by extreme poverty, absence of services and jobs, and a large proportion of black residents. Canadian cities do not tend to follow this pattern). The association between the degree of spatial clustering or ghettoization of low-income neighborhoods in Canadian and U.S. cities paints a stark picture of contrast between the urban environments of the two countries (fig. 8.11). Canadian cities tend to cluster around 1 of White's Spatial Proximity Index,[7] which indicates that low-income urban neighborhoods in Canada tend to be distributed fairly randomly, like a checkerboard pattern, across the cities. American low-income urban neighborhoods tend to measure further away from the neutral score of 1 toward scores that represent the clustering of low-income neighborhoods into large, contiguous ghettos.

There are still more questions than answers regarding the influence of urban structure on health. However, there is certainly enough evidence already at hand to suggest that it may play a much more significant role than has generally been assumed in explaining the different relationships, in Canada and the United States, between urban income inequality and mortality.

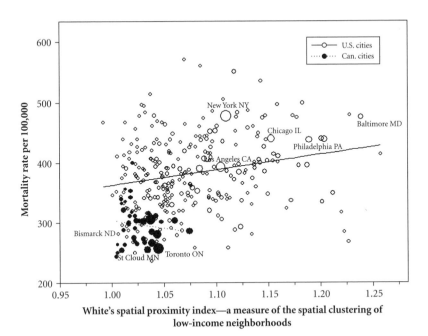

Figure 8.11. Relationship between working-age mortality and clustering of low income neighborhoods in Canadian and U.S. metropolitan areas, 1990–1991

Acknowledgments to Christian Houle at Statistics Canada for generating the index values.

Conclusions and Conjectures

It is now widely accepted that an individual's income or socioeconomic position is a major determinant of health. The evidence reviewed in this chapter further suggests that, beyond individual income, the degree of income inequality may be an independently important factor.[8] The strongest evidence of this comes from recent analyses of U.S. states and cities, though even this is still not universally accepted.

Much more intriguing, however, is the fact that Canada and the United States show fundamentally different patterns in the income inequality—mortality relationship. Income inequality may be a significant determinant of health in the United States and Great Britain, but this does not appear to be the case in Canada, Australia, or Sweden. This does not mean that economic inequality in Canada is unimportant to the health of individuals. Income inequality in Canada does reflect disparities in economic resources at the individual level, and there is a well-established individual-level relationship between income and health. But it does *not* appear that the additional contextual effect of income inequality on health found in the United States also plays out in Canada. If further scrutiny substantiates this result, such an outcome will be tremendously important because it will point to the possible existence of something implicit in Canada's social structure that successfully buffers Canadians against the adverse health effects of income inequality as observed in the United States.

Three possibilities for this difference have been canvassed. One is Canada's approach to financing core health services. With universal publicly funded health insurance for hospital care and medically necessary physician services, Canadians can access care without financial barriers. Although Roos et al., chapter 5 in this volume, demonstrate that the overall effects of health care on population health are less important than many other factors, it may be that the availability of primary care, inversely correlated with income inequality, is an important part of the pathways through which income inequality affects health. In addition, though, Canada's universal health insurance increases disposable income equality in ways that are not picked up in the income inequality data that have been used in comparative analyses to date. Canada's system also removes a major source of the personal stress and uncertainty that plague many individuals in the United States. Another major possibility is the different character of income inequality in Canada and the United States. Not only is inequality higher in the United States than Canada, but it has also been trending differently. For family disposable income, inequality was falling in Canada between the early 1970s and 1997, whereas it was increasing in the United States. The magnitudes of the changes are also larger in the United States. The analysis here suggests that there may be a health-equity tradeoff, where higher inequality may be retarding improvements in health.

Another facet of income inequality is economic segregation within urban areas. U.S. cities, for a given level of family income inequality, are more spatially segregated along economic lines, whereas Canadian cities are composed of more economically heterogeneous neighborhoods. In turn, there are several reasons to expect that such heterogeneity may be better for health. A primary one is that such urban structures are better able and more likely to produce an array of high-quality public goods (e.g., education) that give residents of all social backgrounds more even opportunities, especially when health is considered as an outcome of processes operating over the entire life course (Davey Smith et al. 2000).

It appears possible that Canadian cities, through various (perhaps inadvertent) combinations of municipal zoning and investments in transportation infrastructure, for example, have evolved in ways that are much more supportive of population health than their U.S. counterparts. Canadian cities are fundamentally more "public" than U.S. cities, and Canadian cities' aversion to both income dispersion and the compartmentalization into homogeneous spaces of local control might be a crucial part of the underlying explanation for the Canada—U.S. differences in the income inequality—population health relationship.

Health, however measured, in Canada is clearly patterned by income. We showed at the outset of this chapter that life expectancy for both men and women is lowest for the poorest groups and increases through the income quintiles with the most affluent having the highest life expectancies. Mortality after retirement is, furthermore, strongly graded by midcareer earnings. Although this chapter is principally about income inequality as a health determinant, it is important not to lose sight of the fact that health inequalities by income are very evident and arguably problematic in the Canadian context even though income *inequality* does not account for the way health is patterned across Canadian provinces and cities. Canadian cities are remarkably different contexts for the production of population health than are American cities. Canadian cities have more equal income distributions, their neighborhoods are less segregated, and they have better population health records than their American counterparts. We now need to figure out the specifics of the public choices that create urban environments that are supportive of healthier societies.

Notes

1. This conclusion derived from an examination of the subset of individuals (more than 200,000) whose earnings were increasing every year up to age 65, not only in dollar terms, but also relative to the mean earnings of the cohort. Even in this subpopulation, there was a clear gradient in mortality after age 65 with respect to earnings prior.

2. The OECD "groups 30 member countries sharing a commitment to democratic government and the market economy." For more details see http://www.oecd.org.

3. The Gini coefficient is an overall measure quantifying the degree of income inequality of a particular income distribution and can be derived directly from the Lorenz curve. The

Lorenz curve represents the cumulative distribution of households against the cumulative distribution of income. For example, in a situation of perfect equality, 10% of population has 10% of income. In reality, the actual cumulative shares of income possessed by the cumulative shares of the population will fall below this line of perfect equality. It is this Lorenz curve that allows the estimation of the Gini coefficient, a global income inequality measure explained below. As is true for any measure of proportions, the Gini coefficient lies between 0 and 1, where a Gini coefficient close to 0 indicates a more equal income distribution, whereas a coefficient close to 1 indicates a more unequal income distribution.

4. See Wolfson and Murphy (1998) for complete details on sample sizes and sampling variability of the surveys.

5. Detailed examination of the trends within each quantile group shows that the pictures are not unambiguous with regard to inequality trends. In technical terms, we see indications of crossing Lorenz curves. For example, in Canada the bottom quintile improved its position, whereas the second and third quintiles saw their income shares decline.

6. The greater Pittsburgh metropolitan area, for example, has 442 municipalities with at least land-use planning powers (Orfield, personal communication; see also Orfield 1998).

7. Massey et al. (1996) recommend White's Spatial Proximity Index as the preferred measure of clustering of low-income neighborhoods. The details of its calculation can be found in Massey and Denton 1988a.

8. Wealth inequality may also be important. However, data on the distribution of wealth are not nearly as prevalent as income distribution data.

References

Altshuler, A. A., ed. 1999. *Governance and Opportunity in Metropolitan America. Report of the Committee on Improving the Future of U.S. Cities through Improved Metropolitan Area Governance.* Washington, DC: National Academy Press.

Backlund, E., J. W. Lynch, G. Davey Smith, P. Sorlie, and G. A. Kaplan. n.d. Income inequality and mortality: A multilevel study of 521,247 individuals in 50 U.S. states. Unpublished manuscript.

Berkman, L. F., and L. S. Syme. 1979. Social networks, host resistance, and mortality: A nine-year follow-up study of Alameda County residents. *American Journal of Epidemiology* 109:86–204.

Bezruchka, S. 2001. Societal hierarchy and the health Olympics. *Canadian Medical Association Journal* 164:1701–1703.

Brunner, E. 1997. Stress and the biology of inequality. *British Medical Journal* 314:1472–1476.

Daly, M. C., G. J. Duncan, G. A. Kaplan, and J. W. Lynch. 1998. Macro-to-micro links in the relation between income inequality and mortality. *Milbank Memorial Fund Quarterly* 76:303–304.

Davey Smith, G., D. Gunnell, and Y. Ben-Shlomo. 2000. Lifecourse approaches to socioeconomic differentials in cause-specific adult mortality. In *Poverty, Inequality and Health,* ed. D. Leon and G. Walt. Oxford: Oxford University Press.

Deaton, A., and D. Lubotsky. 2003. Mortality, inequality and race in American cities and states. *Social Science and Medicine* 56:1139–1153.

Department of Health and Social Security (DHSS). 1980. *Inequalities in Health: Report of a Working Group Chaired by Sir Douglas Black.* London: DHSS.

Diez-Rouz, A. V. 1998. Bringing context back into epidemiology: Variables and fallacies in multilevel analyses. *American Journal of Public Health* 88:216–222.

Diez-Roux, A. V., S. S. Merkin, and D. Arnett. 2001. Neighborhood of residence and incidence of coronary heart disease. *New England Journal of Medicine* 345:99–106.

Evans, R. G., M. L. Barer, and T. R. Marmor, eds. 1994. *Why Are Some People Healthy and Others Not?* New York: Aldine de Gruyter.

Farley, R., H. Schuman, S. Bianchi, D. Colasanto, and S. Hatchett. 1978. Chocolate city, vanilla suburbs: Will the trend toward racially separate communities continue? *Social Science Research* 7:319–344.

Fiscella, K., and P. Franks. 1997. Poverty or income inequality as predictor of mortality: Longitudinal cohort study. *British Medical Journal* 314:1724–1727.

Fronstin, P. 2001. Sources of health insurance and characteristics of the uninsured: Analysis of the March 2001 Current Population Survey. *EBRI Issue Brief* 240:1–31.

Glazerman, S. 1998. School quality and social stratification: The determinants and consequences of parental school choice. Paper presented at annual meeting of the American Education Research Association, April 13–17, San Diego, CA.

Goldberg, M. A., and J. Mercer. 1986. *The Myth of the North American City.* Vancouver: University of British Columbia Press.

Gravelle, H. 1998. How much of the relation between population mortality and unequal distribution of income is statistical artefact? *British Medical Journal* 316:382–385.

Gray, A. M. 1982. Inequalities in health: The Black Report, a summary and comment. *International Journal of Health Services* 12:349–380.

Jargowsky, P. A. 1996. Take the money and run: Economic segregation in U.S. metropolitan areas. *American Sociological Review* 61:984–998.

———. 1997. Metropolitan restructuring and urban policy. *Stanford Law and Policy Review* 8 (2):47–60.

———. 2003. Stunning progress, hidden problems: The dramatic decline of concentrated poverty in the 1990s. The Living Cities Census Series, May 2003: The Brookings Institution.

Judge, K. 1995. Income distribution and life expectancy: A critical appraisal. *British Medical Journal* 311:1282–1285.

Kaplan, G. A. 1995. Where do shared pathways lead? Some reflections on a research agenda. *Psychosomatic Medicine* 57:208–212.

Kaplan, G. A., and J. W. Lynch. 2001. Is economic policy health policy? *American Journal of Public Health* 91:351–353.

Kaplan, G. A., E. R. Pamuk, J. W. Lynch, R. D. Cohen, and J. L. Balfour. 1996. Inequality in income and mortality in the United States: Analysis of mortality and potential pathways. *British Medical Journal* 312:999–1003.

Karasek, R., D. Baker, F. Marxer, A. Ahlbom, and T. Theorell. 1981. Job decision latitude, job demands, and cardiovascular disease: A prospective study of Swedish men. *American Journal of Public Health* 71:694–705.

Kautto, M., H. Uusitalo, J. Fritzell, B. Hvinden, and J. Kvist, eds. 2001. *Nordic Welfare States in the European Context.* London: Routledge.

Kennedy, B. P., I. Kawachi, R. Glass, and D. Prothrow-Smith. 1998. Income distribution, socioeconomic status, and self-rated health in the United States: Multilevel analysis. *British Medical Journal* 317:917–921.

Kennedy, B. P., I. Kawachi, and D. Prothrow-Stith. 1996. Income distribution and mortality: Cross sectional ecological study of the Robin Hood index in the United States. *British Medical Journal* 312:1004–1007.

Kohen, D., C. Hertzman, and J. Brooks-Gunn. 1999. Neighborhood affluence and school readiness. *Educational Quarterly Review* 6:44–52.

LeClere, F. B., and M. J. Soobader. 2000. The effect of income inequality on the health of selected U.S. demographic groups. *American Journal of Public Health* 90:1892–1897.

Levi, L., M. Bartley, M. Marmot, R. Karasek, T. Theorell, J. Siegrist, R. Peter, K. Belkic, C. Savic, P. Schnall, and P. Landsbergis. 2000. Stressors at the workplace: Theoretical models. *Occupational Medicine* 15:69–106.

Lochner, K., E. Pamuk, D. Makuc, B. P. Kennedy, and I. Kawachi. 2001. State-level income inequality and individual mortality risk: A prospective, multilevel study. *American Journal of Public Health* 91:385–391.

Lynch, J., G. Davey Smith, S. Harper, M. Hillemeier, N. Ross, G. Kaplan, and M. Wolfson. 2004. Is income inequality a determinant of population health? Part 1. A systematic review. *Milbank Quarterly* 82:5–99.

Lynch, J., G. Davey Smith, M. Hillemeier, M. Shaw, T. Raghunthan, and G. Kaplan. 2001. Income inequality, the psychosocial environment, and health: Comparisons of wealthy nations. *Lancet* 358:194–200.

Lynch, J., G. Davey Smith, G. A. Kaplan, and J. S. House. 2000. Income inequality and mortality: Importance to health of individual income, psychosocial environment, or material conditions. *British Medical Journal* 320:1200–1204.

Lynch, J., and G. A. Kaplan. 1997. Understanding how inequality in the distribution of income affects health. *Journal of Health Psychology* 2:297–314.

Lynch, J., G. A. Kaplan, E. R. Pamuk, R. D. Cohen, K. E. Heck, J. L. Balfour, and I. H. Yen. 1998. Income inequality and mortality in metropolitan areas of the United States. *American Journal of Public Health* 88:1074–1080.

Macintyre, S. 1997. The Black Report and beyond: What are the issues? *Social Science and Medicine* 44:723–746.

Marmot, M. G., H. Bosma, H. Hemingway, E. Brunner, and S. Stasfeld. 1997. Contribution of job control and other risk factors to social variations in coronary heart disease incidence. *Lancet* 350:235–239.

Marmot, M. G., G. Rose, M. Shipley, and P. J. Hamilton. 1978. Employment grade and coronary heart disease in British civil servants. *Journal of Epidemiology and Community Health* 32:244–249.

Marmot, M. G., M. J. Shipley, and G. Rose. 1984. Inequalities in death: Specific explanations of a general pattern? *Lancet* 1:1003–1006.

Massey, D. S., and N. A. Denton. 1988a. The dimensions of residential segregation. *Social Forces* 67:281–315.

———. 1988b. Hypersegregation in U.S. metropolitan areas: Black and Hispanic segregation along five dimensions. *American Journal of Sociology* 94:592–626.

Massey, D. S., M. J. White, and Phua Voon-Chin. 1996. The dimensions of segregation revisited. *Sociological Methods and Research* 25:172–206.

Mellor, J. M., and J. Milyo. 1999. *Income Inequality and Health Status in the United Sates: Evidence from the Current Population Survey.* Princeton, NJ: Robert Wood Johnson Foundation.

Mercer, J., and K. England. 2000. Canadian cities in continental context: Global and continental perspectives on Canadian urban development. In *Canadian Cities in Transition*, 2nd ed., ed. T. Bunting and P. Filion. Toronto: Oxford University Press.

Omran, A. 1971. The epidemiological transition: A theory of the epidemiology of population change. *Milbank Quarterly* 64:335–391.

———. 1983. The epidemiological transition theory: A preliminary update. *Journal of Tropical Pediatrics* 29:305–316.

Orcott-Duleep, H. 1995. Mortality and income inequality among economically developed countries. *Social Security Bulletin* 58:34–50.

Orfield, M. 1997. Metropolitics: Coalitions for regional reform. *Brookings Review* (winter):6–9.

———. 1998. *Metropolitics: A Regional Agenda for Community and Stability.* Washington, DC: Brookings Institution Press and the Lincoln Institute of Land Policy.

Osler, M., E. Prescott, M. Gronbaek, U. Chritensen, P. Due, and G. Engholm. 2002. Income inequality, individual income, and mortality in Danish adults: Analysis of pooled data from two cohort studies. *British Medical Journal* 324:13–16.

Preston, S. H. 1975. The changing relation between mortality and the level of economic development. *Population Studies* 29:231–248.

Rodgers, G. B. 1979. Income and inequality as determinants of mortality: An international cross section analysis. *Population Studies* 33:343–351.

Rogers, R. G., R. A. Hummer, and C. B. Nam. 2000. *Living and Dying in the USA. Behavioral, Health and Social Differentials of Adult Mortality.* San Diego: Academic Press.

Rogot, E., P. D. Sorlie, and N. J. Johnson. 1988. *A Mortality Study of One Million Persons by Demographic, Social and Economic Factors: 1979–1981 Follow-up.* U.S. Department of Health and Human Services, National Institutes of Health publication no. 88-2896, March. Bethesda, MD: National Institutes of Health.

Rose, G. 1985. Sick individuals and sick populations. *International Journal of Epidemiology* 14:32–38.

Rose, G., and M. G. Marmot. 1981. Social class and coronary heart disease. *British Heart Journal* 45:13–19.

Ross, N. A., D. Dorling, J. R. Dunn, G. Henriksson, J. Glover, J. Lynch, and G. Ringbäck Weitoft. 2005. Metropolitan income inequality and working-age mortality: A cross-sectional analysis using comparable data from five countries. *Journal of Urban Health* 82:101–110.

Ross, N. A., C. Houle, J. R. Dunn, and M. Aye. 2004. Dimensions and dynamics of residential segregation by income in urban Canada, 1991–1996. *Canadian Geographer* 48:433–445.

Ross, N. A., K. Nobrega, and J. R. Dunn. 2002. Economic segregation and mortality in North American metropolitan areas. *The Geography of Health and Environment. Geojournal* 53:117–124.

Ross, N. A., M. C. Wolfson, J. R. Dunn, J.-M. Berthelot, G. Kaplan, and J. Lynch. 2000a. Relation between income inequality and mortality in Canada and the United States: Cross-sectional assessment using census data and vital statistics. *British Medical Journal* 320: 898–902.

———. 2000b. Income inequality and mortality in Canada and the United States. Third explanation is possible. Author's reply. *British Medical Journal* 320:1533–1534.

Sanmartin, C., N. A. Ross, S. Tremblay, M. C. Wolfson, J. R. Dunn, and J. Lynch. 2003. Labour market income inequality and mortality in North American metropolitan areas. *Journal of Epidemiology and Community Health* 57:792–797.

Sapolsky, R. 1998. *Why Zebras Don't Get Ulcers.* New York: Freeman.

Shi, L., and B. Starfield. 2000. Primary care, income inequality, and self-rated health in the United States: A mixed-level analysis. *International Journal of Health Services Research* 30:541–555.

Shi, L., B. Starfield, B. Kennedy, and I. Kawachi. 1999. Income inequality, primary care, and health indicators. *Journal of Family Practice* 48:275–284.

Shibuya, K., H. Hashimoto, and E. Yano. 2002. Individual income, income distribution, and self-rated health in Japan: Cross-sectional analysis of nationally representative sample. *British Medical Journal* 324:16–19.

Soobader, M.-J., and F. B. LeClere. 1999. Aggregation and the measurement of income inequality: Effects on morbidity. *Social Science and Medicine* 48:733–744.

Starfield, B. 2000. Is U.S. health really the best in the world? *Journal of the American Medical Association* 284:483–485.

Subramanian, S. V., and I. Kawachi. 2003. The association between state income inequality and worse health is not confounded by race. *International Journal of Epidemiology* 36: 1022–1028.

Subramanian, S. V., I. Kawachi, and B. P. Kennedy. 2001. Does the state you live in make a difference? Multilevel analysis of self-rated health in the U.S. *Social Science and Medicine* 53:9–19.

van Rossum, C., M. J. Shipley, H. van de Mheen, D. E. Grobbee, and M. G. Marmot. 2000. Employment grade differences in cause specific mortality. A 25-year follow up of civil servants from the first Whitehall study. *Journal of Epidemiology and Community Health* 54:178–184.

Wagstaff, A., and E. van Doorslaer. 2000. Income inequality and health: What does the literature tell us? *Annual Review of Public Health* 21:543–567.

Waitzman, N. J., and K. R. Smith. 1998. Separate but lethal: The effects of economic segregation on mortality in metropolitan areas. *Milbank Quarterly* 76:341–373.

Weich, S., G. Lewis, and S. P. Jenkins. 2002. Income inequality and self-rated health in Britain. *Journal of Epidemiology and Community Health* 56:436–441.

Wilkins, R., J.-M. Berthelot, and E. Ng. 2002. Trends in mortality by income in urban Canada from 1971 to 1996. *Health Reports–Supplement 13:1–28*. Ottawa: Statistics Canada Catalogue no. 82-003-XPE.

Wilkinson, R. G. 1992. Income distribution and life expectancy. *British Medical Journal* 304: 165–168.

———. 1994. The epidemiological transition: From material scarcity to social disadvantage? *Daedalus* 123 (4):61–78.

———. 1996. *Unhealthy Societies: The Afflictions of Inequality*. London: Routledge.

Wilson, T. W., G. A. Kaplan, J. Kauhanen, R. D. Cohen, M. Wu, R. Salonen, and J. T. Salonen. 1993. Association between plasma fibrinogen concentration and five socioeconomic indices in the Kuopio Ischemic Heart Disease Risk Factor Study. *American Journal of Epidemiology* 137:292–300.

Wilson, W. J. 1987. *The Truly Disadvantaged. The Inner City, the Underclass, and Public Policy*. Chicago: The University of Chicago.

Wolfson, M. C., G. Kaplan, J. Lynch, N. A. Ross, and J. Backlund. 1999. The relationship between income inequality and mortality is not a statistical artefact—an empirical assessment. *British Medical Journal* 319:953–957.

Wolfson, M. C., and B. B. Murphy. 1998. New views on inequality trends in Canada and the United States. *Monthly Labor Review*, April 3–23.

Wolfson, M. C., G. Rowe, J. F. Gentleman, and M. Tomiak. 1993. Career earnings and death: A longitudinal analysis of older Canadian men. *Journal of Gerontology: Social Sciences* 48:S167–S179.

World Bank. 1999. *World Development Indicators 1999*. Washington, DC: World Bank.

Yeates, M. 1998. *The North American City*. 5th ed. New York: Harper & Row.

Chapter 9

Role of Geography in Inequalities in Health and Human Development

James R. Dunn, Katherine L. Frohlich, Nancy Ross, Lori J. Curtis, and Claudia Sanmartin

At one level, it is almost trite to say that location matters in explaining population health. If one were to compare the average life expectancy of Japan in 1997, for example, at 77.6 years for males and 84.3 for females, to that of Sierra Leone, at 33.2 for males and 35.4 for females, there can be little doubt that it was far better, in health terms, to be in Japan than in Sierra Leone (see table 9.1). Factors that could explain the health differences between the two countries, at least superficially, are not difficult to imagine. An obvious difference is that Japan is a much wealthier country than Sierra Leone and, for reasons thought to be partly attributable to its wealth, does not suffer the same burden of endemic infectious disease, especially AIDS, that has been particularly devastating in a country like Sierra Leone. Circumstances vary from place to place, the argument goes, and since some of those circumstances influence health, health status should vary from place to place, too.

A quick perusal of statistical tables from the World Health Report (WHO 2000) allows for the construction of an even more complete account of factors differing between Japan and Sierra Leone that might be responsible for the health differential. But the task of explaining health differences becomes more complicated if one starts to compare countries of similar wealth but differing health status. Indeed, the remarkable performance of Japan in increasing life expectancy over a very short period of time, relative to other developed countries, was a key observation motivating studies in population health (Evans, Barer, and Marmor 1994). Before World War II, life expectancy in Japan was in the midrange for a developed country, whereas now it leads the world. It has been speculated (e.g., Marmot and Mustard 1994) that differences in diet and factors related to the quality of the social environment have been critical to Japan's long life expectancy, although these factors alone are unlikely to explain the speed of improvement and the wide extent

Table 9.1. Life expectancy at birth, selected countries, 1997

Country	Life expectancy	
	Males (1999)	Females (1999)
Japan	77.6	84.3
Sweden	77.1	81.9
Canada	76.2	81.9
United States	73.8	79.7
Cuba	73.5	77.4
Botswana	39.5	39.3
Malawi	37.3	38.4
Sierra Leone	33.2	35.4

Source: World Health Organization 2000, pp. 192–195.

of the health gains, showing up as they did in a shallow socioeconomic gradient in health (Marmot and Mustard 1994). Indeed, it is likely that a unique conjunction of social, economic, cultural, historical, and biological factors underlies the particular health circumstances observed at a given time and place. In other words, something about the qualities of *place* in particular locations seems to matter. The "effect" of location is not simply due to the coordinates at which one resides but is much more a matter of place and the uniquely place-bound social and economic relations that exist at a given time to produce observed patterns.

Some might dismiss as a superficial tautology the proposition that the specificities of time and place matter in the social production of health, but doing so would obscure an important new insight in population health research with potentially valuable public health implications. If the systematic patterning of an individual's health status is shaped partly by the contexts, places, and locations in which individuals live, in addition to their own individual attributes, this may open up new avenues of intervention, over the long run, that differ fundamentally from traditional individually based interventions. An immediate challenge, however, is to abstract from the concrete circumstances of specific places more general attributes of place that may act as causal factors in the social (and geographical) production of population health. The tension between the uniqueness of places and the desire to draw inferences about "places in general" is made even more challenging when one encounters the multiple possible definitions of place. At a simple level, place can be considered a "bounded setting in which . . . social relations are constituted," but usually also refers to the material circumstances that constitute a place (e.g., its natural and built landscape, its economy, culture) as well as the social and emotional meanings that both individuals and collective social groups usually invest in places (e.g., the "sense of place") (Johnston et al. 2000, 582).

As a first step in this journey, if we change the magnification of the spatial lens and focus on smaller units of aggregation, the evidence that geography matters in explaining variations in health becomes more compelling, although not without its problems of interpretation (Pickett and Pearl 2001). Despite evidence that points toward an influence of both national-level and neighborhood-level factors on health, paradoxes emerge. It is frequently observed, for example, that the life expectancy of young black men in Harlem trails behind that of similarly aged men in Bangladesh (Marmot 2001; McCord and Freeman 1990), despite the fact that United States is the richest country in the world; that the Kerala region of India enjoys unusually good health by developing country standards (Sen 1993), even though India is a relatively poor country; and that Cuba has achieved an unusually high life expectancy at birth (73.5 years for men and 77.4 years for women) despite its relative national poverty (a gross domestic product of roughly $1,700 per capita).[1] Without understanding much more about the specific character of these places, the disjuncture between national poverty (or wealth) and health does occur as a paradox. Taken from another perspective, the health status of these places is anomalous and defies analysis with the methods commonly used in social epidemiology and population health. So what is it about these places that make them unusually (un)healthy, what kind of conceptual and methodological principles should guide research on such questions, and what policy implications follow?

The foregoing suggests that there is justification for further inquiry into the ways in which social environments, contexts, places, or locations—terms that are used interchangeably—matter in the production of health. The salience of this issue is reflected in population health literature's growing focus on the independent influence of place on health and in recent high-profile publications that have underscored its currency (Mayer and Jencks 1989). An empirical analysis recently published in the *New England Journal of Medicine* showed strong and significant place effects (at the level of the census tract) on the incidence of coronary heart disease across the United States (Diez-Roux et al. 2001). Such high profile enthusiasm for this issue exists despite a recent systematic review that found consistent but only modest effects of places on health, independent of individual level attributes (Pickett and Pearl 2001).

The empirical evidence, in short, is compelling but perhaps not yet convincing. To make further progress, we argue that there is a need to go back to the beginning and revisit the scientific basis for asking questions about the influence of places on health. What kinds of evidence would make a more convincing case—either for or against—the independent influence of place-level attributes on health? Is the evidence inconsistent because place effects do not exist or because they cannot be detected with conventional conceptual and methodological tools?

In this chapter we address the conceptual question, offering two perspectives from the past (one from sociology and one from epidemiology) that clarify the motivations for studying place effects and that help to chart a path forward. Emile Durkheim, the early-twentieth-century sociologist well-known in the health literature for his study of suicide, originally distinguished between "social facts" and "individual facts" as scientifically legitimate entities of study. Social facts, Durkheim claimed, are effectively epiphenomena (or emergent properties) of relations between individuals in a society—phenomena that reside neither in the characteristics of individuals nor in the aggregate characteristics of populations but, instead, in social relations. Although his "rules of sociological method," including the notion of social facts, were developed for use in studying whole societies, in this chapter we explore the value of applying Durkheim's approach to the neighborhood as a unit of analysis (Durkheim 1938, 1951).

More recently, path-breaking British epidemiologist Geoffrey Rose created an epidemiological corollary to Durkheim's distinction between social and individual facts: the distinction between sick individuals and sick populations (Rose 1985, 1992; see also Schwartz and Diez-Roux 2001). Rose's key insight was that traditional epidemiology, based on the analysis of variations in individual-level attributes, can provide insights *only* into putative causal agents that are unequally distributed *within* populations, and it is blind to putative causal agents to which a whole population may be equally exposed. Interventions that address the latter, he argued, may make a far greater public health impact than interventions aimed at altering individual risk factors. The insights of Durkheim and Rose go directly to the heart of an inherent paradox of place that remains vexing for analysts. The specificity of places (their character, their history, their "feel") in some ways defies generalization. Indeed, the tension between the specificity of places and the desire to make general statements about place-based phenomena is a tension—a paradox of place—with deep roots in geography. But the nature of the social facts underlying the uniqueness of a specific place, especially those aspects of a place that influence the sickness or health of the population, are the underlying phenomena that we most need to understand—and in ways that are relevant to a global discussion of population health.

The way forward, we argue, is not simply more multilevel analyses of cross-sectional, secondary datasets. Most such studies contain little or no theoretical or conceptual account of the relationship between specific dimensions of places and population health (O'Campo 2003), partly because of the data constraints inherent in multilevel modeling techniques. Multilevel studies typically use secondary datasets with variables that are not of the investigator's choosing and independent and dependent must be selected from the secondary sources to meet the requirements of hierarchical and multi-level modeling analyses. But even in the most skillfully executed empirical studies, the authors can do little more than conjecture about the reasons why, for example, neighborhood-level social structural and built-environment factors help explain variations in individual-level health status. This implies a need for better conceptual and theoretical development of the possible pathways between place and health, not simply more studies that "prove" (or disprove) the hypothesis that variation in individual-level health outcomes can be explained by "place-level" socioeconomic factors in multilevel models.

We argue that new approaches are needed to complement the multilevel model. As has been shown in the West of Scotland-07 Study[2] in Glasgow (Macintyre, Maciver, and Sooman 1993; Macintyre and Ellaway 1998; Macintyre 2000), in-depth, grounded studies of socially contrasting neighborhoods can provide compelling evidence of specific causal mechanisms that shape health both directly and indirectly through systematic constraints on engaging in healthful behaviors. These studies can identify social facts that may go unidentified by the attributes of place that enter multilevel models of routinely collected data. In some studies, the findings of contextually rooted, qualitative place attributes have been quantified to characterize more places, with provocative results (Frohlich et al. 2002b). Another possible approach is to look closely for insights about the operation of place-level factors during the course of changes to relevant social, economic, and health policies that occur in some places but not others. If natural experiments such as these can be marshaled for research, the changes in the characteristics of specific places may reveal systematic tendencies in collective behavior and thought that structure the everyday life and shape population health (Frohlich, Corin, and Potvin 2001). These tendencies, in turn, may be important social facts pointing to the mechanisms by which place matters in the production of health (Macintyre, Maciver, and Sooman 1993; Macintyre and Ellaway 1998; Macintyre 2000).

Location and Health: What Is Known?

What do we currently know about the role of place on health? Despite the fact that there have been relatively few theoretically rich studies of locational effects on health outcomes, there is widespread interest and enormous potential in questions related to the pathways by which locations matter to the social production of health inequalities. In a recent review, Pickett and Pearl (2001) identified twenty-five multilevel studies of socioeconomic factors and physical or mental health in developed countries published before June 1998. They excluded studies of community effects on fertility and sexual behavior, as well as studies that investigated the effect of income inequality on health. (The authors excluded studies that used income inequality as the area-level variable, because such studies have "methodological issues deserving of separate treatment" [p. 112]. Such issues are addressed in chapter 8). Of the twenty-five studies reviewed, twenty-three showed an effect of area-level socioeconomic factors on the health outcome under study, beyond the influence of individual-level factors. Health outcomes analyzed in this group of studies included all-cause mortality (eight studies), heart disease mortality (one study), other mortality causes (one study), low birth weight (three studies), child respiratory conditions (one study), adult chronic illness (nine studies—including ones on chronic ill health, self-rated health, heart disease and associated risk factors, hypertension), mental health (one study), and health behaviors (seven studies— on smoking, alcohol, physical activity, and domestic violence).

A follow-up search of articles published since the date of Pickett and Pearl's review, using the same search criteria, produced additional articles with similar results. Cubbin, LeClere, and Smith (2000), using data from the National Health Interview Study ($n = 472,364$) showed that neighborhood deprivation contributed to injury mortality (homicide, suicide, motor vehicle deaths, and other external causes) in addition to individual socioeconomic characteristics. Van Os and colleagues (2000) found that the proportion of divorced persons in a neighborhood made a modest but statistically significant independent contribution to schizophrenia incidence in thirty-five neighborhoods in Maastricht, suggesting that the neighborhood environment, particularly as it contributes to experiences of social isolation, may modify individuals' risk for schizophrenia. Duncan, Jones, and Moon (1999) investigated the influence of a U.K. ward-level deprivation score computed from four census variables on smoking behavior, independent of individual characteristics. Measures of neighborhood deprivation had an independent effect on smoking behavior but still left a large proportion of the between-ward variation unexplained.

One of the most convincing recent studies of social contextual effects was the widely publicized, large prospective study of Diez-Roux and colleagues that appeared in the *New England Journal of Medicine* in the summer of 2001 (Diez-Roux et al. 2001). This group demonstrated a threefold risk of coronary heart disease incidence among poor people living in poor neighborhoods compared with affluent people living in affluent neighborhoods in four U.S. study sites. Following individuals through time was a chief methodological strength of this work in terms of attributing causality to neighborhood characteristics. The researchers isolated three important neighborhood characteristics with implications for health: wealth and income, education, and occupation.

Neither the studies included in Pickett and Pearl's review nor those more recently published, however, can fully explain the popularity and intellectual appeal of the idea that geography matters in the social production of health. Much of the appeal can be traced back to earlier work in the United Kingdom and the United States. Four investigations have been particularly influential. First, in a fifty-year study of heart disease in Roseto, Pennsylvania, investigators sought to explain unusually low heart disease rates in Roseto (compared with those in neighboring towns) in terms of highly supportive and cohesive social relations (Wolf et al. 1973; Wolf and Bruhn 1993; see also Wilkinson 1996). A phenomenological study seeking evidence of social relations in Roseto that could account for the Roseto health advantage revealed a relatively horizontal social structure and tight social bonds within the community, attributes that were predicted to decline in the next generation, and with them, the Roseto health advantage (Wolf et al. 1973). A follow-up study confirmed the prediction, showing that mortality rates from myocardial infarction and congestive heart failure came to resemble those of Bangor, a neighboring town, by the decade between 1975 and 1984 (Egolf et al. 1992). Second, the Alameda County Study (Haan, Kaplan, and Camacho 1987) was one of the first studies to show a convincing link between residence in a poverty area and heightened chance of mortality. Third, Phillimore, Townsend, and Beattie (1988) examined the role of social class in long-standing differences in mortality rates between the north and south of England. They found that social class explanations were insufficient to explain the north–south health divide and that there was considerable variability between places within the north and south regions of England, suggesting the importance of regional social and economic factors. Fourth, Blaxter (1990), in her comprehensive analysis of the British Health and Lifestyle Survey, noted several important interactions between class, area of residence and general self-rated health, psychosocial health, and unhealthy behaviors. In general, people living in cities and industrial areas had poorer health and healthier behavior patterns than people living in rural areas and high-status areas. That said, within small areas there were very large differences in health indicators that raised questions about more complex interactions between place, class, and health—alcohol consumption, for example was higher among men in the higher occupational classes than the lower grades in high-status areas, but the reverse was true in industrial areas. These four seminal studies laid the foundation for contemporary research attempting to explain the role of place in the production of health inequalities.

These landmark studies provided concrete accounts of the potential role that location and place may play in producing health inequalities. Although some may complain that these studies lacked the statistical power and precision of "true" multilevel studies (i.e., studies that use hierarchical or multilevel statistical techniques to statistically isolate context-level effects from individual-level effects), it is these more descriptive studies that provided the greatest insights into the pathways and mechanisms that could account for relationships between location, place, and health, until recently. These studies are important to the development of more theoretically robust quantitative measures of the health-enhancing or health-diminishing features of locations and places.

Location, Place, and Children's Health and Development

Some of the most influential work on the idea of places exerting an independent influence on human outcomes comes from research on child development. One of the cornerstones of research into child health and well-being, in turn, has been a focus on the influence of family and household characteristics on such outcomes (e.g., Dooley and Lipman 1996; Dooley et al. 1998; Kohen, Hertzman, and Brooks-Gunn 2001; Chase-Lansdale and Brooks-Gunn 1994). Recently, however, compelling results have come from paying attention to the influence of factors within contexts at different scales, for example, the role of school and neighborhood attributes in shaping child development outcomes. Multilevel studies have examined the effects of place on child outcomes thought to be early indicators of future health, well-being, and competence (Mayer and Jencks 1989; Molnar et al. 2004; Caughy, O'Campo, and Muntaner 2003; Saelens et al. 2003; Roosa et al. 2003). The works of Brooks-Gunn and colleagues (1993) and Willms (2001) are excellent examples of the potential for analysis of the independent influence of place on children's outcomes. Brooks-Gunn and colleagues' efforts have been influential in showing that poor children living in mixed-income neighborhoods typically have better developmental outcomes than poor children living in homogenously poor neighborhoods. Willms (2001) offers three hypotheses for explaining community effects on child outcomes: the hypothesis of community differences, which suggests that different communities will have different outcomes even after controlling for individuals' socioeconomic status (SES); the hypothesis of converging gradients, which argues that SES gradients in child development for different communities will converge at the upper ends of the SES spectrum and that successful communities are ones that redress differences between lower-SES individuals; and the hypothesis of double jeopardy, which specifies that individuals from lower-SES backgrounds are disadvantaged and that they will be doubly disadvantaged if they also live in a low-SES neighborhood. He argues that there is mixed evidence for all three hypotheses but that data limitations, especially in Canada, prevent complete testing of all three hypotheses.

Using two large U.S. datasets of national scope, Brooks-Gunn and colleagues (1993) investigated the effects of neighborhood characteristics on child and adolescent development and found that neighborhood effects were significantly associated with child and adolescent outcomes. Growing up in an affluent neighborhood, measured by the proportion of families with annual incomes greater than $30,000, had a "powerful" association with children's cognitive and emotional well-being. However, the authors found only a small, negative association between residing in an impoverished neighborhood, measured by the fraction of families with annual incomes of less than $10,000, and the same childhood cognitive and emotional well-being outcomes. The associations did not differ by poverty status but were stronger for whites than for blacks. High occupational status was found to be significantly associated only with fewer behavioral problems in young children, and the fraction of female-headed households was significantly related to higher school dropout rates at the census tract level. Several other measures of neighborhood characteristics—for instance, fraction black, fraction on public assistance, fraction of males in the labor force—were not found to be significant after controlling for family characteristics. A similar result was found by Chase-Lansdale and colleagues (1997). Low-SES neighborhoods were associated with higher rates of cognitive problems in three- to four-year-olds than in high-SES neighborhoods.

However, once an adjustment was made for individual family characteristics, only the influence of high-SES mix in neighborhoods remained significant.

Several recent studies have demonstrated that the neighborhoods in which a child and his or her family live have strong associations with child health, after controlling for family and child characteristics. Two of these studies linked the Canadian National Longitudinal Survey of Children and Youth (NLSCY) with data from census enumeration areas (EAs). First, Boyle and Lipman (1998) examined emotional, conduct, and hyperactive disorders among four- to eleven-year-olds using three EA-based measures: the proportion of one-parent families in the EA; the proportion of poor families in the EA; and an aggregate measure of neighborhood socioeconomic disadvantage based on the level of neighborhood income, education, and unemployment. They found that children living in EAs with a higher proportion of lone-parent families were more likely to demonstrate poorer outcomes, but the EA-level proportion of poor two-parent families was not associated with child development outcomes. They obtained inconsistent results with an aggregate measure of neighborhood socioeconomic disadvantage.

Second, Kohen, Hertzman, and Brooks-Gunn (1998) focused on neighborhood influences on developmental outcomes for children younger than six, by census enumeration area (EA). They found that four- to five-year-olds living in neighborhoods with a higher proportion of lone-parent families were more likely to have behavioral problems and lower levels of receptive language development. Neither outcome was associated with the proportion of poor families in the EA, but a higher proportion of high-income families (those making more than $50,000) was correlated with fewer behavioral problems. Safer and more cohesive neighborhoods were also associated with positive outcomes. The high–neighborhood-income effect was mediated by family characteristics for the young children, but the associations remained for preschoolers.

Curtis, Dooley, and Phipps (2004) also found consistently significant negative associations between neighborhood problems—such as the presence of uncontained garbage, groups or gangs hanging out, drinking in the neighborhood—and child health. Significant positive relationships were found with indicators of social cohesion, such as the proportion of parents who felt that there were other adults in the neighborhood who would look out for their child if they were not home or who would act as mentors. However, the magnitude of the relationship between social cohesion and health was only one-half to one-third that of the negative relationship between neighborhood problems and child health. Family characteristics, low income, and lone-parent status were significant factors and were associated with poorer child health.

In a large multilevel study of Ontario third-grade students' performance, Tremblay, Ross, and Berthelot (2001) identified a significant contribution of neighborhood context on school outcomes for young children. Although the bulk of the variation in outcomes could be accounted for by the characteristics that students "brought with them to school" (i.e., some combination of early developmental experiences and factors such as natural abilities or intrinsic motivation), a surprisingly large amount of variation was attributable to school context. The school-level variation was similar to that found in U.S. studies, although income inequality is much smaller in Canada than in the United States.

Durkheim and the Place of Social Facts

There are important intellectual and philosophical underpinnings to research on the influence of place on health and early child development. These are seldom acknowledged, but they are important for steering future inquiry along a coherent path that avoids past errors. Durkheim is known in sociological circles for his development of the notion of "social facts" (as noted earlier) and in the population-health world for his analysis of suicide among different religious groups in nineteenth-century Europe (Durkheim 1951). The study of suicide, in fact, was one of Durkheim's major demonstrations of the notion of social facts. It began with the proposition that "society is not a mere sum of individuals. Rather, the system formed by their association represents a specific reality which has its own characteristics" (Durkheim 1938, 103). Durkheim took this proposition very seriously and parlayed it into a broader theory of the ways in which attributes and characteristics of whole societies shape the actions and outcomes of their constituent parts. In this way, measures such as marriage rates, suicide rates, and mortality rates become epiphenomena *sui generis* of whole societies—that is, social facts.

By "social facts," Durkheim did "not mean any facts having to do with society, as understood in common parlance" (Caitlin 1964, xv). Instead, he argued that there are "ways of acting, thinking and feeling that present the noteworthy property of existing outside the individual consciousness" that are valid objects of scientific study (Durkheim 1938, 2). Social facts, according to Durkheim (3), represent a special and unique category of facts with very distinctive characteristics: they consist of ways of acting, thinking, and feeling, external to the individual, and endowed with a power of coercion, by reason of which they "control him [sic]." These ways of thinking could not be confused with biological phenomena, since they consist of representations of actions; not with psychological phenomena, which exist only in the individual consciousness and through it. They constitute, thus, a new variety of phenomena; and it is to them that the term "social" ought to be applied.

There are "two empirical tests for the existence of a 'social fact' ":

1. It has the property of "being general throughout the extent of a given society" (Durkheim 1938, 13). By implication, Durkheim distinguished a social fact from a psychological fact, which is universal to human nature. In addition, he did "not mean that the [social] fact is existent without exception—e.g.,

that all men are suicides or drunkards—but that it is potentially universal in the sense that, granted given conditions, it will anywhere be set up. Its incidence is general" (Caitlin 1964, xv).

2. A social fact is marked by "any manner of action, whether of a set nature or otherwise, capable of exercising over the individual exterior constraint" (13). He argues that "a social fact is to be recognized by the coercive power which it exercises or is capable of exercising over individuals" (10).

A social fact, therefore, "is every way of acting, fixed or not, capable of exercising on the individual an external constraint, or again, every way of acting which is general throughout a given society, while at the same time existing in its own right individual of its own manifestations" (13).

In his initial formulation of the social facts notion in 1938, Durkheim offered few concrete examples or illustrations. The argument was primarily a logical one that used the foils of other disciplines to sustain it. Consider the juxtaposition of the notion of social facts with the reasoning typically employed in the psychology of his time. Durkheim (1938, 104) argued that it is

> in the nature of this collective individuality, not in that of the associated units, that we must seek the immediate and determining causes of the facts appearing therein. The group thinks, feels, and acts quite differently from the way in which its members would were they isolated. If, then, we begin with the individual, we shall be able to understand nothing of what takes place in the group. In a word, there is between psychology and sociology the same break in continuity as between biology and the physiochemical sciences. Consequently, every time that a social phenomenon is directly explained by a psychological phenomenon, we may be sure that the explanation is false.

Durkheim's investigation of suicide (1951) helped to validate the idea of social facts. He began with the observation that the rates of suicide *within* individual European societies were reasonably stable over time, despite upwards of fourfold differences in the rates *between* these same societies in the latter half of the nineteenth century (see table 9.2). He argued that even though the causes of suicide had to be found in the specific life histories of individuals, there was a patterned regularity in suicide rates among population groups, over time, even as individuals moved in and out of these groups. He suggested that there had to be something about the social environment that promoted a characteristic suicide rate for a given group. As Syme and Frohlich 2002 noted, these population characteristics do not determine which individuals in the group commit suicide, but they do help explain the group differences in rates over time.

The stability of national suicide rates is a remarkable finding, especially when the nature of suicide itself is considered. As Durkheim (1951) put it: "Since the

Table 9.2. Rate of suicides per million inhabitants in the different European countries

	Period			Numerical position in the period		
	1866–70	1871–75	1874–78	1 period	2 period	3 period
Italy	30	35	38	1	1	1
Belgium	66	69	78	2	3	4
England	67	66	69	3	2	2
Norway	76	73	71	4	4	3
Austria	78	94	130	5	7	7
Sweden	85	81	91	6	5	5
Bavaria	90	91	100	7	6	6
France	135	150	160	8	9	9
Prussia	142	134	152	9	8	8
Denmark	277	258	255	10	10	10
Saxony	293	267	334	11	11	11

Source: Reprinted with the permission of The Free Press, a Division of Simon & Schuster Adult Publishing Group, from SUICIDE: A Study in Sociology by Emile Durkheim, translated by John A. Spaulding and George Simpson. Edited by George Simpson. Copyright © 1951 by The Free Press. Copyright © renewed 1979 by The Free Press. All rights reserved.

handful of people who kill themselves annually do not form a natural group, and are not in communication with one another, the stable number of suicides can only be due to the influence of a common cause which dominates and survives the individual persons involved" (313). Ultimately, for Durkheim, these findings reinforced the veracity of the notion that social facts are a real and legitimate object of social scientific study:

> Not only are there suicides every year, but there are as a general rule as many each year as in the year preceding. The state of mind which causes men to kill themselves is not purely and simply transmitted, but—something much more remarkable—transmitted to an equal number of persons, all in such situations as to make the state of mind become an act. How can this be if only individuals are concerned? The number as such cannot be directly transmitted. Today's population has not learned from yesterday's the size of the contribution it must make to suicide; nevertheless, it will make one of identical size with that of the past, unless circumstances change. . . . (308)

The conclusion from all these facts is that the social suicide rate can be explained only sociologically. At any given moment the moral constitution of society establishes the contingent of voluntary deaths. There is, therefore, for each people a collective force of a definite amount of energy, impelling men to self-destruction. The victim's acts which at first seem to express only his personal temperament are really the supplement and prolongation of a social condition which they express externally. (299)

Durkheim's focus was on differences between whole societies in the social production of suicide. However, it is also well understood that there is important and noticeable variability between groups within a given society, for example, by region of a country, by neighborhood area, or by urban–rural distinction (Marmot 2001). The scale of the phenomenon of social facts is something that Durkheim never addressed. Yet it follows from the importance of social facts at the societal level, for individual outcomes, that social facts at other levels of social and spatial aggregation could be as influential (although different facts may be influential at different levels of aggregation). Consider the way Durkheim (1951, 302, 313–314) described the reasoning behind the belief that social factors shape individual outcomes independently of individual factors:

> Shall we suppose that the general condition of the social environment, being the same for most individuals, affects nearly all in the same way and so partially bestows a common appearance on them. But the social environment is fundamentally one of common ideas, beliefs, customs and tendencies. For them to impart themselves to individuals, they must somehow exist independently of individuals; and this approaches the solution we suggested. For thus is implicitly acknowledged the existence of a collective inclination to suicide from which individual inclinations are derived, and our whole problem is to know of what it consists and how it acts. . . .
>
> It is not true that society is made up only of individuals; it also includes material things, which play an essential role in common life. The social fact is sometimes so far materialized as to become an element of the external world. For instance, a definite type of architecture is a social phenomenon; but it is partially embodied in houses and buildings of all sorts which, once constructed, become autonomous realities, independent of individuals. . . . Social life, which is thus crystallized, as it were, and fixed on material supports, is by just so much externalized and acts upon us from without.

Despite the emphasis that he placed on the independent influence of social facts on individual outcomes, Durkheim was remarkably silent and agnostic about what sorts of social facts should be investigated in the social production of suicide. Neither in *Suicide* (1951) nor in *The Rules of Sociological Method* (1938) did he give much guidance. His major contribution, however, was to underscore the difficulties in approaching social scientific research from the perspective of social facts, and the impact of that contribution has been profound. As we argue shortly, Durkheim's limited claims concerning the specific social facts to which suicide can be attributed (e.g., marriage rates and religion) is likely a testament to the difficulty of identifying them. In summary, Durkheim's work is helpful for two key reasons. First, it gives us confidence in the logic of place and context effects on human phenomena through the notion of social facts and through Durkheim's study of suicide. Second, his arguments suggest the need to link individual life histories with social factors—something that has not yet been achieved in the study of population health and health inequalities.

Scaling Rose: Beyond Individual-level Approaches

The epidemiological approach to the study of location and health draws from the seminal paper "Sick Individuals and Sick Populations," in which Rose (1985) distinguished between the determinants of individual cases and the determinants of the incidence rate for a given condition in a given population. Rose illustrated the shortcoming of epidemiological research that seeks to answer only which individual-level characteristics explain why some people are healthy and others not. Rose (1985, 33) cautioned that "we should not forget that the more widespread a particular cause, the less it explains the distribution of cases. The hardest cause to identify is the one that is universally present, for then it has no influence on the distribution of disease."

Drawing on the example of serum cholesterol levels among Japanese and Finnish men, Rose argued that if one were to explore the role of diet on cholesterol levels *within* any one of these two countries alone, the results would be inconclusive, as each of these populations was homogenous and most people within them had similar diets (Rose 1992). Only when exploring the reasons for the differences in cholesterol levels *between* the two countries could one understand the etiology of serum cholesterol levels from an aggregate level, as only then could one discover that the diets were different.

Rose used the example of hypertension to further distinguish between two types of etiological questions: "Why do some individuals have hypertension?" and "Why do some populations have much hypertension, while in others it is rare?" He compared the shape and position of the distribution of systolic blood pressure in two populations—British civil servants and Kenyan nomads—and found that although the shape of the distribution (standard normal, bell-shaped) was nearly identical in the two populations, the curve for the British civil servants was shifted significantly to the right of that of the Kenyan nomads (reflecting higher systolic blood pressure, in general). "Why is hypertension absent in the Kenyans and common in London?" asked Rose (1985, 34):

> The answer to that question has to do with the determinants of the population mean; for what distinguishes the two groups is nothing to do with the characteristics of individuals, it is rather a shift of the whole distribution—a mass influence acting on the population as a whole. To find the determinants of incidence and prevalence rates, we need to study characteristics of populations, not characteristics of individuals.

But what exactly do we mean by the term *population* in this context? Surely Rose meant the term to imply more than simply the sum of individual character-istics within a population (its composition). Indeed, using a simple summation of individuals' characteristics to serve as the sole attribute of a population would seem to defeat the purpose of emphasizing population-level determinants of health. Al-though he did not explicitly say it, Rose implied that the key issue concerns some-thing akin to Durkheim's social facts. The only specific social facts he discussed, however, concern the ways in which lifestyle characteristics, such as eating, smok-ing, and exercise, are "constrained by social norms" (Rose 1985, 37). He rightly pointed out the influence that social norms exert on behaviors traditionally ad-dressed from an individualistic perspective:

> If we try to eat differently from our friends it will not only be inconvenient, but we risk being regarded as cranks or hypochondriacs. If a man's work environment encourages heavy drinking, then advice that he is damaging his liver is unlikely to have any effect. No-one who has attempted any sort of health education effort in individuals needs to be told that it is difficult for such people to step out of line with their peers. (37)

Rose's observations implicate the nature of social relations that exist within a population—in the case of one's peers or coworkers that population may be a network more so than a place or location, but it is governed by a set of social practices nevertheless. Indeed, Duncan, Jones, and Moon (1996) demonstrated that both the proportion of smokers in electoral wards in Britain and the number of cigarettes consumed daily by these smokers varied across communities when con-trolling for place composition (age, gender, social class, and marital status). Not only did people tend to be smokers in places where others smoked, but they also tended to smoke similar amounts to those around them. Thus, the ways in which the people around an individual behave seem to strongly influence their own be-havior.

Scaling Rose to the Neighborhood Level

If the lens of magnification is changed, however, and one zooms in from the level of Great Britain and Kenya, it becomes possible to "scale" Rose's insights. In both the United States and Canada, government organizations now routinely produce reports documenting aggregate health patterns at various geographic scales, from the regional health authority to the province in Canada and, typically, at the county or state level in the United States (e.g., Statistics Canada 2002; Barnett et al. 2001). Similarly, public health departments within smaller regions, such as metropolitan areas and cities, routinely produce reports on health statistics by neighborhood areas. These kinds of reports vaguely invoke a geographical approach, raising non-specific references to the social, economic, and political conditions that may coexist with a particular patterning of health status in a particular place. Yet the "place" invoked in such reports is often little more than a container for the extant population and not fundamentally implicated in the production of health in that place.

But what if, in addition to zooming in to smaller geographic units of analysis, one were to employ what we might call a "Rose-colored lens" and to analyze neighborhood differences in health as a product of local social facts? Consider figure 9.1, a map of the city of Vancouver, divided into twenty-three neighborhood areas. The data displayed on this map show Early Development Instrument (EDI) scores (see Janus 2002)[3] for all 3,666 (non–special needs) kindergarten children attending public schools in the city of Vancouver in February 2000 (Hertzman et al. 2002). But the data are presented in two different ways. The underlying chloropleth map (area-based shading of each region) represents the percentage of high-risk children in each neighborhood area—defined as the percentage of children falling in the bottom decile of EDI scores (measured against norms developed from a dataset representing the accumulation of all administrations of the EDI to date). This, of course, illustrates the high-risk, individualistic approach Rose criticized. A further analysis of the data shows a Pearson's correlation coefficient between child's household income and EDI score to be 0.194 ($P < .001$).[4] Using a traditional analysis, one would identify high-risk children to be those with low incomes.

The histograms superimposed on top of each neighborhood, however, add an extra dimension to the picture. These show Rose's insight at a different scale: The distribution of scores is substantially different between populations or, in this case, neighborhoods. The shapes of the distributions are not perfectly normal, as in the comparison between British civil servants and Kenyan nomads, because the distribution of people belonging to each neighborhood is governed by the operation of urban land markets.[5] Skewed shape notwithstanding, the pattern is striking: The distribution is shifted to the right (relative to the grand mean) in the higher-SES neighborhoods on the west side of the city, suggesting a greater frequency of children with better scores. The mean EDI in neighborhoods of relatively low SES in east Vancouver is shifted to the right relative to the EDI grand mean (suggesting poorer readiness for school), and the mean EDI of relatively high-SES neighborhoods in west Vancouver is shifted to the left (suggesting better readiness for school). In other words, the fact of being high-risk, although the property of an individual child, cannot be understood solely as an individual fact of that child. It is also tied to the social fact of the neighborhood level of readiness for school.

Applying Rose's Insights to Public Health Interventions

Equally striking are the implications of using a Rose-colored lens when thinking about public health interventions. An individualistic approach to reducing disparities in EDI scores would use risk-factor information such as household income,

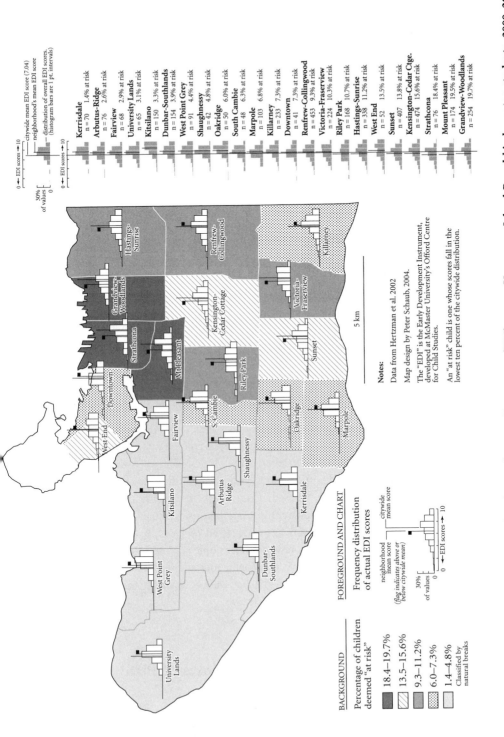

Figure 9.1. Frequency distribution of Early Development Instrument (EDI) scores, Vancouver School Board kindergarten students, 2000–2001

253

parents' educational attainment, or parenting style to identify children living in families at high risk. This would lead along a well-traveled road to individualistic family-based interventions emblematic of what the British call the nanny state. It would miss the opportunity to identify those neighborhoods where higher-risk children live and to put community-based supports in place. The objective of a Rose-based approach, however, would be to put in place supports (e.g., drop-in programs for mothers and their infants or toddlers, reading programs with picture books for preschoolers), along with community development strategies (to link individuals to supports), to shift the distribution of readiness for school (and its determinants) across the neighborhood. By encouraging and cultivating social practices that incorporate those supports into the daily lives of local preschoolers, all children in the area would automatically receive, in the course of routine activity, the kind of stimulation required to narrow the gap between their own and other neighborhoods' developmental trajectories, also narrowing the gap between EDI scores. Not only should this type of intervention be more acceptable than nannyism, but if local norms and local social facts are altered (as well as the material conditions and collective resources that support them), then in-migrants and subsequent generations would potentially benefit, making for sustainability—a radical proposition, Rose would say.

The prospect of implementing environmental or contextual interventions, rather than just individual-based ones, is doubly radical. Another of Rose's fundamental points was that we should examine entire population distributions rather than just those at "high risk," since it is the average rate that is of import, not the extremes of the distribution. Rose (1992) observed that when a risk factor is normally distributed within a population, lowering everyone's risk even by a modest amount has a greater overall effect than changing the risk profiles of only those at high risk. Change comes about by influencing entire populations and the conditions to which these populations are exposed. Community interventions therefore, may have more of an impact on population change than individual-level interventions.

What both Rose and Durkheim have suggested to us is that something about the social environment—that is, the ways that people act and interact in the places they live, work, and grow up—influence behaviors and, ultimately, disease rates. This basic idea has been taken up in the population health literature in the past decade under the rubric of location and health.

Generalizability and Paradoxes of Place

The ability to investigate the independent effects of place depends crucially on being able to identify, define, and characterize places in ways that are, first, consistent with theoretical links between socioeconomic environments and health and, second, geographically sensitive and robust. This is problematic for both practical and conceptual reasons.

Practical Challenges in Studying Place

From a practical standpoint, researchers are often constrained in their research by the geographic boundaries used by census agencies or other producers of aggregate data (such as government agencies). This constraint can pose difficulties because the data may not be at the correct scale for the questions being asked, or the researcher may want to characterize places using aggregate data from different policy sectors (e.g., crime, education, health, voting, census) to ask questions about the broad determinants of health, only to find that different agencies use different boundaries, even if they happen to aggregate to a similar scale.

What can be done about these problems? Relatively little, unfortunately, from a strictly quantitative perspective. As Willms (2001) has argued, any definition of *community* is open to attack. That said, the questions that need to be addressed in the study of the effects of location, contexts, and places on health can proceed, albeit with these and a few other more philosophical caveats in mind.

One important way that researchers could improve their practices in this kind of work is to spend more time and effort "ground truthing" their large-scale empirical observations about places from secondary data, as well as conducting research from the opposite direction: from the ground up. Although census data and other secondary data sources allow us to make standardized observations about the character of individual places, these are blunt instruments that also conceal a great deal of information about actual practices and relations relevant to the social production of health in specific places. These observations may be crucial in the causal pathway between the characteristics of a place and health, but they may not be generalizable across all times and all places.

Frohlich and colleagues (2002a, 2002b) encountered just this issue in their study of the role of neighborhood social norms on smoking initiation among youth. They found a pattern of significant correlations between socioeconomic disadvantage and smoking-encouraging resources (agents selling tobacco, restricting/permitting smoking in public places, providing information discouraging smoking, etc.) across thirty-two areas in Québec, Canada. Focus group discussions with youths from these same areas, however, revealed that social practices of people within the neighborhoods did not necessarily reflect the "objectified" measures of social structure; that is, despite some neighborhoods being socioeconomically advantaged and having few measurable smoking-encouraging resources, youths in these areas described rampant smoking practices. The ironic lesson from this study is that interventions based on generalized causal mechanisms will not function similarly in every location. Instead, the general principle is that interventions should be tailored to local variations in social practices and social relations.

Conceptual Challenges in Studying Place

The key conceptual problem for place and health research just described—that is, the limited appropriateness of local interventions based on generalizing causal mechanisms—resonates with one of the central dilemmas of geographical theory and methodology. Geographers, perhaps more so than other social scientists, have been routinely thwarted in their attempts to specify general theories, explanations, and laws that apply at all times and all places—perhaps rightly so. As Harvey (1993, 5) observed, "The incorporation of space into social theory, of whatever sort, always seemed to disrupt its power. The innumerable contingencies, specificities and 'othernesses' which geographers encountered could be (and often were) regarded by geographers as fundamentally undermining . . . of all forms of social scientific metatheory."

If one adopts a particularly cautious perspective, in other words, it is impossible to say anything about "places in general" or to generalize across places at all. Harvey (1993, 5) further argued:

> The inference, of course, is that geography is not open to universal theory and is the realm of specificity and particularity. My own view, however, is that while too much can be made of the universal at the expense of understanding particularity, there is no sense in blindly cantering off into the other direction into that opaque world of supposedly unfathomable differences in which geographers have for so long wallowed. The problem is to rewrite the metatheory, to specify dialectical processes in time-space, rather than abandon the whole project.

The approach that Harvey alludes to requires more of a very different kind of empirical work from that which has become popular in social epidemiology and population health and a substantial enhancement of what passes for explanation in social epidemiology (Sayer 1992).

Although several researchers (Lochner, Kawachi, and Kennedy 1999; Caughy, O'Campo, and Patterson 2001; Sampson 1991; Cohen, Spear, and Scribner 2000) have recently sought, quite wisely, to develop better methods for characterizing places, with the methods they have been using, these attempts *could not* reach the explanatory heights Harvey suggested—that is, to "specify dialectical processes in time-space." Take, for example, the paper by Cohen, Spear, and Scribner (2000), which examined the relationship between what the authors called "community disorder" and gonorrhea rates in New Orleans neighborhoods. These researchers created a "broken window" index, reflecting neighborhood deterioration, by combining information regarding the sum of the percentage of homes with structural damage; the percentage of streets with trash, abandoned cars, and graffiti; and the number of physical problems in high schools. Their index showed a strong association (by neighborhood) with gonorrhea rates (R^2 = .42). They briefly examined three possible explanations for their findings: individuals with high-risk behaviors might have clustered in deteriorated neighborhoods, deteriorated environments might have encouraged high-risk behavior, or these two explanations might have been mutually reinforcing. Results from this study raise the crucial issue that disease outcomes are not purely individually determined but, rather, that some aspect of the environment surrounding individuals—be it the physical or the social environment—influences individuals' health status. These insights are again very much in line with Rose's reasoning. That said, the measures used are abstractions from specific places, and without recontextualizing them, in the end we are left with relatively little understanding of what it is about neighborhoods with broken windows that could have *produced* higher rates of gonorrhea (i.e., the causal pathways).

But although some devices for characterizing places rightly attempt to break out of the problem of using compositional (i.e., census) data to characterize contexts by proposing "true" contextual effects, each of them also presupposes an implicit (and usually unstated) theoretical account of the way(s) in which a place or location may shape health. These implicit models need to be made explicit, and at the same time, researchers need to specify dialectical processes in time-space. This may involve the use of a concept such as the epidemiology of everyday life (Kaplan and Lynch 1997), but to date few serious attempts to do so have been made in social epidemiology. Breakthroughs in research on the health effects of place will likely require a more balanced mix of "extensive" (e.g., analyses of place characteristics drawn from large secondary databases) and "intensive" (e.g., analyses of actual place-bound social relations and practices in specific places by identifiable agents) research strategies (Sayer 1992). Use of more intensive research methods, although often slow and painstaking, is needed to develop robust measurements and explanations of contextual effects.

What Might the Underlying Contextual-level Effects Be?

Macintyre and other researchers at the Medical Research Council (MRC) Social and Public Health Sciences Unit in Glasgow, Scotland, have sought, by studying two pairs of socially contrasting localities in Glasgow, to characterize area-level factors that may shape health. They have argued that there is poorer provision of a range of "opportunity structures" such as physical recreation facilities, primary care, public transport, and retail food outlets in more deprived areas (Macintyre and Ellaway 1998), which may largely account for the increased rates of poor-health behaviors in these areas. Macintyre (2000) has shown that these opportunity structures may follow a pattern of "deprivation amplification." In the case of physical activity, for instance, they have found that in addition to more deprived individuals in the more socially deprived area, there were fewer formal bowling greens, tennis courts, sports centers; fewer people had access to cars; public transport was less frequent; there were fewer safe, open green spaces for walking or jogging, or for children to play; children's playgrounds were less safe and attractive; and there were more threats to safety, which likely deterred people from using their neighborhood for outdoor activities. This lack of opportunity structures was associated with less physical activity among people in this neighborhood than in the more affluent area.

Recently, Frohlich and colleagues (2002a) explored opportunity structures in relation to the role of material resources on the prevalence of smoking initiation among eleven- to fourteen-year-olds in thirty-two communities across Québec, Canada. They devised a methodology to identify organizations in communities that, through their normal operations, facilitated the uptake, maintenance, or (in contrast) prevention of smoking. Examples of these organizations were stores and restaurants. Next, they developed an inventory of all the smoking-related resources that these organizations made available to local populations. Resources included nonsmoking areas, the selling of cigarettes, and so on. Using hierarchical linear modeling with individual sociodemographic variables at level 1 and the resource and organizational variables at level 2, the researchers found that, after controlling for the individual-level predictors of smoking initiation, 51% of the variance in the prevalence of community smoking initiation was explained by the community-level predictors. That said, the authors' intensive research showed a much more complex relationship between area SES, smoking-related contextual resources, and youth smoking initiation than would have been possible with secondary data on places. Their findings defied simple generalizations about the way that place-bound opportunity structures operate at all times and all places. This example shows that, when careful attention is paid to the construction of contextual variables, the explanatory power of place may be much greater than commonly recognized.

Many questions remain about the influence of place on adult health. First, would we expect that all such effects are mediated by health behaviors, or might there be more direct pathways? (See the discussion of the life of the hypothalamic-pituitary-adrenal axis in society in chapter 2 of this volume). Would we expect that the same place-level factors that shape health behaviors also shape health outcomes along direct pathways, independently of health behaviors, or are there some factors that work only directly and others only indirectly? How can we avoid, methodologically and conceptually, giving undue primacy to the influence of residential environments on adult health (as opposed to work environments, for example), while still recognizing their potential influence? In other words, could it be that locations and places make more of a difference to health for some people than others in some systematic way? Are people of lower SES more vulnerable to place effects than people of higher SES?

The Way Forward

Truly embracing an understanding of the ways in which places independently influence health and its antecedents, along with the implications of such an understanding, would lead to significant policy and practice shifts in population health. Populations would be seen not simply as aggregates of individuals whose behaviors and attributes are the most appropriate target of intervention but, instead, as social objects meaningfully situated in a specific historical and geographical context, with human behavior and experience seen as fundamentally shaped by that context.

At a conceptual level, such a view is all well and good, but what does it mean practically? To carry on the example of early child development, it might mean investments in public resources such as recreational programs and facilities or language-sensitive caregiver–child programs, supported by appropriate community development initiatives to build connections between services and potential recipients. In addition, it might mean changes in land development and urban planning policies to encourage mixed land-use patterns and mixed-income housing developments.

For other potential determinants of health, such as health behaviors, the adoption of a perspective that seeks to alter "collective lifestyles" while acknowledging the territoriality of such lifestyles (Frohlich, Corin, and Potvin 2001; Frohlich et al. 2002a) has considerable promise. For example, Frohlich and colleagues' study of neighborhood-level factors in smoking initiation among Quebec youth showed that socioeconomically disadvantaged communities had a local community structure that facilitated the acquisition of cigarettes and norms around smoking (Frohlich et al. 2002b).

For health outcomes that may be primarily the result of lifelong cumulative disadvantage and stress, yet a different set of population-based interventions may be called for. The provision of affordable resources (e.g., public transit, time-flexible child and elder care, affordable housing, planned mixed-income neighborhoods) to reduce the stresses of everyday life is one approach. Mixed-income and land-use community planning have the further benefit that they may provide socioeconomically disadvantaged individuals with connections to individuals of local and extralocal influence (for finding jobs, acquiring resources, and attracting public services and facilities). Moreover, such environments may help to narrow socioeconomic disparities in early child development, since they provide children from socioeconomically disadvantaged families with a standard peer group with higher cognitive, language and physical abilities. In this way, the attributes of successful childhood from higher-SES children can be passed on to lower-SES children with no transaction costs.

Actions to redress these issues from a population-based public policy have a very large potential public health impact, one that likely exceeds the possibilities of an individual-based approach. Regrettably, the promise of such approaches is hampered by the dominance of individualistic approaches embodied in finely targeted programs and the overall societal discourse of individualism. Leaders in public health, however, should be undaunted by such obstacles and should continue to articulate, evaluate, and practice a geographically informed, population-based approach.

Notes

1. See http://www.cia.gov.
2. The West of Scotland 07 study is a twenty-year study of the social processes producing or maintaining in health by key social positions, like social class, gender, area of residence, age, ethnicity, and family composition. A highly innovative component of the study involves intensive investigation of two pairs of socially contrasting neighborhoods in greater Glasgow, with a focus on differences in the opportunity structures for good health in each. Specific attributes of these places, such as the availability of recreational facilities, affordability and availability of a healthy food basket, social capital/cohesion, and neighborhood reputation have been systematically analyzed for their relationship to relevant health outcomes. See Macintyre 2000; Macintyre and Ellaway 1998; and Macintyre, Maciver, and Sooman 1993 for details.
3. The EDI measures "readiness to learn" among children entering their first formal schooling in kindergarten (usually at age five).
4. Household income was estimated by using median income for the Census of Canada enumeration area in which the child lived as a proxy for the child's household income. Previous studies had shown this to be robust (Mustard et al. 1999).
5. Urban land markets, in short, are very effective sociospatial sorting mechanisms. Through largely informal sorting processes, they tend to sort people of similar SES into similar parts of the city. Assisted by urban planning practices and the extant built environment, this sorting is an enduring feature of industrial cities (Dunn 2000; Badcock 1984; Engels [1844] 1952).

References

Badcock, B. 1984. *Unfairly Structured Cities.* Oxford: Basil Blackwell.
Barnett, E., M. L. Casper, J. A. Halverson, G. A. Elmes, V. E. Braham, Z. A. Majeed, A. S. Bloom, and S. Stanley. 2001. *Men and Heart Disease: An Atlas of Racial and Ethnic Disparities in Mortality.* Morgantown, WV: Office for Social Environment and Health Research, West Virginia University and Centers for Disease Control and Prevention.
Blaxter, M. 1990. *Health and Lifestyles.* London: Routledge.
Boyle, M., and E. Lipman. 1998. *Do Places Matter? A Multilevel Analysis of Geographic Variations in Child Behavior in Canada.* Report no. W-98-16E. Ottawa: Human Resources Development Canada.
Brooks-Gunn, J., G. J. Duncan, P. K. Klebanov, and N. Sealand. 1993. Do neighborhoods influence child and adolescent development? *American Journal of Sociology* 99:353–395.
Caitlin, G. E. G. 1964. Introduction to *The Rules of Sociological Method,* by E. Durkheim. 8th ed. New York: Free Press.

Caughy, M. O., P. J. O'Campo, and C. Muntaner. 2003. When being alone might be better: Neighborhood poverty, social capital, and child mental health. *Social Science and Medicine* 57:227–237.

Caughy, M. O., P. J. O'Campo, and J. Patterson. 2001. A brief observational measure for urban neighbourhoods. *Health and Place* 7:225–236.

Chase-Lansdale, P. L., and J. Brooks-Gunn, eds. 1994. *Escape from Poverty: What Makes a Difference for Poor Children?* New York: Cambridge University Press.

Chase-Lansdale, P. L., R. A. Gordon, J. Brooks-Gunn, and P. K. Klebanov. 1997. Neighborhood and family influences on the intellectual and behavioral competence of preschool and school-age children. In *Neighborhood Poverty*. Vol. 1, ed. J. Brooks-Gunn, G. J. Duncan, and J. L. Aber. New York: Russell Sage Foundation.

Cohen, D., S. Spear, and R. Scribner. 2000. Broken windows and the risk of gonorrhea. *American Journal of Public Health* 90:230–236.

Cubbin, C., F. B. LeClere, and G. S. Smith. 2000. Socioeconomic status and injury mortality: Individual and neighborhood determinants. *Journal of Epidemiology and Community Health* 54:517–524.

Curtis, L. J., M. D. Dooley, and S. A. Phipps. 2004. Child well-being and neighbourhood quality: Evidence from the National Longitudinal Survey of Children and Youth. *Social Science and Medicine* 58:1917–1927.

Diez-Roux, A. V., S. Merkin, D. Arnett, L. Chambless, M. Massing, F. J. Nieto, P. Sorlie, M. Szklo, H. A. Tyroler, and R. L. Watson. 2001. Neighborhood of residence and incidence of coronary heart disease. *New England Journal of Medicine* 345:99–106.

Dooley, M. D., L. Curtis, E. Lipman, and D. Feeny. 1998. Child behaviour problems, poor school performance and social problems: The roles of family structure and low income in cycle one of the National Longitudinal Survey of Children and Youth. In *Labour Markets, Social Institutions, and the Future of Canada's Children*, ed. M. Corak. Ottawa: Statistics Canada.

Dooley, M. D., and E. Lipman. 1996. Child psychiatric disorders and poor school performance: The roles of family type, maternal market work and low income. In *Towards the 21st Century: Emerging Sociodemographic Trends and Policy Issues in Canada*. Ottawa: Proceedings of a symposium of the Federation of Canadian Demographers.

Duncan, C., K. Jones, and G. Moon. 1996. Health-related behaviour in context: A multilevel modeling approach. *Social Science and Medicine* 42:817–830.

———. 1999. Smoking and deprivation: Are there neighbourhood effects? *Social Science and Medicine* 48:497–505.

Dunn, J. R. 2000. Housing and health inequalities: Review and prospects for research. *Housing Studies* 15:341–366.

Durkheim, E. 1938. *The Rules of Sociological Method*. Chicago: University of Chicago Press. 1964 edition.

———. 1951. *Suicide: A Study in Sociology*. Translated by J. A. Spaulding and G. Simpson. New York: Free Press.

Egolf, B., J. Lasker, S. Wolf, and L. Potvin. 1992. The Roseto effect: A 50-year comparison of mortality rates. *American Journal of Public Health* 82:1089–1092.

Engels, F. [1844] 1952. [*The Condition of the Working Class in England in 1844.*] Translated by F. Wischnewtzky. London: Allen and Unwin.

Evans, R. G., M. L. Barer, and T. R. Marmor. 1994. *Why Are Some People Healthy and Others Not? The Determinants of Health of Populations*. New York: Aldine de Gruyter.

Frohlich, K. L., E. Corin, and L. Potvin. 2001. A theoretical proposal for the relationship between context and disease. *Sociology of Health and Illness* 23:776–797.

Frohlich, K. L., L. Potvin, P. Chabot, and E. Corin. 2002a. A theoretical and empirical analysis of context: Neighbourhoods, smoking and youth. *Social Science and Medicine* 54:1401–1417.

Frohlich, K. L., L. Potvin, L. Gauvin, and P. Chabot. 2002b. Youth smoking initiation: Disentangling context from composition. *Health and Place* 8:155–166.

Haan, M., G. A. Kaplan, and T. Camacho. 1987. Poverty and health: Prospective evidence from the Alameda County Study. *American Journal of Epidemiology* 125:989–998.

Harvey, D. 1993. From space to place and back again: Reflections on the condition of postmodernity. In *Mapping the Futures*, ed. J. Bird, B. Curtis, T. Putnam, G. Robertson, and L. Tickner. New York: Routledge.

Hertzman, C., S. McLean, D. Kohen, J. R. Dunn, and T. Evans. 2002. *Early Development in Vancouver: Report of the Community Asset Mapping Project (CAMP)*. Vancouver, BC: Human Early Learning Partnership, University of British Columbia.

Janus, M. 2002. *Validation of the Early Development Instrument in a Sample of First Nations' Children*. Toronto: Canadian Centre for Studies of Children at Risk.

Johnston, R. J., D. Gregory, G. Pratt, and M. Watts, eds. 2000. *The Dictionary of Human Geography*. Oxford: Blackwell Publishers.

Kaplan, G., and J. Lynch. 1997. Editorial: Whither studies on the socioeconomic foundations of population health? *American Journal of Public Health* 87:1409–1411.

Kohen, D., C. Hertzman, and J. Brooks-Gunn. 1998. *Neighbourhood influences on children's school readiness*. Report no. W-98-15E. Ottawa: Human Resources Development Canada.

———. 2001. *Family socio-economic indicators and behavioural readiness to learn*. Ottawa: Human Resources Development Canada.

Lochner, K., I. Kawachi, and B. P. Kennedy. 1999. Social capital: A guide to its measurement. *Health and Place* 5:259–270.

Macintyre, S. 2000. The social patterning of exercise behaviours: The role of personal and local resources. *British Journal of Sports Medicine* 34(1):6.

Macintyre, S., and A. Ellaway. 1998. Social and local variations in the use of urban neighbourhoods: A case study in Glasgow. *Health and Place* 4:91–94.

Macintyre, S., S. Maciver, and A. Sooman. 1993. Area, class and health: Should we be focusing on places or people? *Journal of Social Policy* 22:213–234.

Marmot, M. G. 2001. Editorial: Inequalities in health. *New England Journal of Medicine* 345:134–136.

Marmot, M. G., and J. F. Mustard. 1994. Coronary heart disease from a population perspective. In *Why Are Some People Healthy and Others Not? The Determinants of Health of Populations*, ed. R. G. Evans, M. L. Barer, and T. R. Marmor, 189–214. New York: Aldine de Gruyter.

Mayer, S. E., and C. Jencks. 1989. Growing up in poor neighborhoods: How much does it matter? *Science* 243:1441–1445.

McCord, C., and H. P. Freeman. 1990. Excess mortality in Harlem. *New England Journal of Medicine* 322:173–177.

Molnar, B. E., S. L. Gortmaker, F. C. Bull, and S. L. Buka. 2004. Unsafe to play? Neighborhood disorder and lack of safety predict reduced physical activity among urban children and adolescents. *American Journal of Health Promotion* 18:378–386.

Mustard, C. A., S. Derksen, J.-M. Berthelot, and M. Wolfson. 1999. Assessing ecologic proxies for household income: A comparison of household and neighbourhood level income measures in the study of population health status. *Health and Place* 5:157–171.

O'Campo, P. 2003. Invited commentary: Advancing theory and methods for multilevel models of residential neighborhoods and health. *American Journal of Epidemiology* 157:9–13.

Phillimore, P., P. Townsend, and A. Beattie. 1988. *Health and Deprivation: Inequality and the North*. London: Croom Helm.

Pickett, K. E., and M. Pearl. 2001. Multilevel analyses of neighborhood socioeconomic context and health outcomes: A critical review. *Journal of Epidemiology and Community Health* 55:111–122.

Roosa, M. W., S. Jones, J. Y. Tein, and W. Cree. 2003. Prevention science and neighborhood influences on low-income children's development: theoretical and methodological issues. *American Journal of Community Psychology* 31 (1–2):55–72.

Rose, G. 1985. Sick individuals and sick populations. *International Journal of Epidemiology* 14:32–38.

———. 1992. *The Strategy of Preventive Medicine*. Oxford: Oxford University Press.

Saelens, B. E., J. F. Sallis, J. B. Black, and D. Chen. 2003. Neighborhood-based differences in physical activity: An environment scale evaluation. *American Journal of Public Health* 93:1552–1558.

Sampson, R. J. 1991. Linking the micro- and macro-level dimensions of community social organization. *Social Forces* 70 (1):43–64.

Sayer, A. 1992. *Method in Social Science: A Realist Approach*. 2nd ed. London: Routledge.

Schwartz, S., and A. V. Diez-Roux. 2001. Commentary: Causes of incidence and causes of cases—a Durkheimian perspective on Rose. *International Journal of Epidemiology* 30:435–439.

Sen, A. 1993. The economics of life and death. *Scientific American* 268:40–47.

Statistics Canada. 2002. *How Healthy Are Canadians? Annual Report 2002*. Ottawa: Statistics Canada and the Canadian Institute for Health Information (CIHI).

Syme, S. L., and K. L. Frohlich. 2002. The contribution of social epidemiology: Ten new books. *Epidemiology* 13:110–112

Tremblay, S., N. A. Ross, and J.-M. Berthelot. 2001. Individual and community factors affecting grade three academic performance: A multi-level analysis. *Education Quarterly Review* 7 (4):25–36.

Van Os, J., G. Driessen, N. Gunther, and P. Delespaul. 2000. Neighbourhood variation in incidence of schizophrenia. *British Journal of Psychiatry* 176:243–248.

Wilkinson, R. G. 1996. *Unhealthy Societies: The Afflictions of Inequality*. New York: Routledge.

Willms, J. D. 2001. Three hypotheses about community effects on social outcomes. *ISUMA: Canadian Journal of Policy Research* 2 (1):53–62.

Wolf, S., and J. G. Bruhn. 1993. *The Power of Clan: The Influence of Human Relationships on Heart Disease*. New Brunswick, NJ: Transaction Publishers.

Wolf, S., K. L. Grace, J. Bruhn, and C. Stout. 1973. Roseto revisited: Further data on the incidence of myocardial infarction in Roseto and neighboring Pennsylvania communities. *Transactions of the American Clinical and Climatological Association* 85:100–108.

World Health Organization. 2000. *The World Health Report: Health Systems: Improving Performance*. Geneva: WHO.

Part III

Moving from
Research to Policy

Chapter 10

Social Welfare Models, Labor Markets, and Health Outcomes

Joachim Vogel and Töres Theorell

Both theory and research have suggested that the degree and level of income inequality influence the distribution of health outcomes. Standard economic theory posits that as income increases, there are decreasing marginal returns to health. This assumption implies that raising the income of the poor (at the expense of the rich) will raise average health status, because the improvement in the health of persons at the low end of the income scale, where the returns to a dollar more of income are great, will exceed the reduction in health status among those at the top end of the income scale, where changes in income have smaller effects on health. This theory predicts that at a given level of economic development, the average quality of health will be higher in societies with a narrower range of incomes, all other things being equal (Kawachi 2000). Although not completely consistent in their findings, studies involving data from a range of countries and a variety of methods have provided evidence to support this theory. Studies have shown that income inequality influences several health outcomes, including life expectancy, infant mortality, and average health status. (For a detailed discussion of these studies, see Subramanian and Kawachi 2003.)

The potentially strong link between income inequality and health—and the evidence that globalization is contributing to the increasing income inequalities both between and within countries—suggests the critical importance to public health of addressing the inequalities in material living standards. Of course, many different institutions and methods are used to address such inequalities. Some countries (such as Sweden and Finland) depend on a primarily public sector model, whereby the government uses tax and transfer programs to take responsibility more directly for how income is distributed. At the other end of the spectrum are countries (such as Italy and Spain) in which individual, family, and community norms and actions modify the initial income distribution. Still others (such as the United Kingdom and the United States) depend primarily on the labor market to serve as the vehicle for welfare distribution (although all nations depend on the labor market to some degree). However, all three factors—public policies, the labor market, and families—will likely play a role in any country, but the nature and strength of their roles will vary.

The nations belonging to the European Union (EU)[1] encompass several different configurations of labor market conditions, welfare state arrangements, and family arrangements. In this chapter, we refer to such configurations as welfare production models. The concept "welfare" refers in this chapter to the European usage of this term, focusing on general living conditions within a cluster of some ten social domains, in the tradition of the social indicator movement. The EU can therefore be seen as a natural laboratory for analysis of the link between welfare production strategies and the distribution of health. In this chapter, we explore the link between welfare production strategies and living conditions, focusing on health status. Since variations in wages and other forms of pay typically explain a large portion of the disparities in overall income both within and between countries (Galbraith et al. 1999), we pay close attention to the role of labor market arrangements and conditions. We compare institutional variation in two dimensions: between nations (EU nations) and in a specific time perspective (the Swedish case). We begin with a summary of the welfare production model perspective and describe the institutional arrangements among EU member states. In the second part of this chapter we examine health variations between clusters of EU member states, and we discuss a longitudinal analysis (spanning thirty-five years) of changes in health outcomes and in the labor market within Sweden. This nation is particularly interesting from the point of view of labor market changes that may affect public health, because dramatic structural changes have taken place in Sweden during the past decade.

A Regimes Model of Welfare Distribution

Recent empirical studies of welfare production (Vogel 1997, 1998a, 1998b, 1999) have built on the so-called regimes tradition (welfare state regimes, labor market regimes, gender regimes, family regimes), in a search for similarities and dissimilarities between nations with respect to institutional preconditions that shape the distribution of general living conditions. The regimes tradition, summarized by Vogel (1997, 1999), has been developed in and used as a basis for several studies (Castles and Mitchell 1992; Duncan 1995; Esping-Andersen 1990, 1996, 1999; Hirdman 1990; Lewis 1992; and Rubery, Fagan, and Smith 1994). The basic theoretical assumptions of the regimes approach to welfare production models are as follows. The three welfare delivery institutions—namely, the labor market (employers), the welfare state (politics), and the family (social networks)—represent a functional division of responsibility for welfare delivery. In various proportions, the overall distributive structure of any given society displays the imprint of each of the three institutions, reflecting the distributive principles central to the labor market (competition, competence), the welfare state (collective solidarity), and the family (reciprocity). The character of the distributive outcome (i.e., the level of inequality and the impact of social cleavages) should, according to the theory, correspond to the configuration of the three institutions in any given country. The division of responsibility, as well as the benefits provided by each of the three institutions, can be evaluated with respect to the welfare mix's efficiency in distributing living conditions and reducing poverty, social exclusion, and general inequality. (Definitions of poverty are considered later in this chapter.) The driving forces behind any given country's welfare mix are both external and internal factors, such as national resources, infrastructures, historical and ideological traditions, global competition, power relations, and ideological struggles. Hence, the welfare mix will differ between nations, evolve, and accommodate to economic changes and power relations.

According to the theoretical assumptions, the configuration of institutions, should, for analytical purposes, be reduced to a limited number of logical combinations, or welfare production models. In any such model, the labor market is likely to play the major role, since malfunctioning of the labor market will in theory exhaust both the welfare state and the family, whereas efficient labor markets (i.e., those offering adequate jobs and earnings) will relieve both the welfare state and the family. Conversely, the generous welfare state requires an efficient labor market (i.e., one providing full employment). Likewise, efficient labor markets promote emancipation from the family and, thus, financial independence. At the micro level, people will adapt to the available options within the welfare mix. Through coping behaviors, people can not only avoid poverty and social exclusion but also maximize their general living conditions. Coping behaviors can relate to the labor market (as with seeking jobs or training) and welfare state (as with adjusting to available transfers and services), as well as to the family (as with choosing if and when to leave the parental home, seek a partner, bear children, or separate from a partner).

Recent economic changes have involved major malfunctions of the welfare mix, related to the labor market (with global competition, mass unemployment, and job and wage instability), the welfare state (with recovery policies), and the family (with fragmentation), implying not only a changing institutional configuration but also decreased overall institutional efficiency in providing good and equal living conditions (See Vogel 2002a for a general discussion of these changes). Figure 10.1 contains a schematic model of welfare production that summarizes this regimes perspective.

Although consequences for health are not specified in the general model, the regimes tradition posits that institutional performance will influence the quality of life beyond economic and material living standards, including health status. Re-

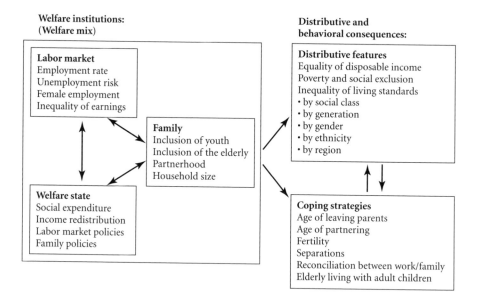

Figure 10.1. Welfare production model

gimes theory suggests that the effects on health may be both direct and indirect through mediating variables such as income, housing, material assets, economic security, job security, social networks, participation in collective organizations, leisure, education, and lifestyle. These hypothesized pathways are as follows. The welfare state provides correctives—in the form of both general and health-related public transfers and services—that directly or indirectly can affect public health. The family provides economic and social supports that can influence health. The labor market provides job opportunities and earnings, and accordingly, various levels of economic security, as well as a lifelong working environment, all of which can affect health. The model also posits that public health should be affected by quantitative, as well as qualitative, characteristics of the labor market. Employment levels and employment security (i.e., the risk of unemployment, the nature of job contracts, etc.) should affect health, as should physical and psychosocial job characteristics. Hence, public health should be influenced by the interplay of the three institutions, with working conditions acting as a mediating variable between the configuration and structure of institutions and the distribution of health outcomes. Applying the welfare regimes model, we thus posited, first, that differences in institutional configurations would be associated with public health differences between EU member states and, second, that the changing institutional performance in Sweden would be related to change in Swedish public health.

Applying the Regimes Model to the European Union and to Sweden

In our research, we have explored, from both comparative and longitudinal perspectives, the relationship between the configuration of the approaches to addressing income inequalities and health. Through the comparative approach, we have sought to identify similarities and dissimilarities between EU member states with respect to their institutional configurations and corresponding distributive outcomes. This approach provides a temporal account of the variation within the EU in the mid-1990s. Through the longitudinal approach, we have sought to capture change in institutional performance, plus the corresponding change in distributive outcomes.

In our research, we followed the Swedish case over two decades, for three reasons. First, the longitudinal approach—in particular, regarding the Swedish case—provides insights about globalization's long-term effects on institutional performance. Second, Sweden has a special role as a global forerunner moving toward a general expansion of the welfare state, an inclusive labor market (i.e., one characterized by active labor market policies, labor protection policies, income compensation transfers, job security legislation, etc.), and a general breakdown of traditional family bonds (see Vogel 2002a for a more detailed discussion). Third, Sweden is one of very few European countries that have amassed high-quality, comprehensive time-series data.

Data for Comparative and Longitudinal Analyses

The studies described here have been based on a large variety of data sources. First, we used data on general living conditions, labor market participation, and health that were gathered by the European Community Household Panel in 1994 (on twelve EU nations) and by three Nordic Social Surveys. The Swedish and Finnish surveys were conducted in 1994, and the Norwegian in 1991. The combined comparative database includes a sample of 143,000 adults (aged sixteen to eighty-four years) in fifteen countries. These data were collected through interviews by the statistical offices or other data-collecting agencies in the participating member states.

Second, we relied on a corresponding longitudinal Swedish database, the Annual Swedish Survey System of Living Conditions (Undersokningar av Levnads-Forhallanden [ULF]), which covered 1975 to 1995 and included a sample of 156,000 adults.[2] The ULF data were collected by Statistics Sweden, the national statistical institute or the Swedish Census Bureau, through mixed interview and register approach (see Vogel 2002a for a detailed presentation of the ULF system). These two databases thus allowed us to analyze the link between institutional performance and distributive outcomes through both comparative and longitudinal

perspectives. For comparative and longitudinal analyses of institutional characteristics, we also used other databases published by international and Swedish statistical institutes.

Results of the Comparative Analysis

Three Approaches to Welfare Production

Recent research using the regimes tradition focusing on the EU (Vogel 1997, 2003)
has revealed a clear clustering of nations in terms of institutional configuration, as
well as the equality of the distribution of various social indicators such as income
and poverty, housing conditions, consumption, assets, family formation, and health
across major social cleavages such as social class, gender, generation, family types,
region, and ethnicity. Specifically, we found the following:

- A Nordic cluster—representing institutional welfare state regimes and including Sweden, Denmark, Finland, and Norway—exhibited high employment and
  social expenditure but weak family ties, coupled with lower poverty rates and
  low levels of income inequality.
- A southern European cluster—representing family welfare regimes and including Italy, Spain, Greece, and Portugal—was characterized by low employment and social expenditure but strong traditional families, coupled with high
  poverty rates and high levels of income inequality.
- A central European cluster—representing intermediate welfare regimes and
  including Germany, France, Belgium, the Netherlands, Luxembourg, (i.e., the
  remaining EU nations)—had intermediate levels of employment, social expenditure, and family ties, coupled with intermediate rates of poverty and
  income inequality. The United Kingdom joined the southern cluster with high
  levels of income inequality and poverty.

Figure 10.2 demonstrates the institutional homogeneity within these three clusters of countries. The institutional configuration between labor market, welfare
state, and family is displayed by combining three central indicators pairwise for
the fifteen nations surveyed. The member states within each cluster exhibited about
the same welfare mix, with very few exceptions from this general pattern. As noted
in figure 10.2, we could order the nations by the labor force participation rate (as
a gauge of the labor market, using the labor force participation rate among fifteen-
to sixty-four-year-olds as of 1995) and social protection expenditure (as a gauge
of the welfare state, using the percentage of the gross domestic product represented
by the social protection expenditure). We identified three clusters along the north–
south axis, although exceptions to the general patterns existed. For example, among

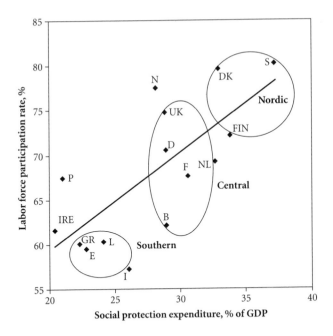

Figure 10.2. The interrelationship between labor market and welfare state in the European welfare mix

Legend: Nordic cluster = *DK*, Denmark; *FIN*, Finland; *N*, Norway; *S*, Sweden; *Central* cluster = *B*, Belgium; *F*, France; *D*, Germany; *IRE*, Ireland; *L*, Luxembourg; *NL*, Netherlands; *UK*, United Kingdom; *Southern* cluster = *SP*, Spain; *GR*, Greece; *I*, Italy; *P*, Portugal. This key applies to all remaining figures in this chapter.

nations in the southern European cluster, Portugal was an outlier regarding employment, and it belonged in this respect to the central cluster. Among nations in the Nordic cluster, Sweden and Finland were in a deep recession in the early 1990s, and the situation as of 1994, which the data under consideration referred to, was therefore not representative of their labor market performance and social protection expenditure over time. Around 1990, as well as again toward the end of the 1990s, both countries had much higher labor force levels and, accordingly, deviated much more sharply from countries in the other clusters (Vogel 1997).

Our analyses indicated how the labor force participation rate (as a measure of the labor market) was related to the traditional family index,[3] again displaying the same three largely homogenous clusters of similar welfare mixes. The outliers were Portugal, which has already been discussed, and Ireland, which seemed close to the southern cluster regarding female employment and the role of the traditional family. The Netherlands was close to the Nordic cluster with respect to family formation. Finally, we ordered the nations by social protection expenditure (welfare state) versus the traditional family index (family). Again, the Netherlands ranked close to the Nordic cluster.

These findings underscore the functional relationship between the three welfare delivery institutions. The welfare state has had its largest impact in the Nordic cluster of countries. All of the Nordic cluster nations also have had the most efficient labor markets, meaning ones that contribute the most to the entire population's material welfare by providing jobs and earnings. Hence, the Nordic cluster nations have combined a generous welfare state with extensive labor market policies that have promoted full employment and equal opportunities. In fact, it is in the Nordic cluster nations that the labor market has played its most efficient role as a welfare delivery system. The labor market also has supported generous welfare state arrangements in the Nordic cluster countries, since it not only has widened the tax base but also has limited the need for social intervention. (Vogel 1997, 1998a, 1998b, 1999, 2000, 2002a, 2002b).

In our analyses, the Nordic and southern European clusters represented two poles in the way welfare was produced. All of the Nordic countries rated low on traditional family support. This finding can be interpreted as resulting from the strong welfare state and market, which open the opportunity for a pluralization of family forms (such as higher rates of singlehood and separations, early partnering, higher fertility rates, early exit from the parents' household). In the southern European cluster, the traditional family has represented the functional alternative when the market and the welfare state have failed to deliver basic living standards (Vogel 2002a).

Welfare Production Models and Distribution of Material Living Standards

Figures 10.3 and 10.4 illustrate the overall distributive outcomes of the three types of welfare production. We found that income inequality (fig. 10.3) and poverty (fig. 10.4) were related to a north–south clustering of nations. These data suggest that inequality and social exclusion are indeed associated with poor labor market and extensive welfare state performance. Other research has shown an association between welfare mix and the distribution of a variety of other social indicators (Vogel 1997, 2003).

We next examined data on social class inequality in which the general material living standards of manual workers were compared with those of upper-level non-manual employees, including managers and employers. On the basis of these data, we computed an inequality index (based on a group of eleven assets),[4] which involved comparing the average proportion in the two categories having these assets. The index was an extension of logistic regression analysis, also controlling for gender, generation, family structure, and region. Class inequality appeared to be the lowest in the Nordic cluster nations, which were characterized by inclusive labor markets and extensive social intervention. Class inequality was the highest in Portugal, the United Kingdom, Luxembourg, and Ireland. The remaining central European countries were in an intermediate position.

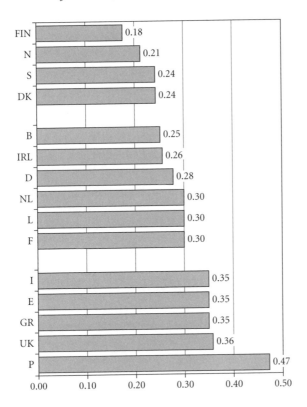

Figure 10.3. Inequality of equivalent disposable income (Gini coefficients) for persons aged 20–84 years

Source: Data from European Community Household Panel and Nordic Social Surveys, around 1994 (ECHP/NSS).

Welfare Production Models and Distribution of Health

As documented in the previous sections, considerable covariation existed between institutional performance and distributive outcome, with respect to material living conditions. In this section, we extend this analysis of European welfare regimes and distributive outcome by exploring health variations. As described earlier, the welfare production model posits that the level and variation in general living standards will also be reflected in health outcomes. In recent decades, northern Europe has developed toward lower levels of inequality in material living standards and, in particular, toward higher material standards for low-income citizens. Applying the welfare regimes perspective, we hypothesized that this trend should be reflected in higher average health status and lower morbidity, as well as lower socioeconomic differences in health status. In southern Europe the family has been a major provider of health care, but this situation may have increased health inequity, since differences in family income have not been buffered. In addition, the health care

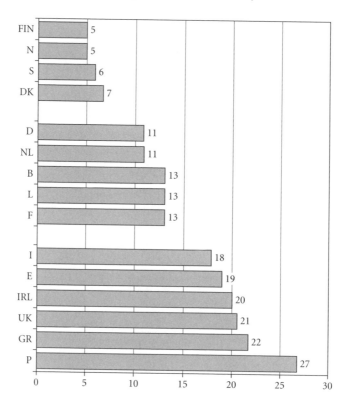

Figure 10.4. Poverty rates in the European Union, in percentages. Poverty limit = 50% of the national average equivalent disposable household income

Source: Data from European Community Household Panel and Nordic Social Surveys, around 1994 (ECHP/NSS).

system has been less extensive and the programs for disease prevention less advanced than in northern Europe. The western parts of the central European countries have occupied an intermediate position. Thus, we hypothesized that, with some exceptions for specific illnesses, higher morbidity and lower average health status, as well as higher levels of health inequity, would exist in the southern European countries. Thus, we also hypothesized that lower average health status and increasing socioeconomic health gaps would exist.

The measure of health status that we examined was morbidity, as measured by two standard questions in health surveys. The first question concerned the respondents' health in general (with six response categories, ranging from very good to very bad), and the other question was linked to daily activities ("Are you severely hampered in your daily activities by any chronic physical or mental health problem, illness, or disability?"). We recognize that these measures of public health status posed fundamental technical problems, in that both indicators had subjective elements and could have led to underestimation of disease and of socially defined health problems. For instance, subjects in chronic dialysis often reported good subjective health (Theorell et al. 1991). We acknowledge that these limitations likely affected the comparability of data between nations and between subgroups, as well as in trend analysis. The second indicator was probably more robust, since it tried to relate health to daily activities. (These issues are further discussed in Vogel 2002a, chapter 6.)

EUROPEAN WELFARE PRODUCTION MODELS AND VARIATIONS IN AVERAGE HEALTH STATUS

With regard to the question on which respondents rated their "general health," we first compared across countries the proportion who said "good" or "very good." The dominant geographical ranking of member states that had been found in relation to other welfare domains was not fully reproduced (fig. 10.5). Specifically, the southern European, central European, and Nordic countries were blended to an extent, but the Nordic countries as a group still tended to perform better (in this case, to reflect better self-reported general health) than those in the central

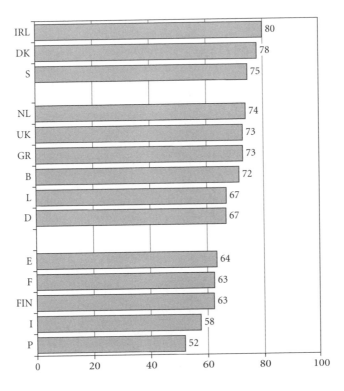

Figure 10.5. Self-ratings of health as *good,* in percentages

Source: Data from European Community Household Panel and Nordic Social Surveys, around 1994 (ECHP/NSS).

and southern European clusters. The Nordic countries of Denmark and Sweden, but not Finland, were located at the upper end, whereas the southern cluster countries were concentrated toward the lower end. However, the subjective elements involved in these ratings, as described earlier, may have influenced the results. Furthermore, a certain national cultural propensity toward taking a more or less positive (or pessimistic) attitude in general subjective ratings in surveys of this character may have existed. For instance, as a general observation, we noted that the Danish sample was overly positive on most subjective indicators measured in the European Community Household Panel (including self-rated health) and that the related results did not always correspond to the objective conditions registered for the same sample.

Using the same interview question, we next focused on the lower end of the distribution, that is, the proportions reporting that their general health was bad or very bad (fig. 10.6). The derived ranking of member states was, of course, similar to that for the previous indicator, but in this case the separation from the neutral categories (i.e., "in between" and "don't know") was more distinct. However, on

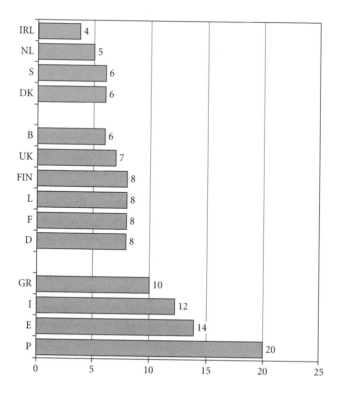

Figure 10.6. Self-ratings of health as *bad*, in percentages

Source: Data from European Community Household Panel and Nordic Social Surveys, around 1994 (ECHP/NSS).

these responses regarding poor health, we got a ranking much closer to the clustering of member states found for other social and economic indicators presented in this chapter and by Vogel (1997), particularly with respect to employment, welfare state provisions, income, poverty, and family structure. Again, all four nations in the southern European cluster (Portugal, Spain, Italy, and Greece) had distinctly higher proportions of people reporting that their health was bad than did the nations in the central European and Nordic clusters. As noted in figure 10.5, two of the Nordic cluster countries were among the nations with the highest percentages of respondents indicating good health. Finland fell out of the Nordic cluster in most classifications on morbidity and mortality, and this finding was probably attributable largely to food habits. The variation between nations on this indicator (i.e., bad general health) was large: whereas 20% of the Portuguese respondents indicated this, 4% of the Irish ones did.

From these analyses, we concluded that the notion of "bad health" used in the interviews was more robust in relation to subjective influences in the measurement process (than the notion of "good health") and that the distribution of health would best be evaluated by using the proportion who had rated their general health as bad.

EUROPEAN WELFARE PRODUCTION MODELS AND UNEQUAL DISTRIBUTION OF HEALTH STATUS

Figure 10.7 depicts the degree to which economic stress and health were found to be related across the different welfare production model clusters, specifically, in relation to poor households. To classify monetary poverty, or a poverty line, we identified those people who were living in a household with less than half of the average national disposable equivalent income. Thus, the poverty line was relative to the national context and varied between nations, and people living in these households represented the lowest part of the respective income structures. (For further discussion of the ways to define poverty, see Subramanian and Kawachi 2003.) We chose poor households for this analysis because poverty is an indicator that overarches other indicators of social exclusion, such as unemployment, poor social networks, poor education, or lower social class affiliation. The health indicator was the self-rated health question presented earlier, and we used, in this analysis, data from those respondents who indicated that their health was bad or very bad.

Figure 10.7 demonstrates again that the highest levels of health problems among the poor were found in the southern European cluster (Portugal, Italy, Spain, and Greece), whereas the lowest levels were found in Sweden, Denmark, and Finland (the Nordic cluster) and in Ireland, the Netherlands, and Belgium (the central European cluster). The fact that we found a clear clustering when we focused on health problems, instead of good health, supports the observation noted earlier that using this strategy yields more robust results.

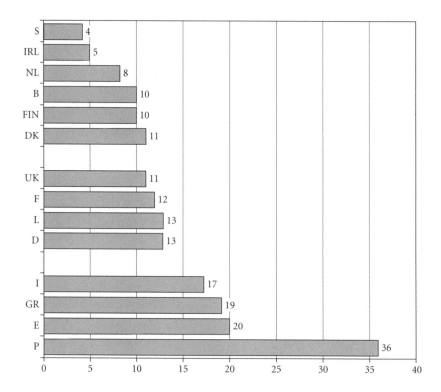

Figure 10.7. Self-ratings of health as *bad* among persons living in poor households, in percentages

Source: Data from European Community Household Panel and Nordic Social Surveys, around 1994 (ECHP/NSS).

We also compared the proportions of people who reported bad health in poor and in higher-income households (with higher income defined as households with more than 150% of the average equivalent disposable income, or three times the poverty line). We found that the variations within the southern European cluster were extreme, whereas the variations within the Nordic and central clusters were more limited. The health variation is rather limited among the rich everywhere, but the health variation between member states among the poor is rather large.

Our analysis of the patterns of variation, however, revealed extremely complex interrelationships. Social and economic exclusion and health were found to be interrelated, with causal links in both directions. Furthermore, the set of relevant processes and health determinants were likely to vary a great deal across member states. Health status was strongly related to age, which also was involved in processes of exclusion. For instance, poverty in Sweden was primarily a matter of early exit from the parents' household, which in Sweden normally occurred before the end of schooling and entry into the labor market around age twenty, whereas in Portugal and Greece it tended to be related to partnering and childbirth about five to ten years later (see Vogel 2003). In future investigations, researchers need to employ integrated and comparative databases and multivariate techniques to explore the causal background and to capture the diverse health determinants in the member states. And finally, health in itself could have influenced social and economic exclusion.

In summary, the results of the comparative analysis, although not altogether consistent, provided partial support for the claim that the configuration of welfare state, labor market, and family arrangements influences health status and morbidity. However, the picture that emerged from our research was not entirely clear. The variation of public health found in EU member states likely reflected not only differences in health-related determinants but also cultural factors and methodological problems related to the limited information gathered and the subjectivity in the measurement process.

Longitudinal Analysis: The Swedish Case

Although good comparative data linking welfare production to working conditions and health are limited, trend analysis in the Swedish case has many strengths because it is based on systematic and long-term data sources that contain coordinated microlevel information on general living conditions, working conditions, and health. To examine the data linking welfare production to working conditions and health in this case, we review, first, the evidence on Swedish institutional performance during the extreme recession of the 1990s, including globalization's general influences on working life, and, second, the long-term performance (from the 1960s through the 1990s) of the Swedish labor market and welfare state.

Recent Trends in Sweden's Labor Market and Their Health Impacts

Sweden can be characterized as a highly developed industrial economy and as a society that emphasizes the state as the key provider of social security and active labor market policies. As noted earlier, Sweden has had a special role over the past decades as a forerunner in the general expansion of the welfare state, promotion of an inclusive labor market, and movement toward a general breakdown of traditional family bonds.

Sweden differed from many other countries in the late 1980s, since Swedish social and labor market policies had, to some extent, protected the labor force from the social effects of work globalization. According to ULF national surveys of general living conditions (Vogel and Häll 1997), employees' personal decision-making authority (regarding the influence over the pace and planning of work) and intellectual discretion (i.e., whether the employee had "opportunities to learn new things at work") improved between 1975 (when the surveys began asking about the psychosocial work environment) and 1989. Decision-making authority and intellectual discretion were the cornerstones of the psychosocial work environment that were associated with improved health (Belkic et al. 2000; Karasek and Theorell 1990, Theorell 2004) in the 1970s and 1980s. The prevalence of psychological demands at work (rating work as "psychologically strenuous" and identifying feelings of being "rushed"), was relatively unchanged from 1975 to 1989; measures of these psychological demands increased slightly for women and evidenced no change for men. On balance, therefore, the psychosocial work environment appeared to improve during the 1970s and 1980s in Sweden. Swedish surveys have reported higher levels of democratic codetermination at work, union membership, and intrinsic work orientation (as opposed to instrumental work orientation) than have been found in other EU member states (Vogel 2003). Hence, in a longer time perspective, one would expect the Nordic model to produce environmental conditions—at work as well as outside of work—favorable to public health and, more specifically, workers' health.

However, in the late 1980s and early 1990s a series of events occurred that diminished this likelihood of protection. First, Sweden planned to enter the EU in the 1990s and, in fact, did so in 1996. In preparation for that shift, some of Sweden's financial policies and taxation systems had to be adjusted to fit with the EU's policies. A tax reform launched in 1991 created a huge budget deficit, which was remedied by broad recovery policies. The change in economic policies caused a dramatic decline in the employment rate: The proportion of unemployed increased from a steady level of 1% to 3% during the 1970s and 1980s to about 10% during the early 1990s. During the late 1990s, the unemployment rates again decreased but never returned to the pre-1990 levels. In addition, the proportion of temporarily employed workers increased steadily during the 1990s.

Recovery policies hit most of the public transfer systems and services during the 1980s and 1990s. For instance, governmental support of the occupational health care system (including the entities that monitored health, agencies that conducted surveys of psychosocial work environment and health outcomes, as well as medical and psychological health care) was withdrawn during the late 1980s. Since this support constituted 30% of the funding for occupational health care, this change markedly affected the subsequent development of occupational health care, and it led to both a decreased emphasis on prevention and psychosocial factors and a greater emphasis on conventional health care (Theorell 1999). Between 1993 and 1998, Sweden extensively consolidated the budget and, among other things, reduced the social protection expenditure from 37% to 33% of the gross domestic product. Through such actions, Sweden shifted from a 12.3% deficit to a 2.1% surplus during those five years (Scharpf 2000).

The health care and education systems, which had previously been financed almost entirely by taxes, were under constant debate in the 1990s. Some aspects of health care, particularly of primary care, became to some extent privatized, as did the medical care of elderly people. However, these were not the major consequences of the demands on increased effectiveness. The main effects were substantial downsizing—on average, by 20% of the staff in Swedish hospitals—and repeated reorganizations. Consequently, health personnel (and teachers), who previously had viewed their occupations as involving both high demands and high levels of decision-making latitude, more often perceived their jobs as straining ones involving high demands and limited decision-making latitude, compared with most other occupations (Arbetsmiljöverket 2000). Among health personnel, as well as teachers, symptoms related to anxiety and fatigue increased; for instance, the proportion of individuals who reported feeling "tired and listless" increased during 1993 and 1999 (Petterson and Arnetz 1998; Swedish National Board of Health and Social Security [SNBHSS] 2001). Many in health and education sought other jobs. The changes during these years have been further described by the Swedish Welfare Commission (Palme et al. 2003).

These same changes held true among women and youth in general. The proportion of individuals reporting "worry and anxiety" increased by 11% among women and by 8% among men aged 16 to 34 between 1988–1989 and 1998–1999. There was virtually no change in the corresponding proportion reporting these symptoms among men and women aged 65 to 84 (no change and a decrease of 3%, respectively) over the same time period. The proportion of individuals reporting a "sleep disturbance" increased by 8% in both men and women aged 16 to 34 and showed no change in men or women aged 65 to 84 over the same period (SNBHSS 2001). In fact, during the 1990s, decision-making authority declined for most Swedish employees, and particularly for female public sector employees (mainly health care employees) during the mid- and late 1990s (Arbetsmiljöverket 2001). Among individuals employed in the public sector at the county and community levels, the proportion of employees who reported having little opportunity to influence working conditions (a combined index based on a question regarding possibilities for influencing working hours, planning, and pacing of work) increased by 11% among both men and women. The proportion of individuals reporting few possibilities for influencing working conditions was particularly high among women working for counties (mainly health care staff). A parallel—though much smaller—change was seen in the private sector, where the proportion increased by 3% to 6%. At the same time, psychological demands, feelings of being rushed, and the number of hours at work increased (SNBHSS 2001).

STRUCTURAL CHANGES IN WORK AND CHANGES IN HEALTH
OUTCOMES: UNDERLYING FACTORS

Are there plausible biological mechanisms that would explain the connections between structural changes in work and changes in health outcomes? Demand–control theory posits that increasing demands and decreasing decision-making latitude would be associated with increasing levels of sleep disturbance and anxiety in the population and, as a consequence, increasing incidences of physiological disturbance, with rising blood pressures and long-lasting states of physiological exhaustion (Karasek and Theorell 1990; Belkic et al. 2000). When anxiety increases, and particularly if this change affects sleep, there are several physiological consequences, the two most important being that the ability to mobilize energy is disturbed and that the capacity to restore and repair worn-out cells and tissues (regeneration) is inhibited. Both of these consequences are important in the pathogenesis of several stress-related disorders such as metabolic syndrome (which is strongly related to an increased risk of developing cardiovascular disease) and myocardial infarction (Belkic et al. 2000, 2004). Research has also shown that these consequences likely are related to an inhibited capacity to recover after an acute episode of a musculoskeletal disorder such as low back pain (Hasselhorn et al. 2001). Thus, theory and research would predict that after experiencing long periods of downsizing, reorganization, and insecurity, workers would be more likely to develop serious conditions such as chronic fatigue syndrome and cardiovascular disease. If such increased problems were to occur, the use of long-term sick leave would also be hypothesized to increase.

Many of these hypotheses have, in fact, been investigated in Sweden. For example, burnout-related mental disorders have been discussed extensively in the Swedish mass media since the late 1990s (Barklöf 2000). Since that time, the rates of people taking long-term sick leave have increased dramatically. The prevalence of sick leave increased by 4% among men and 9% among women from 1996 to 1999 and has continued to increase. A parallel increase in the number of early retirements was observed up to 1998. These trends continued in 2000 and 2001 (SNBHSS 2001). The increase in long lasting episodes of sick leave during this period was particularly pronounced among subjects who reported low decision authority (Wikman 2004).

During the 1970s and 1980s, while the welfare state and the labor market were still effectively providing welfare delivery, the symptom levels of anxiety, tiredness, and sleep disturbance were relatively stable among Swedish adults. However, during the first half of the 1990s, these levels increased among both men and women by approximately 7% and 10%, respectively, and more so among younger than older people, as previously discussed (Vogel and Häll 1997). The proportion of subjects who reported symptoms caused by stress, psychological problems, or bullying at work increased steadily during the late 1990s (Arbetsmiljöverket 2001), from 3.6% to 6.6% among men and from 5.8% to 11.2% among women between 1996 and 2001.

However, data on morbidity and mortality have not shown dramatic increases since the 1990s. For example, the incidence of completed suicides has continued to decrease during this period, due in part to the increased clinical use of effective antidepressive medications, which has prevented many suicides (SNBHSS 2001).

As another example, the incidence of myocardial infarction has continued to de-crease since the 1990s. One potential explanation for this change is the effectiveness of smoking-cessation campaigns and other efforts in reducing smoking rates, par-ticularly among middle-aged men, who traditionally have had the highest incidence of myocardial infarction. Since smoking is one of the most important cardiovas-cular risk factors, the effects of decreased smoking in the population could, how-ever, conceal possible effects on cardiovascular illness risks caused by psychosocial factors. In addition, differences in cardiovascular mortality between European countries may be particularly hard to interpret (Kunst et al. 1999). The social pattern has been different in southern and northern European countries.

In summary, some of the hypotheses have been confirmed in the statistics. In particular, the mental health of the Swedish working population has been shown to have deteriorated since the beginning of the structural changes. However, actual health outcomes have not been shown to have been affected. It is possible that effects on mortality and morbidity take longer to develop than do effects on per-ceptions about health. As noted earlier, there may also be competing mechanisms that could conceal effects of labor market changes on myocardial infarction and suicide incidence, such as reduced cigarette smoking and greater use of effective antidepressive medications, respectively.

The health effects of the dramatic changes in Sweden's social situation are of interest to other countries, since the pronounced structural changes in the late 1980s and early 1990s rapidly pushed Sweden into some of the drawbacks of a global working world, such as increasing rates of temporary employment and more flexible employment contracts. The Swedish case could be regarded almost as a natural experiment. The surveys described earlier revealed that mental problems had increased substantially in some parts of the population affected by the changing institutional performance, especially health care personnel and teachers, plus younger men and women in general. The most pronounced deterioration was observed among female health care staff.

The serious consequences of these changes, including the increasing use of long-term sick leave, were not visible immediately but rather during the late 1990s and early 2000s. Accordingly, there may be social and physiological delay mechanisms of several years. Physiological changes were illustrated in a recent study of health care staff in a regional hospital. After the last downsizing and reorganization de-cision was made in 1998, a random sample of female staff were followed physio-logically during the year when they had to adapt to the situation. Researchers found evidence of an early stage physiological exhaustion and signs of immunological exhaustion (specifically, the lower blood concentration of immunoglobulin G); decreased protection against atherosclerosis (evidenced by the reduced content of protective cholesterol); and lowered concentrations of the female sex hormone estradiol, which is central to the body's regenerative capacity and ability to protect against the effects of stress (Hertting and Theorell 2002).

Long-term Changes in the Swedish Labor Market and Their Health Impacts

Our examination of the Swedish case from 1980 through 1998 points to the importance of the institutional context in determining the distribution of general living conditions, as well as health. Up to the 1980s there was a steady increase in employment and welfare state provisions (transfers and public services)—in short, a continuous expansion of the Nordic model. We suggest that the consequences affected public health both directly and indirectly, through influences on economic security, housing, access to material resources, and a sense of solidarity and trust in what might be labeled citizens' rights (as provided and guaranteed by the political system). In addition, up to the 1980s Sweden provided publicly financed health care and had in place labor protection legislation, as well as governmental transfers related to work absenteeism, health problems and conditions, and retirement. According to the theory and research described thus far, these policies, exercised over decades, should produce feelings of personal security, social support, personal independence, and general embeddedness and trust—which should, in theory, contribute to good health.

However, as noted earlier, the dramatic changes in the 1990s—with decreased employment, increased unemployment, and increased job and income insecurity—have reversed the long-term advancement of contributions from both the labor market and the welfare state, thereby affecting public health in different ways. Various data sources have shed light on the health-related effects. For example, trend analysis of public health has been part of the regular social reporting program of Statistics Sweden, which is based on the ULF survey system that has been conducted annually since 1974 (Vogel and Häll 1997). The ULF system also includes a large annual health survey module, a standard element in a larger survey instrument. (See Vogel 2002b for more details on the ULF and the health module.)

HEALTH-RELATED TREND ANALYSIS

Vogel and colleagues (2000) conducted a trend analysis using a recent report that had compared cross-sections from the pooled data (for a total sample size of 60,000) yielded by eight annual ULF surveys (1980–1983 and 1994–1997). The partial findings, based on a more limited set of health indicators than those analyzed overall, are presented in figure 10.8. The method involved a logistic regression analysis, with age (in five-year groups), gender, social class, family type, and region as independent variables. For this chapter, we are interpreting Swedish health variations and health trends with reference to the changes in aspects of the welfare mix, particularly regarding the demand and opportunity structure offered by the labor market.

First, we examined the change in self-rated health problems over fourteen years within five-year age groups. Overall, self-rated health problems decreased after age sixty-five (possibly due to reduced stress at normal retirement age), whereas a new

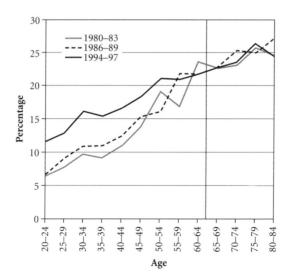

Figure 10.8. Insomnia in Sweden, by period and age (controlled for sex, social class, family type, and region), in percentages

Source: Data from Undersökningen av Levnadsförhållanden (Swedish Survey of Living Conditions; ULF).

rise in health problems was found after age seventy-five (possibly due to the effects of biological aging). Since the early 1980s, there was a general decrease in the rate of health problems among people aged fifty or older. This decrease could have been due to many influences, including improved health technology, improved working environments, and earlier ages for retirement. On the other hand, among those thirty-five or younger, an increase in health problems had occurred since the early 1980s. Although no causal relationship was demonstrated, these findings are consistent with our hypotheses regarding the role of the labor market regimes that would predict an increase in health problems among workers due to the changing demand structure related to the labor market, including delayed labor market entry, increased job stress, and insecurity of employment and income since the 1980s as indicated by Swedish Labor Force and general ULF surveys. Sweden experienced an extraordinary and dramatic decline of employment (by 15%) and a fourfold increase in unemployment rates between 1991 and 1994, which primarily hit the youngest workers (Vogel 2000, 2002a, 2003). Similar trends were recorded for a larger set of morbidity indicators applied in Statistics Sweden's annual health survey measurement, and many of those related to psychosomatic stress. For example, detailed analysis revealed that young adults reported the highest insomnia rates (see fig. 10.8).

Figure 10.9 reflects our analysis of the data for men and women. Younger women reported a larger increase in health problems than did younger men. In midlife, men reported larger improvements in health than did women. Although other

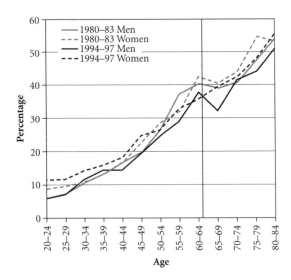

Figure 10.9. Self-rated health problems in Sweden, by period, age, and sex (controlled for social class, family, and region), in percentages

Source: Data from Undersökningen av Levnadsförhållanden (Swedish Survey of Living Conditions; ULF).

explanations cannot be ruled out, this finding could be explained by the changing demand structure that women have been facing during recent decades, including increased employment rates.

Figure 10.10, comparing data for manual workers with those for intermediate- and upper-level nonmanual professionals, shows that health problems came earlier in life for manual workers. Young adults aged twenty to forty-five in both social classes (i.e., as proxied by manual and nonmanual work) had experienced losses, whereas the adults aged fifty-five and older had experienced a decrease in health problems. Health improvements were particularly large among manual workers in retirement age (after age sixty-five). Again, while there are many plausible explanations for these findings, they are consistent with our hypotheses predicting that the long-term humanization of working conditions reflected in ULF time-series data on job conditions over three decades would produce health improvements among older workers. Among the oldest age groups, biological aging catches up and reduces health variations between social classes.

Finally, we compared the health problems reported for single persons and for pairs. In addition to the underlying trends already addressed, we found clear differences between singles and couples. For all age groups, except the oldest (i.e., those approximately eighty or older), we found higher levels of reported health problems among single persons, suggesting either that partnerhood improved health or that health problems were an impediment to partnerhood. The trends

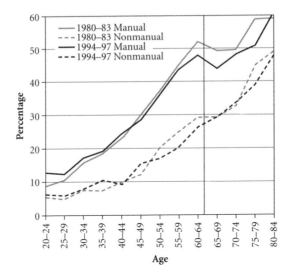

Figure 10.10. Self-rated health problems in Sweden, by period, age, and social class (controlled for sex, family, and region), in percentages

Source: Data from Undersökningen av Levnadsförhållanden (Swedish Survey of Living Conditions; ULF).

for younger persons in the age range before partnering would normally have been completed (thirty to forty) were especially interesting. In particular, we found a clear increase in health problems among singles in this age group, which should indicate increased stress related to the partnering process, including sorting, increased competition, increased separation rates, and higher rates of singlehood.

Our next analysis concerned long-term illness that had reduced the working capacity of workers in their then-current jobs or, for retirees, in their daily activities. This measure was more likely to have reflected the impact of increased job demands on health. The analysis revealed a more distinct picture of an increase in health problems using this indicator. Furthermore, the health improvement reflected by this indicator was found to be more marked after retirement age. Although it was not possible with these analyses to draw conclusions regarding explanations for these trends, we hypothesized that these findings reflected the role of job demands that increased during the mid-1990s, according to ULF time-series data, and that disappeared at retirement. The findings shown in figure 10.11—the increase in long-standing illness for women—were also hypothesized to be reflecting the special changes in women's labor market experiences between the 1980s and 1990s: increased employment rates and working hours among women, in addition to the increased job demands of the 1990s, as indicated by Swedish Labour Force Surveys and general ULF surveys. Figure 10.12 reveals an increase in health problems among pre–retirement-age manual workers. However, after retirement,

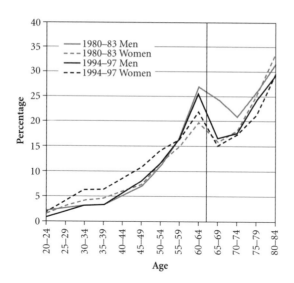

Figure 10.11. Long-standing illness with reduced working capacity in Sweden, by period, age, and sex (controlled for social class, family, and region), in percentages

Source: Data from Undersökningen av Levnadsförhållanden (Swedish Survey of Living Conditions; ULF).

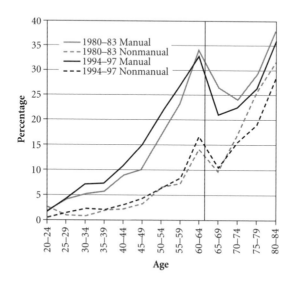

Figure 10.12. Long-standing illness with reduced working capacity in Sweden, by period, age, and social class (controlled for sex, family, and region), in percentages

Source: Data from Undersökningen av Levnadsförhållanden (Swedish Survey of Living Conditions; ULF).

manual workers to a greater degree reported marked improvements in their health, according to this indicator. We found similar, though much weaker, trends for nonmanual workers. Finally, for this indicator we also found the same trends as for health problems.

Conclusions and Recommendations

The configuration of a nation's welfare mix is likely influenced by many factors, including national resources, historical notions about the role of family and government, the distribution of political power, and economic conditions. As major changes in any one of these factors occur, the welfare mix will accommodate. In the 1990s, economic changes—including rising global competition and integration, mass unemployment, and job and wage flexibility—caused many European countries to make major shifts in how they addressed poverty and inequalities in living conditions through their institutional configurations and their overall institutional efficiency (see Subramanian and Kawachi 2003). Given the growing body of evidence suggesting that inequalities in living standards also have important public health impacts, it is critical to understand how and to what degree variations in the strategies used to address income inequalities influence health status.

Comparisons between European states regarding strategies to address inequalities in the distribution of general living standards and their impact on health could be performed in many ways. Comparative studies of morbidity using representative samples of the populations are expensive and technically demanding. Questionnaire studies of self-rated health are difficult to interpret because of differences in verbal formulations and in the culturally determined meaning of words, differences in access to health care (which may influence the participants' awareness of symptomatic medical conditions and reports of specific diagnoses), and differences in insurance systems and social security regulation.

We have surveyed health variations against the background of variations in welfare production strategies, focusing on differences in labor market performance, welfare state provisions, and family tradition. Our analyses covered a comparative study (involving EU member states) and a longitudinal study of Sweden's welfare production model over thirty years. From a technical point of view, empirical proof of the specific links between welfare regimes, working conditions, and health have been hard to come by. Although in the Swedish case we had extensive long-term surveys and time-series data, we generally had access to only fragments of the needed information, which limited verification of causal relations.

Despite all these technical difficulties, comparative and longitudinal analyses provide some evidence that the labor market and welfare state interact to shape not only general living conditions but also public health. More specifically, our findings suggest that public health is optimal (i.e., at the lowest levels of general health problems and lowest levels of inequality in health) when there is an efficient sym-

biosis between the labor market and the welfare state—that is, where responsibilities for public health are shared by the labor market (in the form of job opportunities, equality in earnings, job security and economic security, labor protection
policies), and the welfare state (as reflected in extensive public services/transfers,
including publicly financed comprehensive health insurance with total population
coverage). In direct comparisons between EU member states we found that in
Nordic countries, which long have emphasized the state's role in providing welfare
in general and in stimulating the inclusive labor market (as described earlier),[5]
survey respondents have tended to report good self-rated health and lower rates
of ill health. Furthermore, these countries also have been more successful in providing employment opportunities for a larger share of their working-age populations.

Our data for the Swedish case, studying health trends in relation to the changing
welfare mix during the 1990s, also revealed the link between the labor market
conditions and morbidity. There was clear evidence of negative health effects in
the 1990s, when, compared with the 1980s, there was a marked reduction in employment levels, a fourfold increase in unemployment, increased job-related stress
and insecurity, and a subsequent reduction in welfare state provisions. Claims of
a causal relationship between the welfare production strategy and health outcomes
may not be warranted on the basis of these epidemiological studies, but the observed associations are, at a minimum, suggestive and can be explained by biological mechanisms illustrated in physiological process studies.

In this chapter we have pursued three research strategies in linking variations
in institutional configurations to variations in health—namely, variations between
nations (EU member states), variations over time (the Swedish case), and variations
between groups (social class, sex, age, family type). The expansion of official statistics, along with new comparative research–driven surveys, offers new research
opportunities in the study of potential health determinants. The EU is building up
new longitudinal comparative time-series data for its member states at the micro
level (i.e., individual- and household-level data), as well as at the aggregate level
(i.e., data available at the national, regional, and institutional levels). Some of the
member states, and particularly the Nordic countries, already have a long tradition
in building integrated statistical systems that incorporate simultaneous information
on social and economic conditions, which also include extensive data on morbidity
and mortality.

The EU is a natural laboratory for the study of social and economic determinants
of health. With increased access to and therefore potential use of comparative
statistics and with growing cross-cultural coordination of policies, the merits and
consequences of various welfare production strategies pursued by EU member
states will be raised in policy discussions, and health inequities within and between
nations will likely be put on policy-making agendas.

The analysis presented in this chapter has still been restricted to the aggregate level. The new data sources will provide openings for moving on to the next frontier, the micro level. The Swedish ULF system (Vogel 2002b)—which combines integrated, multilevel data (on individuals and/or households, institutional characteristics, and area characteristics) and true longitudinal sample design—is just one example of the data sources in Europe to be exploited in further research on the social determinants of health.

Notes

1. At the time of this writing, the EU nations were Sweden, Denmark, Finland, Germany, Austria, France, Belgium, Netherlands, Luxembourg, UK, Ireland, Greece, Italy, Spain, and Portugal.

2. Details are reported in Vogel 1997, 1999.

3. This is a composite index based on six indicators, including household size, the rate of single adults aged thirty to sixty-four, the proportion of adults living in consensual unions, the proportion of adults younger than thirty who are still living with their parents, and the percentage of adults aged seventy to eighty-four years who are living with their children aged thirty or older. The index is calculated as the average ranking of each nation on these indicators. For other details about the index, see Vogel 2003.

4. The index equals the average percentage difference between manual and upper-level nonmanual workers, with respect to the absence of poverty; an income exceeding 150% of the average; high standard of housing space (defined as a greater-than-average amount of housing space); ownership of a car, a videotape player, a boat, a dishwasher, or a freezer; and subscription to a daily newspaper.

5. Our data revealed that this strategy was most clearly demonstrated in the Nordic states. However, other nations displayed similar welfare production strategies; and in all cases, nations with extensive welfare states also had inclusive labor markets. In addition, all nations with highly inclusive labor markets had high tax and social expenditure levels. In fact, there were no nations that rated high on only one of these two institutional configurations among the EU member states.

References

Arbetsmiljöverket (Board of Work Safety and Health). 2000. *Arbetsmiljön 1999* [*The work environment 1999*]. Stockholm: Board of Work Safety and Health.

———. 2001. *Arbetsmiljön 2001* [*The work environment 2001*]. Stockholm: Board of Work Safety and Health.

Barklöf, K., ed. 2000. *Smärtgränsen? En antologi om hälsokonsekvenser i magra organisationer Rådet för arbetslivsforskning* [*Pain threshold? An anthology about health consequences in lean organizations*]. Stockholm: Council for Working Life Research.

Belkic, K., P. Landsbergis, D. Baker, P. Schnall and D. Baker. 2004. Is job strain a major source of cardiovascular disease risk? *Scandinavian Journal of Work and Environmental Health* 30:85–128.

Belkic, K., P. Landsbergis, P. Schnall, D. Baker, T. Theorell, J. Siegrist, R. Peter, and R. Karasek. 2000. Psychosocial factors: Review of the empirical data among men. In *Occupational Medicine: The Workplace and Cardiovascular Disease*, ed. P. L. Schnall, K. Belkic, P. Landsbergis, and D. Baker. Philadelphia: Hanley and Belfus.

Castles, F. G., and D. Mitchell. 1992. Identifying welfare states regimes: The links between politics, instruments and outcomes. *Governance* 5:1–26.

Duncan, S. 1995. Theorising European gender systems. *Journal of European Social Policy* 5 (4):263–284.

Esping-Andersen, G. 1990. *The Three Worlds of Welfare Capitalism.* Cambridge: Polity Press.

———, ed. 1996. *Welfare States in Transition.* National Adaptations in Global Economies. London: UNRISD and Sage.

———. 1999. *Social Foundations of Postindustrial Economies.* Oxford: Oxford University Press.

Galbraith, J. K., L. Jiaqing, and W. Darity. 1999. *Measuring the Evolution of Inequality in the Global Economy.* Austin: University of Texas.

Hasselhorn, H. M., T. Theorell, E. Vingård, and the MUSIC-Norrtälje Study Group. 2001. Endocrine and immunological parameters indicative of 6-month prognosis after the onset of low back pain or neck/shoulder pain. *Spine* 26:E24–E29.

Hertting, A., and T. Theorell. 2002. Physiological changes associated with downsizing of personnel and reorganisation in the health care sector. *Psychotherapy and Psychosomatics* 71: 117–122.

Hirdman, Y. 1990. Genussystemet (the gender system). In *Demokrati Och Makt I Sverige [Democracy and Power in Sweden].* Maktutredningens huvurapport. Stockholm: SOU.

Karasek, R. A., and T. Theorell. 1990. *Healthy Work.* New York: Basic Books.

Kawachi, I. 2000. Income inequality and health. In *Social Epidemiology,* ed. L. F. Berkman and I. Kawachi. New York: Oxford University Press.

Kunst, A. E., F. Groenhof, O. Andersen, J. K. Borgan, G. Costa, G. Desplanques, H. Filakti, M. R. Giraldes, F. Faggiano, S. Harding, C. Junker, P. Martikainen, C. Minder, B. Nolan, F. Pagnanelli, E. Regidor, D. Vagero, T. Valkonen, and J. P. Mackenbach. 1999. Occupational class and ischemic heart disease mortality in the United States and 11 European countries. *American Journal of Public Health* 89:47–53.

Lewis, J. 1992. Gender and the development of welfare regimes. *Journal of European Social Policy* 2 (3):159–173.

Palme, J., A. Bergmark, O. Backman, F. Estrada, J. Fritzell, O. Lundberg, O. Sjoberg, L. Sommestad, and M. Szebehely. 2003. Swedish Welfare Commission. A welfare balance sheet for the 1990s. Final report of the Swedish Welfare Commission. *Scandinavian Journal of Public Health* (suppl. 60):7–143.

Petterson, I. L., and B. B. Arnetz. 1998. Psychosocial stressors and well-being in health care workers—the impact of an intervention program. *Social Science and Medicine* 47:1763–1772.

Rubery, J., C. Fagan, and M. Smith. 1994. *Changing Patterns of Work and Working-time in the European Union and the Impact of Gender Divisions.* Report to the Equal Opportunities Unit, DG5. Commission of the European Communities.

Scharpf, F. 2000. Economic changes, vulnerabilities, and institutional capabilities. In *Welfare and Work in the Open Economy,* vol. 1, ed. F. Scharpf and V. Schmidt. New York: Oxford University Press.

Subramanian, S. V., and I. Kawachi. 2003. Wage poverty, earned income inequality, and health. In *Global Inequalities at Work: Work's Impact on the Health of Individuals, Families, and Societies,* ed. J. Heymann. New York: Oxford University Press.

Swedish National Board of Health and Social Security. 2001. Folkhälsorapport 2001 (Public health report 2001). *Socialstyrelsen,* 12–23.

Theorell, T. 1999. How to deal with stress in organizations—a health perspective on theory and practice. *Scandinavian Journal of Work and Environmental Health* 25:616–624.

———. 2004. Democracy at work and its relationship to health. In Vol. 3, *Research in Occupational Stress and Well Being. Emotional and Physiological Processes and Positive Intervention Strategies,* ed. P. Perrewé and D. Ganster. Amsterdam: Elsevier.

Theorell, T., J. K. Konarski-Svensson, J. Ahlmén, and A. Perski. 1991. The role of paid work in Swedish chronic dialysis patients—a nation-wide survey. *Journal of Internal Medicine* 230:501–509.

Vogel, J. 1997. *Living Conditions and Inequality in the European Union.* Population and Social Conditions report no. E/1997-3. Luxembourg: Eurostat.

———. 1998a. Coping with the European welfare mix. Welfare delivery systems, family formation and material inequality between types of families in the European Union. Paper presented at the 1998 Siena Group Meeting on Families at the End of the Twentieth Century, December 7–12, Sydney, Australia.

———. 1998b. Three types of European society. Nordic News Network. Available from http://www.nnn.se.

———. 1999. The European welfare mix: Institutional configuration and distributive outcome in Sweden and the European Union. A longitudinal and comparative perspective. *Social Indicators Research* 48:245–297.

———. 2000. Welfare production models and income structure. A comparative and longitudinal perspective: European Union, Mid 1990s, and Sweden, 1963–1998. Paper prepared for the Rich–Poor Conference of ISA Working Group 6, October 20–21, Berlin.

———. 2002a. Strategies and traditions in Swedish social reporting: A 30-year experience. In *Assessing Quality of Life and Living Conditions to Guide National Policy: The State of the Art,* ed. M. Hagerty, J. Vogel, and V. Meller. Social Indicators Research, vol. 53, no. 1–3, special issue.

———. 2002b. [Towards a typology of European welfare production]. In *Sozialer Wandel und gesellschaftliche Dauerbeobachtung,* W. Glatzer, R. Habich, and K. U. Mayer, eds. Opladen, Germany: Leske and Budrich.

———, ed. 2003. *European Welfare Production: Institutional Configuration and Distributional Outcome.* Amsterdam: Kluwer.

Vogel, J., and L. Häll, eds. 1997. *Välfärd och ojämlikhet i 20-årsperspektiv, 1975–95 [Living Conditions and Inequality, 1975–95].* Levnadsförhållanden [Living conditions] series, report no. 91. Stockholm: Statistics Sweden.

Vogel, J., L. Häll, S. E. Johansson, and C. Skjöld. 2000. *Äldres levnadsförhållanden, 1980–1998 [Living Conditions of the Elderly, 1980–1998].* Levnadsförhållanden [Living conditions] series, report no. 93. Stockholm: Statistics Sweden.

Wikman, A. 2004. Arbetsliv och sjukfrånvaro [Working life and sick leave]. In *Den höga sjukfrånvaron—sanning och konsekvens [The High Sick Leave Prevalence—Truth and Consequence].* Statens folkhälsoinstitutet (National Institute for Public Health) 2004:15.

Chapter 11

Changing Trends in Economic Well-being in OECD Countries: What Measure Is Most Relevant for Health?

Lars Osberg and Andrew Sharpe

The connection between health and economic well-being has become a growing area of research, and there has been much debate about how best to measure "health." In this discussion we look at the other side of the issue—how best to measure economic well-being—to better understand the relationship between economic well-being and health.

The most commonly used measure of economic well-being at the national level has been average money incomes—specifically, per capita gross domestic product (GDP). However, this measure is blind to many things that people clearly care about. Money income from market transactions omits consideration of the goods and services produced outside the market, as well as any changes in life span and in leisure. In general, economic well-being also depends on the size of the bequest this generation will leave for the benefit of future generations, which current money incomes do not reveal. Average money income also does not indicate how unequally incomes are distributed and, therefore, does not indicate how likely it is that any particular individual will share in average prosperity. Finally, average money incomes do not reflect the degree of anxiety and insecurity with which individuals contemplate their own futures.

We therefore argue that a better index of a society's economic well-being should be composed of four components:

- current effective per capita consumption flows
- net societal accumulation of stocks of productive resources
- income distribution
- economic security

In this chapter we develop such an index of economic well-being for selected Organization for Economic Cooperation and Development (OECD) countries for the period 1980–1999 and compare trends in economic well-being to trends in GDP per person. Estimates of the overall index and the subcomponents are presented for 1980 through 1999 for the United States, the United Kingdom, Canada, Australia, Norway, and Sweden. In every case, growth in economic well-being proved less than growth in GDP per capita, although to different degrees in different countries. We conclude with a discussion of why the connection between health and trends in economic well-being might be stronger than the relationship between health and GDP per person.

Economic Well-being, GDP per Capita, and Health

In 1980 Ronald Reagan, then campaigning for election as U.S. president, asked the American people a seemingly simple question: "Are you better off today than you were four years ago?" Although U.S. per capita GDP was, in 1980, some 9.2% higher than in 1976 when measured in constant (after-inflation) dollars, his audiences answered "No!" More recently, when Canadians were asked in 1998 how the overall financial situation of their generation compared with that of their parents at the same stage of life, only 44% thought that there had been an improvement—despite an increase of approximately 60% in real gross domestic product (GDP) per capita over the previous 25 years (Angus 1998). Evidently, national income accounting measures may not necessarily be a good guide to popular perceptions of trends in economic well-being. Are such popular perceptions unreasonable? And if GDP per capita is not a good measure of economic well-being, is it possible to find a better measure, conceptually and practically?[1]

In measuring GDP, national income accountants attempt to get an accurate count of the total money value of goods and services produced for sale in the market in a given country in a given year. This measure is clearly important for many purposes, but it is equally clear that it omits consideration of many issues (e.g., leisure time, length of life) that are important to individuals' well-being. All the same, for many years the System of National Accounts (SNA), developed by the United Nations and several international organizations to standardize methods for calculating the output and economic growth of countries, has been the accounting framework within which most discussions of trends in economic well-being have been conducted, and GDP per capita has often been used as a summary measure of economic trends.[2]

The compilers of the national accounts have sometimes protested that their attempt to measure the aggregate money value of marketed economic output was never intended as a full measure of economic well-being—*but* it has often been used as such. If an inappropriate measure of economic well-being is used, both policy and analysis are likely to suffer. Economic policy makers may want to increase economic well-being, but if they are aiming at the wrong target, they are unlikely to be fully successful in hitting the right one. Also, there is good reason to believe that the issues omitted from consideration in GDP accounting are especially relevant to health, so analysts of the relationship between health and economic well-being are likely to be misled if they focus on trends in per capita GDP.

Early economists (such as Adam Smith, Karl Marx, and Alfred Marshall) were fairly broad (and a bit vague) in their conception of "prosperity," but they were in no doubt that it had many positive implications (including better health). More recently, the measure of economic success (GDP per capita) has been both narrower and more precise. It now falls to critics to show that alternative measures to GDP per capita are possible, plausible, and more reflective of true economic well-being. In this chapter we therefore present for selected OECD countries an index of economic well-being based on four dimensions or components of economic well-being: consumption, accumulation, income distribution, and economic security.

In identifying these dimensions of economic well-being, we recognize explicitly that reasonable people may disagree in the relative weight they would assign to each dimension—that is, some will argue that inequality in income distribution is highly important, whereas others will argue the converse. For this reason, specifying *explicit* weights of the components of economic well-being is important because it enables others to assess whether, by their personal values of what is important in economic well-being, they would agree with an overall assessment of trends in the economy.

Of course, some events have qualitatively similar impacts on all four dimensions of well-being. A major recession will, for example, usually produce lower average consumption, more inequality, more insecurity, and less accumulation of capital for the benefit of future generations. In such a case, differences among people in the values that determine the relative weights to be assigned to the components of well-being are of secondary concern. However, in other instances (e.g., environmental policy concerning global warming) the relative weights assigned to different dimensions of economic well-being (e.g., current consumption versus the bequest to future generations) may be crucial. A major reason for being explicit about the weights to be assigned to the dimensions of well-being is to be clear about when there is, and when there is not, a difference of values large enough to matter in the assessment of aggregate social trends.[3]

In everyday life, it is common to observe that debates about values, facts, and economic policies are hopelessly intermingled. However, the hypothesis underlying this chapter is that democratic discourse is likely to be more productive if issues of values, fact, and analysis can be separated as much as possible. Issues of fact can be seen as answers to the question "Where are we?" Discussions of values can be seen as answering the query "Where do we want to go?" There remains the crucial question of policy: "How do we get there?" But in principle these are separable questions.

This chapter is about the "Where are we?" issue. Its basic hypothesis—that a society's well-being depends on total consumption and accumulation and on the individual inequality and insecurity that surround the distribution of macroeconomic aggregates—is consistent with a variety of theoretical perspectives. We therefore avoid a specific, formal model.[4] The rest of the chapter is divided into three main parts. In the following section, we discuss how we have developed estimates of the four key components or dimensions of the index—consumption flows, stocks of wealth, inequality, and insecurity. Next, we present preliminary estimates of the overall index and its components for the United States, the United Kingdom, Canada, Australia, Norway, and Sweden from 1980 to 1999, and we compare trends in the index and its components.[5] In the final section, we conclude by discussing the linkage between health and trends in economic well-being.

An Index of Economic Well-being

If people typically derive pleasure both from their own consumption and from the prospect of future generations' well-being, they will want to consume part of their current income and save the rest. Economic well-being will therefore depend on the proportion of income saved for the future, but GDP is a measure of the aggregate market income of a society that does not reveal the savings rate. Furthermore, there is little reason to believe that the savings rate is automatically optimal—particularly if some assets (like the environment) do not have market prices. Hence, to estimate the economic well-being of society, one must measure both current consumption and the bequest this generation will leave for the benefit of future generations. In addition, although trends in average income are important, individuals are justifiably concerned about the degree to which they personally will share in prosperity and the degree to which their personal economic future is secure.[6] Therefore, four components or dimensions of economic well-being are

1. effective per capita consumption flows, which include consumption of marketed goods and services, government services, effective per capita flows of household production, leisure, and changes in life span.
2. net societal accumulation of stocks of productive resources, which includes net accumulation of tangible capital, housing stocks, and net changes in the value of natural resources stocks; environmental costs; net change in the level of foreign indebtedness; and accumulation of human capital and R&D investment.
3. income distribution—the intensity of poverty (incidence and depth) and the inequality of income.

4. economic security from job loss and unemployment, illness, family breakup, and poverty in old age.

Each dimension of economic well-being is itself an aggregation of many underlying trends, on which the existing literature is of variable quality—and often differs across countries. By contrast, the System of National Accounts has had many years of development effort by international agencies (particularly the United Nations and the International Monetary Fund) and has produced an accounting system for GDP that is rigorously standardized across countries. Internationally comparable statistics on other dimensions of economic well-being are far less complete. However, using GDP per capita as a measure of well-being would implicitly (1) assume that the aggregate share of income devoted to accumulation (including the value of unpriced environmental assets) is automatically optimal and (2) set the weight of income distribution or economic insecurity to zero, by ignoring entirely either's influence. Neither assumption seems justifiable.

Average Consumption Flows

Current consumption is certainly an important component of economic well-being, and the objective of this section is to estimate its average effective level. The easiest part to measure is purchased consumer goods and services. Data on aggregate real personal consumption per capita expressed in national currency units and in constant prices are available from the OECD national accounts. All countries experienced increases in real per capita marketed personal consumption over the 1980–1999 period, but there were large variations in the increase, ranging from a high of 59.4% in the United Kingdom to a low of 19.4% in Sweden. The increases in the other countries were: Norway (44.7%), Canada (30.2%), the United States (48.7%), and Australia (43.3%).

However, several other factors also influence effective consumption flows, such as leisure, household size, regrettables, the underground economy, and life expectancy. We discuss these and other factors later, with approximate estimates of their value, in some cases. At this stage in the development of the Index of Economic Well-being, our preference is to include (wherever possible), rather than exclude, imprecise measures. Omitting a variable would implicitly set its value to zero. Hence, an imprecise measure of a variable is likely to embody a smaller error than complete omission. However, there is no estimate available at all for some countries, and omission is sometimes unavoidable.

In some instances, however, assessment of aggregate trends in economic well-being may not be very sensitive to the omission of a particular variable. The so-called underground economy is an example.[7] Since there always has been some level of underground activity, the issue for the measurement of trends in well-being is whether or not the prevalence of the underground economy has changed substantially over time. Some trends may encourage an expansion (e.g., rising tax rates), but other factors have worked in the opposite direction (e.g., the increased penetration of franchise systems in the small business sector and the greater computerization of business records). However, whatever the direction of the trend, it is from a small base. Credible benchmark estimates of the prevalence of underground activity put it at a relatively small percentage of GDP. Gervais (1994), for instance, estimated the upper limit of unmeasured production at 2.7% of GDP in Canada in the early 1990s. When the level is this small to start with, the absolute size of a change is even smaller. Because comparable estimates of the underground economy were not available over time and across countries, we omitted this variable.

We also omitted any adjustment for the fraction of consumption expenditures that are arguably an "intermediate input" in the production of income (like commuting expenses) or a "defensive necessity" to offset the impact of adverse social trends (like expenditures on antiburglary measures due to higher crime rates). This class of expenditure has been labeled regrettable expenditures on the grounds that increases do not indicate greater utility for consumers. In our earlier estimates of the Index of Economic Well-being for Canada and the United States (Osberg and Sharpe 1998, 1999), we subtracted estimates for regrettable expenditures from personal consumption. However, such data were unavailable for other countries; and since there was little *trend* in the amount of such expenditures in North America, the omission of these data may not be crucial.

By contrast, we had good data on the significant increase in life expectancy in recent years in all the countries examined, and we have every reason to believe that having a long life is an important component of well-being. If one wants to measure the current consumption of this generation, the economic value of these extra years of life should be included in the total consumption flows of individuals, since, presumably, people care about both how much they consume per year and how many years they get to consume.[8]

Although a longer life span is valuable to people, GDP numbers will not reveal its importance and may, in fact, move in a contrary direction. If people can make more money by assuming more risk,[9] increases in marketed output that come from greater risk taking will have costs in decreased longevity that should be counted in an index of economic well-being. Ideally, a full appraisal of the value of increased longevity should consider trends in morbidity and health-adjusted life expectancy (HALE).[10] However, one also must face the issue that the value of more years of healthy life may look very different, the closer one actually is to death. Changes in life expectancy and morbidity are occurring "in real time" and are affecting the well-being of everyone now alive. In aggregating over the population now alive, one is aggregating over individuals at very different points in the life course. For the purposes of this chapter, we adopted the simple expedient of adjusting per capita consumption flows in each year upward by the percentage increase in average life expectancy relative to the base year (1980).[11] However, we do recognize the crudity of this measure of an existential issue.

Our data on life expectancy were taken from the OECD Health Data CD-ROM.[12] Between 1980 and 1999, all countries enjoyed increased life expectancy, but there was a significant variation across countries in the size of the increase, as follows: Australia, 5.9%; Canada, 4.8%; Norway, 3.4%; Sweden, 4.9%; the United Kingdom, 4.5%; and the United States, 4.1%.

The old saying "Two can live as cheaply as one" is romantic, but it is also a bit of an exaggeration of the fact that when individuals cohabit in households, they save money because they benefit from economies of scale in household consumption (e.g., see Burkhauser, Smeeding, and Merz [1996] or Phipps and Garner [1994].) Because households have shrunk in average size in all countries, people have lost some of the savings in cost of living that come from sharing a household.[13] Trends in average per capita consumption should, therefore, be adjusted for the average loss in economic well-being over time due to lessened economies of scale in household consumption.

As well, countries differed markedly in the average size of households. The average family size for the most recent year available (year in parentheses) was 2.46 in Australia (1994); 2.51 in Canada (1994); 2.19 in Norway (1995); 1.85 in Sweden (1992); 2.55 in the United Kingdom (1986); and 2.58 in the United States (1997). All countries had experienced a long-term decline in average family size since the 1970s. We applied the Luxembourg Income Study's (LIS) equivalence scale (i.e., the square root of family size) to average family size in each year and used an index of these data (1980 = 100) to adjust personal consumption per capita. Australia had the largest downward adjustment in 1999, relative to 1980 (4.1%).

A major defect of GDP as a measure of well-being is that because it counts only market income, it effectively assigns a zero value to leisure time. Among OECD countries there are major differences in both the initial level and trends over time in the average annual number of hours worked. For example, in 1980 average working hours per adult (ages 15–64) were 1,224.5 in the United States and 1,154.9 in Germany. These differences were greatly magnified by 1997. Working hours per adult rose by 204 hours in the United States, to 1,428.5, while falling by 173 hours in Germany, to 981.9. Since these differences in working hours are large—equivalent to about 8.6 hours per week—it seems important to take them into account in a measure of economic well-being.

To account for the value of these differences, we adjusted the value of consumption for differences in paid hours relative to a benchmark, namely the value in the United States in 1980. Specifically, countries with average annual hours worked less than the benchmark had a positive adjustment to consumption, and countries with more working time than the benchmark had a negative adjustment. Our methodology was equivalent to saying that at the margin, individuals ascribe a value equal to the after-tax average wage to changes in nonworking time that are not due to unemployment fluctuations. However, unemployment does not constitute leisure. To account for involuntary leisure, we subtracted average annual hours of unemployment per working-age person from the relative nonworking-time estimate.

Between 1980 and 1997 most of the countries for which we had data experienced declines in working time, although Sweden and the United States experienced increases.[14] By 1997, U.S. per-adult working hours were 204 hours above their 1980 level of 1,225 hours. Between 1980 and 1997, working hours per working-age person declined by 54 hours in Norway, 52 hours in the United Kingdom, and 38 hours in Canada. Since some of these changes were large (204 hours is equivalent to 4 hours per week), they represented substantial changes in economic well-being. Such changes should be reflected in a reasonable measure of economic progress.

A strong case can be made that some hours of unemployment, which are included in nonwork or leisure time, are not by choice and do not contribute to economic well-being. (Indeed, if there are psychological costs to unemployment, such hours may have strong disutility associated with them [Clark and Oswald 1994].) In the calculation of the imputations for the value of nonworking time, we deducted hours of unemployment[15]—that is, assigned such hours zero value. Compared with a 1980 U.S. base, the imputation for changing nonworking time was, by 1999, worth +$700.70 per capita in Norway (1995 U.S. dollars), +$113.40 for Sweden, −$41.60 for the United Kingdom, −$242.00 for Canada, −$467.90 for Australia, and −$1,473.00 for the United States.

To measure the value of consumption, we needed to count the provision of nonmarketed or heavily subsidized services by the government as part of the consumption flow. Current expenditure data on all levels of government, including defense and capital consumption allowances but excluding debt service charges and transfer payments, were taken from the OECD national accounts, expressed in constant prices in national currency units. The importance of government expenditures in our total adjusted consumption measure differed markedly among OECD countries. In 1996, it ranged from a high of 54.2% in Sweden to a low of 24.3% in the United States. The figures for the other countries, in descending order of the relative importance of government expenditure, were as follows: Norway, 41.5%; United Kingdom, 32.7%; and Canada, 29.1%. In addition, from 1980 to 1999 there were major differences across countries in the rate of growth of real per capita government final consumption expenditures.

TOTAL CONSUMPTION FLOWS

Total per capita consumption is defined as the sum of personal consumption (adjusted for changes in average household size and longevity of life), government services, and the adjusted relative value of leisure. Between 1980 and 1999 the increase in real per capita total consumption flows was 23.8% in Sweden but much higher in the United Kingdom (62.6%), the United States (54.4%), Australia (45.5%), and Norway (41.1%). Canada (32.2%) was an intermediate case (see table 11.1).

Accumulation, Sustainability, and the Intergenerational Bequest

If individuals today care about the well-being of future generations, then the measurement of trends in current well-being should include consideration of probable changes in the well-being of those generations. This consideration of future generations can also be justified on the grounds that a concept of "society" should include both present and future generations. The economic well-being of future generations depends on their inheritance of real productive assets—not on the financial instruments that will determine the *allocation* of the returns from those assets. It is the stocks of real wealth, broadly conceived to include not only natural

Table 11.1. Consumption—components of average personal consumption

Country and year	Personal consumption per capita ($95 U.S.) (A)	Index of life expectancy 1980 = 1.00 (B)	Average family size, persons (C)	Index of equivalent income 1980 = 1.00 (D) = index of the square root of (C)	Adjusted personal consumption per capita ($95 U.S.) E = A*B*D	Index of adjusted personal consumption per capita 1980 = 1.00 (F)
Australia						
1980	10,167	1.000	2.68	1.000	10,167.4	1.000
1999	14,571	1.059	2.46	0.959	14,793.7	1.455
Canada						
1980	10,729	1.000	2.68	1.000	10,729	1.000
1999	13,974	1.048	2.51	0.969	14,188	1.322
Norway						
1980	8,541	1.000	2.48	1.000	8,541	1.000
1999	12,363	1.034	2.19	0.942	12,049	1.411
Sweden						
1980	8,918	1.000	1.89	1.000	8,918	1.000
1999	10,648	1.049	1.85	0.988	11,039	1.238
U.K.						
1980	8,260	1.000	2.68	1.000	8,260	1.000
1999	13,170	1.045	2.55	0.976	13,430	1.626
U.S.						
1980	14,084	1.000	2.59	1.000	14,084	1.000
1999	20,950	1.041	2.58	0.997	21,747	1.544

Sources: Data appendix posted at http://www.csls.ca; personal consumption per capita, Table A2; population, Table A1; life expectancy, Table A3; average family size, LIS database.

and human resources but also physical capital stock, left to the next generation that will determine whether a society is on a sustainable long-run trajectory of aggregate consumption, irrespective of the distribution of claims on those consumption flows at the individual level.

The physical capital stock includes residential and nonresidential structures, machinery, and equipment in both the business and government sectors. The greater the capital stock, the greater are the future productive capacity, future potential consumption flows, and economic well-being. We took from the OECD publication *Flows and Stocks of Fixed Capital* (1998) data for the current net fixed capital stock, expressed in constant prices and national currency units. We assumed that the estimates were internationally comparable, although the use of different depreciation rates by statistical agencies may have reduced comparability for both level- and rate-of-growth comparisons.[16] Between 1980 and 1999, the increase in the fixed capital stock, on a per capita basis, was notably less in the United States (30.8%) and Australia (27.5%) than in the United Kingdom (41%), Norway (39.9%), Canada (33%), and Sweden (32.5%).

In a knowledge-based economy, the stock of skills embodied in the workforce is a crucial determinant of current and future economic well-being. There is a strong relationship between educational attainment and individual income, and there is substantial evidence that education yields significant social benefits, beyond its impact on individual earnings. Although school retention and participation in postsecondary education have increased dramatically in many countries over the past three decades, human capital is intangible and is not now counted in balance sheet estimates of national wealth.[17]

In our analyses, we used an admittedly crude and incomplete (but feasible) method of estimating investment in human capital—the cost per year of education expenditures at the primary, secondary, and postsecondary levels. OECD data on the educational attainment of the population aged twenty-five to sixty-four and expenditure per student (available in both local currency and U.S. dollars) for the early childhood, primary, secondary, nonuniversity-tertiary-level, and university-level education were used to estimate the per capita stock of human capital. In order to distinguish clearly intercountry differences in the quantity of education obtained, as opposed to differences in its cost of production, we applied a common cost base (the cost of education in the United States) to all countries.

In an era of rapid technological change, expenditure on research and development (R&D) is also a crucial ingredient in society's ability to innovate and create wealth. Statistical agencies do not produce R&D stock data, but OECD data on annual flows of total business enterprise expenditure on R&D can be accumulated into a stock of R&D capital valued at the cost of investment, with a depreciation rate of 20% on the declining balance assumed. Between 1980 and 1999, the per capita real business enterprise R&D stock increased proportionately quite rapidly in Australia and Canada—but from a relatively small base. The United States started with the greatest absolute stock of R&D investment, and the absolute size of the increase in R&D capital in the United States ($1,274) was much larger than in Norway ($626), Australia ($567), Canada ($720), and the United Kingdom ($337).[18] Only Sweden came close, at +$1,010.

Current consumption levels could be increased by running down stocks of non-renewable natural resources or by exploiting renewable resources in a nonsustainable manner, but this would be at the cost of the consumption of future generations. A key aspect of the wealth accumulation component of economic well-being is net changes in the value of natural resources. From an intergenerational perspective, it is the value of the natural resources, not their physical extent, that counts.

The World Bank (1997) has produced estimates for one year (1994) of natural capital, or "the entire environmental patrimony of a country," for nearly 100 countries. *Natural capital* is defined to include pastureland, cropland, timber resources, nontimber forest resources, protected areas, and subsoil assets. Unfortunately, the single year of data availability would preclude the use of this variable in our proposed index of economic well-being. World Bank estimates of natural capital for OECD countries, on a per capita basis expressed in 1994 U.S. dollars, were $36,590 for Canada; $35,340 for Australia; $30,220 for Norway; $16,500 for the United States; $14,590 for Sweden; and $4,940 for the United Kingdom.

In general, a financial instrument can be seen from two angles: It is an asset to the holder and a liability to the issuer. If both persons are residents of the same country, these assets and liabilities offset each other. With our index, we therefore did not count the gross level of government or corporate debt as a "burden" on future generations, and we did not count as part of the intergenerational bequest the value of paper gains in the stock market. Although the distribution of financial assets and liabilities will play a major role in *allocating* the future returns to the capital stock, the issue at this point is the aggregate value of the intergenerational bequest. However, net debt to foreigners is another issue. Since interest payments on the net foreign indebtedness of citizens of one country to residents of other countries will lower the aggregate future consumption options of those citizens, increases in the level of foreign indebtedness reduce economic well-being within a given country.

Estimates of the net investment position, expressed in current U.S. dollars, have been published in the International Monetary Fund's *International Financial Statistics Yearbook* (2002). We converted these estimates to current-price national currencies at market exchange rates and then deflated by the GDP deflator and adjusted for population to obtain real per capita estimates in the net international investment position, expressed in national currency units.

Like the excess depletion of natural resources, current consumption can be increased at the expense of the environment's degradation, reducing the economic well-being of future generations. Consequently, changes in the level of air and water pollution should be considered an important aspect of wealth accumulation. Probably the best-known environmental change is global warming, which has arisen from increased emissions of greenhouse gases—most commonly, carbon dioxide (CO_2) emissions (Intergovernmental Panel on Climate Change [IPCC] 2001). Fortunately, data are available on these emissions, and it is possible to estimate the costs of these emissions. These costs can then be subtracted from the stock of wealth to obtain an environmentally adjusted stock of wealth.[19] Since global warming affects all countries, we estimated world total costs of emissions and allocated these costs on the basis of a country's share of world GDP.

Fankhauser (1995) has estimated the globalized social costs of CO_2 emissions (with no adjustment for different national costs) at $20 U.S. per ton in 1990. According to data from the International Energy Agency (IEA), world CO_2 emissions in 1997 were 22,636 millions of metric tons (2003). Based on the $20 U.S. per ton cost of CO_2 emissions, the world social cost of CO_2 emissions was $452,720 million. We allocated this amount on the basis of a country's share of nominal world GDP, expressed in U.S. dollars. We then converted it into national currency at the purchasing power parity exchange rate[20] and divided by population. As these costs represent a loss in the value of the services provided by the environment, they can be considered a deduction from the total societal stock of wealth. For example, in 1999, per capita stocks of wealth in Canada were reduced by $317 (U.S. dollars) because of the social costs imposed by CO_2 emissions, according to this methodology.

ESTIMATES OF TOTAL WEALTH

As the estimates of the physical capital stock, the R&D capital stock, net foreign debt, and environmental degradation are expressed in value terms, they can be aggregated and presented on a per capita basis. Net foreign debt per capita is a negative entry, and the social costs of CO_2 emissions are subtracted from the stocks of wealth.

For the 1980–1999 period, estimates for the five components of the wealth stock included in this chapter indicated that per capita real wealth stocks increased by 18.0% in the United States, much less than Norway's 55.7%. Sweden (20.1%), the United Kingdom (28.2%), Australia, (30.5%) and Canada (35.8%) were intermediate cases (see table 11.2).

Income Distribution—Inequality and Poverty

Would economic well-being in a society in which everyone had a $500 income remain the same if income were redistributed so that half the population had $999 and the other half had $1? Average income would be the same in both cases, but the more equal situation would be likely to generate more aggregate utility.[21] The

Table 11.2. Accumulation—stocks of wealth, 1995 U.S. dollars

Country and year	Total net fixed capital per capita	Total business enterprise expenditures on R&D per capita	Total net international invest. position per capita	Human capital stock per capita	Greenhouse gas emission cost per capita	Total real per capita wealth	Index of total real per capita wealth 1980 = 1.00
Australia							
1980	44,827.5	179.4	−8,536.7	18,562.4	−299.8	54,732.8	1.0000
1999	57,188.5	746.4	−10,838.0	24,663.8	−318.6	71,442.1	1.3053
Canada							
1980	22,578.6	336.7	−6,491.5	20,563.7	−333.5	36,654.0	1.0000
1999	30,043.7	1,057.6	−6,342.3	25,347.5	−317.2	49,789.3	1.3584
Norway							
1980	51,037.4	386.6	−8,041.8	19,570.4	−301.0	62,651.7	1.0000
1999	71,425.8	1,012.9	−2,312.6	27,747.4	−339.9	97,533.6	1.5568
Sweden							
1980	43,345.3	1,593.9	−3,953.1	22,057.6	−311.8	62,731.9	1.0000
1999	57,442.7	2,604.0	−8,085.6	23,693.1	−294.0	75,360.1	1.2013
U.K.							
1980	40,111.4	850.6	1,320.8	20,055.8	−264.4	62,074.2	1.0000
1999	56,567.9	1,188.1	−3,506.2	25,629.4	−282.7	79,596.6	1.2823
U.S.							
1980	50,414.2	1,324.9	1,931.6	24,443.9	−779.4	77,335.2	1.0000
1999	65,956.9	2,599.0	−5,022.5	28,709.8	−1,006.7	91,236.5	1.1798

Source: Data appendix posted at http://www.csls.ca.

idea that "social welfare" depends, in general, on *both* average income and the inequality of incomes has a long tradition in welfare economics (e.g., Arrow 1951; Sen 1970). However, in measuring the level of social welfare, the exact relative weight to be assigned to changes in average incomes, compared with changes in inequality, cannot be specified by economic theory.

Furthermore, poverty is not quite the same issue as inequality. Since the population's economic well-being is affected both by inequality in the distribution of income among all people and by the adequacy of incomes for the least well-off (i.e., the extent of poverty), there are two issues: (1) one's perspective on the importance of inequality/poverty compared with trends in average income and (2) one's view of the relative weight to be placed on poverty compared with inequality. We therefore suggest that a compound subindex that explicitly recognizes these issues would place some weight (β, a parameter between zero and unity) on a measure of inequality in the aggregate distribution of income and the remaining weight $(1 - \beta)$ on a measure of poverty.

The most popular measure of inequality in the distribution of income is undoubtedly the Gini index.[22] For the construction of the Index of Economic Well-being, we have chosen the Gini coefficient of after-tax household income, calculated from the Luxembourg Income Study micro-data files. For the most recent year for which data were available for each country, income inequality as measured by the Gini coefficient was largest (and, hence, income inequality greatest) in the United States (0.387) and lowest in Norway (0.222).

Recently, Osberg and Xu (2000) noted that the Sen-Shorrocks-Thon measure of poverty intensity is not only theoretically attractive as a measure of poverty but also convenient, since it can be decomposed as the product of the poverty rate, the average poverty gap ratio, and the inequality of poverty gap ratios. The *poverty rate* is the proportion of persons who fall below the poverty line, defined here as half the median equivalent after-tax family income. The *poverty gap ratio* is defined as the percentage gap between the poverty line and the income of those below the poverty line. Furthermore, since the inequality of poverty gap ratios is essentially constant, changes in poverty depend on changes in the poverty rate and the average poverty gap ratio.

We observed from the LIS data that the poverty rate varied greatly among each of the countries. For the most recent year for which micro-data tapes were available for each country, it ranged from a high of 18.0% in the United States and 17.5% in Australia to 12.4% in Canada, 9.7% in the United Kingdom, 9.2% in Norway, and 8.9% in Sweden. There was much less variation across countries in the average poverty gap ratio: Sweden, 36.6%; the United States, 34.9%; Canada, 31.0%; Norway, 28.5%; the United Kingdom, 28.5%; and Australia, 27.7%.

For our overall index of equality, we used a weighted average of the indices of poverty intensity for all units or households and the Gini coefficient, with equal weights. We multiplied the index by -1 in order to reflect the convention that increases are desirable. Unfortunately, the LIS database allows calculation of income distribution estimates for several years over a long time period for only a few countries. Hence, values of the income distribution and poverty variables in the years before the first LIS estimate for that country are assumed equal to the estimate for the first year of LIS data, and the values for the years after the last LIS estimate are assumed equal to the estimate of the last year of LIS data (see table 11.3). This is obviously an inadequate method and may lead to unreliable estimates for countries for which LIS estimates are only available for a small number of years over a short time period.

Insecurity

If individuals knew their own economic futures with certainty, their welfare would depend only on their actual incomes over their lifetimes, since there would be no reason to feel anxiety about the future. However, uncertainty about the future will decrease the economic welfare of risk-averse individuals. Individuals can try to avoid risk through social and private insurance, but such mechanisms do not

Table 11.3. Distribution—economic inequality and poverty

Country and year	Gini coefficient (A)	Poverty rate (B)	Average poverty gap (% of poverty line) (C)	Poverty intensity D = B*C	Poverty intensity index D'	Gini coeff. (income after tax), index A'	Overall index of inequality E = (−1)* (D'* 0.5 + A'*0.5)
Australia							
1980	0.3040	15.48	26.73	0.0414	1.0000	1.0000	−1.000
1999	0.3378	17.48	27.66	0.0484	1.1685	1.1112	−1.140
Canada							
1980	0.3099	15.36	30.93	0.0475	1.0000	1.0000	−1.000
1999	0.3019	12.37	30.99	0.0383	0.8068	0.9743	−0.891
Norway							
1980	0.2500	6.35	34.66	0.0220	1.0000	1.0000	−1.000
1999	0.2659	9.15	28.53	0.0261	1.1866	1.0636	−1.125
Sweden							
1980	0.2139	5.49	36.02	0.0198	1.0000	1.0000	−1.000
1999	0.2530	8.65	36.64	0.0317	1.6024	1.1832	−1.393
U.K.							
1980	0.2903	9.20	19.93	0.0183	1.0000	1.0000	−1.000
1999	0.3430	13.20	28.49	0.0376	2.0512	1.1816	−1.616
U.S.							
1980	0.3314	17.96	34.80	0.0625	1.0000	1.0000	−1.000
1999	0.3869	17.93	34.94	0.0627	1.0023	1.1677	−1.085

Note: Poverty line = one half of median equivalent income; equivalent income = net family income after taxes adjusted by equivalence scale (square root of family size), negative or zero income excluded; average poverty gap = ratio of the gap (between poverty line and mean equivalent income of those under poverty line) to poverty line.

Source: Authors' calculations from LIS database.

completely eliminate economic anxieties, which have to be considered a subtraction from well-being.

Although public opinion polling can reveal that many feel themselves to be economically insecure, and that such insecurity decreases their subjective well-being, there is no generally agreed-upon definition of *economic insecurity*. Osberg (1998) has argued that economic insecurity is, in a general sense, the anxiety produced by a lack of economic safety—i.e., by an inability to obtain protection against subjectively significant potential economic losses. Ideally, one would measure trends in economic security with data that included (for example) the percentage of the population who had credible guarantees of employment continuity and the adequacy of personal savings to support consumption during illness or unemployment. However, such data are not widely available.

For these reasons, rather than attempt an overall measure of economic insecurity, we have adopted a "named risks" approach, and we have addressed the change over time in four key economic risks. More than fifty years ago, the United Nations' *Universal Declaration of Human Rights* (1948) stated:

> Everyone has the right to a standard of living adequate for the health and well-being of himself and of his family, including food, clothing, housing and medical care and necessary social services, and the right to security in the event of unemployment, sickness, disability, widowhood, old age or other loss of livelihood in circumstances beyond his control. [Article 25][23]

For this discussion, we constructed measures of the percentage change over time in the economic risks associated with unemployment, illness, "widowhood" (interpreted here as single-female parenthood), and old age. In each case, we modeled the risk of an economic loss associated with the event as a conditional probability, which can itself be represented as the product of several underlying probabilities. We weighted the prevalence of the underlying risk by the proportion of the population that it affected. The core hypothesis underlying the measure of economic insecurity we propose is that changes in the subjective level of anxiety about a lack of economic safety are proportionate to changes in objective risk.

Security from the economic risk associated with unemployment can be modeled as dependent on the risk of unemployment and the extent to which people are protected from the income losses of unemployment. We took as a proxy for the risk of unemployment changes in the employment rate (employment/population ratio). Changes in this ratio reflect changes in the unemployment rate and changes in the participation rate (both cyclical and structural). The extent to which people have been protected by unemployment insurance (UI) from the financial impacts of unemployment can be modeled as the product of (1) the percentage of the unemployed who claim regular UI benefits and (2) the percentage of average weekly wages replaced by UI. Internationally comparable data on these two variables, particularly the first, have proven very difficult to obtain. Hence, when calculating the risk of unemployment, we used an unpublished OECD series on the gross replacement rate for the unemployed. This series showed a markedly different trend than the UI coverage rate for certain countries such as Canada in the 1990s.[24]

We did not attempt to model the psychological insecurities associated with health or confront the issue of whether more education and greater knowledge of potential health risks (even ones of very small probability, such as mad cow disease) produce more or less anxiety. Our focus was on the economic losses associated with illness, which certainly dropped considerably with the introduction of universal health insurance in many countries. However, data limitations forced us to ignore trends in the risk of loss of earnings. Historically, a portion of the labor force has had some income-loss protection through sick leave provisions in their individual or collective employment contracts. One implication of a trend to short-term contract employment and self-employment in developed economies is an increase in the fraction of the population whose employment income ceases totally in the event of ill health.

Instead, we focused on the financial risk associated with health care costs, assuming that risk to be proportional to the share of uninsured private medical care expenses in disposable income. The OECD Health Data CD-ROM provided us with data for a long period on medical care expenses as a proportion of disposable income (excluding medical insurance premiums and net of all insurance reimbursement for medical expenses), which ranged from a high of 14.0% in the United States to a low of 1.1% in the United Kingdom in 1996. The proportion in the other countries was 5.5% in Australia, 3.2% in Canada, 2.0% in Norway, and 1.6% in Sweden.

To follow the convention that increases in the subcomponents of the index of economic security are improvements, we wanted an index of "security" and not an index of "insecurity." Hence, since increases in health costs are negative for economic well-being, we multiplied the financial risk due to illness by −1. An increased negative value therefore represented a decline in well-being.

When the UN Universal Declaration of Human Rights was drafted in 1948, the percentage of single-parent families was relatively high in many countries, partly as a result of World War II. At that time, widowhood was the primary way in which women and children lost access to male earnings. Since then, divorce and separation have become the primary origins of single-parent families. However, it remains true that many women and children are "one man away from poverty," since the prevalence of poverty among single-parent families is extremely high (e.g., OECD 2003, 53). To model trends in this aspect of economic insecurity, we applied the following formula: (the probability of divorce) × (the poverty rate among single-female-parent families)[25] × (the average poverty gap ratio among single-female-parent families).[26] The product of these last two variables is the intensity of poverty.

We stress that in constructing a measure of the economic insecurity associated with single-parent status, we were *not* constructing a measure of the social costs of divorce. Economic well-being is only part of social well-being, and divorce has emotional and social costs (e.g., for the involved children) that are not considered here. Arguably, over time the social costs associated with divorce (e.g., stigma) have changed, as the institution of marriage itself has changed—but such issues lie well beyond the scope of this chapter.

Data on divorce rates come from the UN's *Demographic Yearbook* (1997) and estimates of the poverty rate and poverty gap ratio for single-female parents were calculated from the LIS micro-data tapes. The annual divorce rate in 1996 (or the most recent year before 1996 for which data were available) was 4.33% of legally married couples in the United States—significantly higher than in the United Kingdom (2.89%), Australia (2.86%), Canada (2.62%), Sweden (2.42%), and Norway (2.28%).

The data indicate that international differences in the economic consequences of single-parent status reinforce differences in its probability. The poverty rate for single-female parents in the most recent year (in parentheses) from LIS micro-data files ranged from a high of 44.0% (1997) in the United States to a low of 2.8% (1992) in Sweden. In between were Australia, 40.7% (1994); Canada, 40.7% (1994); the United Kingdom, 13.8% (1986); and Norway, 11.3% (1995). The average poverty gap ratio for single-female parents in the same year was 41.6% in Norway, 39.6% in the United States, 27.5% in Canada, 24.5% in Australia, and 23.6% in the United Kingdom.

Again, to follow the convention that increases in the subcomponents of the index of economic security are improvements, we wanted an index of "security" and not an index of "insecurity." Hence, we multiplied the financial risk associated with single-parenthood, where increases were negative for economic well-being, by −1. A negative sign, therefore, indicated that an increased negative value represented a decline in well-being.

Since income in old age is the result of a lifelong series of events and decisions, which we cannot hope to disentangle in this chapter, we modeled the idea of "insecurity in old age" as dependent on the chance that an elderly person would be poor, and the average depth of that poverty. The poverty rate for the elderly in the most recent year (in parentheses) for LIS micro-data files ranged from a high of 33.1% (1994) in Australia to 24.4% (1997) in the United States; 12.0% (1995) in Norway; 6.0% (1992) in Sweden; 5.4% (1986) in the United Kingdom; and 4.8% (1994) in Canada. The average poverty gap ratio for the elderly in the same years ranged from a low of 9.3% in Norway to 27.6% in Australia. The United States (24.4%), Canada (13.4%), Sweden (12.7%), and the United Kingdom (11.7%) were in between.

Again, to follow the convention that increases in the subcomponents of the index of economic security are improvements; we wanted an index of "security" and not an index of "insecurity." Hence, we multiplied the risk of elderly poverty by −1.

OVERALL INDEX OF ECONOMIC SECURITY

We aggregated the four risks discussed thus far into an index of economic security using as aggregation weights the relative importance of the four groups in the population:

- for unemployment, the proportion of the population aged fifteen to sixty-four in the total population
- for illness, the proportion of the population at risk of illness—100%
- for single-parent poverty, the proportion of the population comprised of married women with children younger than eighteen

- for old-age poverty, the proportion of the population in immediate risk of poverty in old age, defined as the proportion of the population aged forty-five to sixty-four in the total population

As indicated in table 11.4, these proportions were normalized for all years to 1.0. For example, the weights for Canada in 1997 were the following: unemployment, 0.2779; illness, 0.4160; single parenthood, 0.2158; and old age, 0.0904.[27] Implicitly, by expressing changes as proportionate to an initial base, we were assuming that individuals habituated to a given level of background stimulus but responded similarly to proportionate changes in stimulus.

Estimates of Trends in the Overall Index of Economic Well-being

Trends in any index are determined by the choice of variables included in the index, the trends in those variables, and the weights those variables receive. Since the four main dimensions of average consumption, intergenerational bequest, inequality/poverty, and insecurity were separately identified, it is easy to conduct sensitivity analyses of the impact on perceived overall trends of different weighting of these dimensions.[28] Also, it would be straightforward to use these estimates to determine which component of economic well-being had the largest impact on which dimension of "health." It may be that all dimensions of health—mortality from different causes, morbidity of different types—respond similarly to each of these four components of economic well-being, but this supposition remains to be proven.

For discussion purposes, our "standard" weighting gave each component an equal weight of 0.25. Since the subcomponents of the consumption flows and wealth stocks were expressed in dollars, there was no need for explicit weighting. Their dollar values represented implicit weights. In terms of the inequality/poverty subcomponents, we assigned equal weight to each. The subcomponents of the economic security index were weighted by the relative importance of the specific population at risk in the total population (see table 11.5).

Economic Well-being over Time

We are acutely conscious that the data sources available to us were far from what we would have liked. We know that restricting ourselves to internationally comparable data series has meant that we have neglected issues (such as the decline in UI coverage in Canada) important for some countries. We also know the reliance on interpolation between the LIS data points implies, necessarily, that we cannot detect year-to-year fluctuations in some components of our index. However, we

Table 11.4. Economic security

Country and year	Index 1, unemployment	Index 2, health (÷2)	Index 3, single-parent poverty (÷2)	Index 4, old-age poverty (÷2)	Weighted index 1, unemployment	Weighted index 2, health	Weighted index 3, single-parent poverty	Weighted index 4, old-age poverty	Average weighted index of economic security
Australia									
1980	1.0000	1.0000	1.0000	1.0000	0.2729	0.4189	0.2283	0.0799	1.0000
1999	1.1656	0.9329	1.3656	-0.6293	0.3210	0.3830	0.2875	-0.0652	0.9262
Canada									
1980	1.0000	1.0000	1.0000	1.0000	0.2791	0.4114	0.2316	0.0779	1.0000
1999	1.2521	0.2926	1.3424	1.8814	0.3471	0.1190	0.2781	0.2051	0.9493
Norway									
1980	1.0000	1.0000	1.0000	1.0000	0.2655	0.4210	0.2231	0.0905	1.0000
1999	1.6829	0.7509	0.5885	1.6596	0.4615	0.3180	0.1204	0.1622	1.0621
Sweden									
1980	1.0000	1.0000	1.0000	1.0000	0.2781	0.4339	0.1902	0.0978	1.0000
1999	1.0031	-0.0637	1.7717	0.7801	0.2771	-0.0274	0.3193	0.0884	0.6575
U.K.									
1980	1.0000	1.0000	1.0000	1.0000	0.2643	0.4127	0.2304	0.0926	1.0000
1999	0.7876	0.0925	1.0955	1.1901	0.2124	0.0383	0.2396	0.1160	0.6064
U.S.									
1980	1.0000	1.0000	1.0000	1.0000	0.2809	0.4238	0.2109	0.0843	1.0000
1999	1.0812	0.4133	1.1736	1.3419	0.3047	0.1771	0.2250	0.1315	0.8384

Source: Data appendix posted at http://www.csls.ca.

Table 11.5. Index of economic well-being

Country and year	Consumption per capita (A)	Wealth stocks per capita (B)	Income distribution (C)	Economic security (D)	Well-being index— equal weighting	Well-being index— alternative weighting	GDP per capita index
Australia							
1980	1.0000	1.0000	1.0000	1.0000	1.0000	1.0000	1.0000
1999	1.4176	1.3053	0.8602	0.9262	1.1273	1.3015	1.4779
Canada							
1980	1.0000	1.0000	1.0000	1.0000	1.0000	1.0000	1.0000
1999	1.2247	1.3584	1.1094	0.9493	1.1604	1.1990	1.3228
Norway							
1980	1.0000	1.0000	1.0000	1.0000	1.0000	1.0000	1.0000
1999	1.4727	1.5568	0.8749	1.0621	1.2416	1.3803	1.5703
Sweden							
1980	1.0000	1.0000	1.0000	1.0000	1.0000	1.0000	1.0000
1999	1.2192	1.2013	0.6072	0.6575	0.9213	1.1001	1.3113
U.K.							
1980	1.0000	1.0000	1.0000	1.0000	1.0000	1.0000	1.0000
1999	1.5215	1.2823	0.3836	0.6064	0.9484	1.2923	1.4873
U.S.							
1980	1.0000	1.0000	1.0000	1.0000	1.0000	1.0000	1.0000
1999	1.3782	1.1798	0.9150	0.8384	1.0778	1.2580	1.4970

Note: Equal weighting well-being index = 0.25 * A + 0.25 * B + 0.25 * C + 0.25 * D. Alternative weighting well-being index = 0.7 * A + 0.1 * B + 0.1 * C + 0.1 * D.

Source: Data appendix posted at http://www.csls.ca.

hope that enough data remain to give a preliminary indication of trends in economic well-being from a broader perspective than that provided by GDP accounting.

Since we wanted to examine the sensitivity of a measure of economic well-being to alternative possible weightings of accumulation, income distribution, and insecurity, figures 11.1 to 11.6 present both our "standard" and an "alternative" weighting. The alternative one is much more heavily weighted to average consumption (0.7) and has much less weight on accumulation (0.1), income distribution (0.1), and insecurity (0.1). For each country, we compared trends in the standard and alternative indices with trends in GDP per capita.

For all countries, consideration of bequest, inequality/poverty, and insecurity reduced the measured rate of growth of economic well-being, compared with the use of the GDP per capita index. Generally, the more heavily current average consumption was emphasized, the closer our index came to GDP per capita. However, in every instance the consideration of a wider range of issues than those recognized in GDP accounting reduced the measured increase in economic well-being.

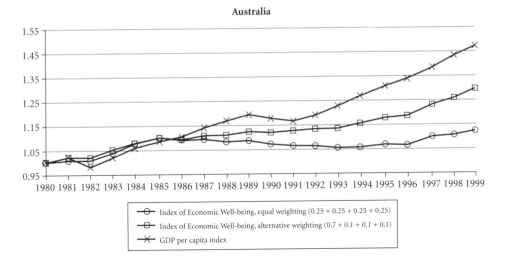

Figure 11.1. The index of economic well-being for Australia, 1980–1999

In some countries, the change in the perception of trends in economic well-being that a broader measure produced was striking. In the United States, GDP per capita increased by approximately 50% from 1980 to 1999, but our standard index was much flatter, with a total increase of 8% over the period. In the United Kingdom, increases in per capita GDP were of similar size (48.7%), but our standard weighting (which had a heavy emphasis on economic inequality and insecurity) showed a decline of about 5%. Both the United States and the United Kingdom were marked by a substantial increase in economic inequality over this

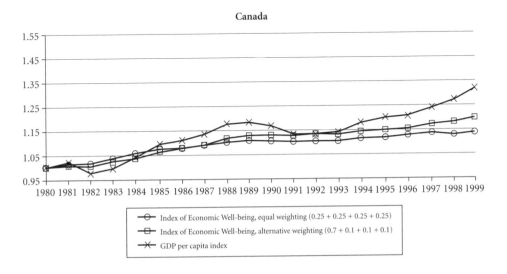

Figure 11.2. The index of economic well-being for Canada, 1980–1999

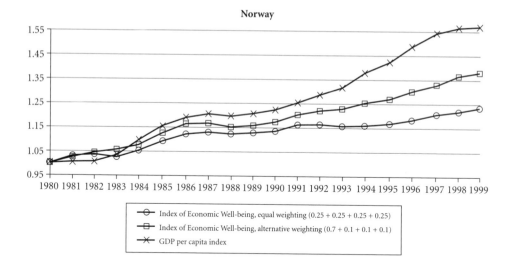

Figure 11.3. The index of economic well-being for Norway, 1980–1999

period, and increases in money income were limited to the top end of the income distribution (see Osberg 1999). In addition, increases in money income in the United States were obtained at the cost of substantial increases in working hours.

For the United Kingdom and Sweden, GDP per capita rose, whereas our standard index of economic well-being declined. In both cases, however, this qualitative result was quite sensitive to the relative weighting of current consumption, compared with distribution and insecurity: The alternative index did not actually decline,[29] although it was almost flat, in the Swedish data. As Osberg and Xu (2000)

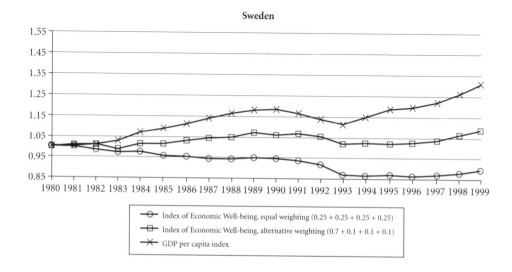

Figure 11.4. The index of economic well-being for Sweden, 1980–1999

United Kingdom

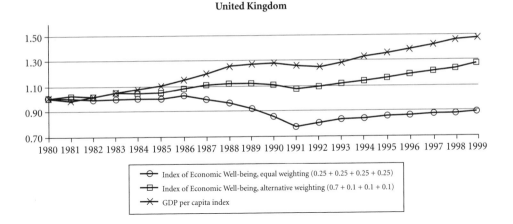

Figure 11.5. The index of economic well-being for the United Kingdom, 1980–1999

have noted, recent years have seen an increase in Swedish poverty intensity. Hence, we were not surprised that an index heavily weighting trends in income distribution and insecurity showed a deterioration.

From 1980 to 1999, Norway had the greatest increase in both GDP per capita and economic well-being, whichever weights were used for calculations. In Norway, trends in economic well-being were, more or less, scaled-down versions of the trend in GDP per capita. In this case, our current estimates of trends in the Index of Economic Well-being could be said to provide relatively little "value added," compared with trends in GDP per capita, since each index moves in much the

United States

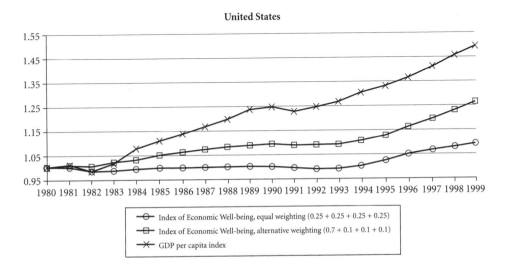

Figure 11.6. The index of economic well-being for the United States, 1980–1999

same way over time (albeit showing much stronger growth in GDP per capita than in economic well-being).

However, Australia and Canada—whose economies share a relative dependence on raw materials production—were noteworthy in showing a greater cyclical sensitivity in GDP per capita than one finds in either measure of economic well-being or in GDP per capita in other countries. In Canada and Australia, the recessions of both the early 1980s and early 1990s show up clearly in per capita GDP fluctuations—to a much greater degree than in Germany or Norway (the early 1980s recession is hard to find in UK or Swedish GDP per capita data). However, in both countries the trend in economic well-being indices is much smoother, because changes in current income can be much more rapid than changes in wealth stocks, income distribution, and insecurity. Canadian trends in economic well-being are also quite similar for "standard" and "alternative" weightings of the index.[30]

Level Comparisons of Economic Well-being

Comparisons of the level of well-being across countries are, in our judgment, inherently much more problematic than comparisons of the trends in various components of economic well-being within countries. In cross-country comparisons, the institutional context of economic data may differ far more than in within-country, longitudinal comparisons. Calculations of purchasing power parity equivalence across several countries appear to have greater uncertainty than comparisons of within-country consumer price levels. Statistical agencies in different countries typically differ in their data availability and data-gathering practices more than they change those practices over time in the same country. For all these reasons, we avoid in this chapter direct commentary on comparative levels of economic well-being.

Conclusion and Implications for Health

Early economists were fairly broad in their conception of "prosperity," but they were in no doubt that it had many positive implications. More recently, however, the measure of economic success has been narrower. Now, it falls to critics of the SNA to show that alternative measures to GDP per capita are possible, plausible, and more reflective of true economic well-being. Therefore, we have developed an index of economic well-being based on four dimensions, or components, of economic well-being for selected OECD countries: consumption, accumulation, income distribution, and economic security. One key finding was that economic well-being, for at least two different sets of relative weights, had increased at a much slower rate over the past twenty years than had real GDP per capita, a widely used indicator of economic well-being.

In Norway, trends in economic well-being are qualitatively, if not quantitatively, similar to trends in GDP per capita. However, in two countries (Australia and Canada), trends in well-being are cyclically dissimilar to GDP per capita trends. In the United States and the United Kingdom the secular trend one perceives in economic well-being depends heavily on whether one uses GDP per capita or a broader index of economic well-being that includes consideration of income distribution and economic insecurity—and the same is even more true of Sweden. In some countries (e.g., Sweden) the trend one perceives in economic well-being is very sensitive to the relative weighting of consumption, accumulation, distribution, and insecurity—but in others this sensitivity is much less pronounced. In short, even with the highly imperfect data available for this study, there is a good deal more information content in using a broader measure of economic well-being than GDP per capita.

Why should someone concerned with health outcomes be concerned with the divergence between trends in economic well-being and trends in GDP? Clearly, the issue depends partly on the definition of *health* being used, and there are several alternatives. However, to ascertain the relationship between health and economic well-being, we should not concentrate solely on health measurement and ignore the issue of accurate measurement of trends in economic well-being.

Some trends are likely to have both a direct link to health and an effect on economic well-being. Obviously, increased life span is directly linked to health, and we have argued for its consideration in a measure of trends in economic well-being. This chapter has also argued that changing household size affects economic well-being, and we know from the work of Wilkinson (1996) and Lavis and Stoddart (2000) that a broad range of health outcomes are closely linked to the social support available to individuals. It is also clear that decreasing household size necessarily implies less shared contact within families and that the availability of time outside of work[31] is a prime constraint on the formation of social links outside of work and family.

We were not able to include in this chapter costs of "regrettable necessities" in our measure of personal consumption, although some such adjustments (such as the increased expenditures necessary to avoid the costs of crime) are linked to aspects of health. Our proposed measure of economic well-being also included a proposal to count the accumulated value of human capital stocks, and it is well known that health outcomes are highly correlated with educational attainment.

We included measures of income distribution and economic insecurity in the proposed index of economic well-being because they directly affect individuals' well-being and because they strongly affect health. Whatever the level of per capita GDP, it clearly matters to individuals both what their personal prospect of lifetime income may be and how uncertain that prospect may be. Insecurity and economic stress have often been linked to mental and physical ill health. Wilkinson (1996) also argued that greater inequality increases the mortality rate. Daly and Duncan

(1998) argued that absolute deprivation reduces life expectancy, and they concluded that policies targeted at increasing the incomes of the poor are likely to have a larger effect on mortality risk than policies designed to reduce inequality more generally. In short, whatever the relationship between health and GDP per capita trends, health probably is more closely linked to a more adequate conceptualization of economic well-being.

Notes

1. For this chapter to be self-contained and provide a full explanation of the methodology used to estimate the index of economic well-being, we have drawn on material from earlier papers in which we developed the index (Osberg 1985; Osberg and Sharpe 1998, 1999). This chapter represents part of the output of an ongoing research agenda. Other articles and the most recent amendments to index methodology—such as those embodied in Osberg and Sharpe (2005)—can be found at http://www.csls.ca/iwb.asp. The sources for the data underlying all charts in the text of this chapter can be found in an Excel database file, posted for free download at http://www.csls.ca.iwb/oecd.asp. Please follow the links for specific charts to find the most recent discussion of sources and any revision of data. Background data for additional OECD countries, as well as for the seven countries that this chapter considers (for which data are more reliable), are also presented.

2. Keunig (1998) reviewed the contributions of Dawson (1996) and Kendrick (1996) and the most recent revisions to the SNA (UN 1993).

3. Furthermore, if we discover that there is disagreement about values and that it does matter for policy purposes, we can focus further discussion on those issues. In a democracy, much of the political process revolves around attempts to persuade others about which values should take precedence.

4. However, a sufficient (but not necessary) set of conditions for the index of economic well-being that we propose would be the following: Societal economic well-being can be represented as the well-being of a "representative agent" *if* (1) such an agent has a risk-averse utility function (i.e., diminishing marginal utility); (2) each person, from behind a "veil of ignorance" as to his or her own characteristics, draws an individual income stream (and prospects of future income) from the actual distribution of income streams; (3) each person has a utility function in which both personal consumption and a bequest to future generations are valued; (4) individual income streams are exposed to unpredictable future shocks; and (5) capital markets and public policies do not always automatically produce a socially optimal aggregate savings rate.

5. Only these countries had a large enough number of public-use micro-data files for construction of reliable long-run time series on the variables we needed. In addition, maintaining international comparability of estimates meant that some data used in our other papers to construct the index for Canada and the United States, but not available for other countries, were not used for this chapter.

6. An extended discussion of the rationale for this framework of consumption, accumulation, distribution, and insecurity can be found in Osberg (1985).

7. The underground economy refers to economic activity that is either illegal, or legal but unreported to the tax authorities.

8. Dan Usher (1980), of Queen's University, has developed a methodology for the estimation of the value of increased longevity.

9. For example, when fishing fleets stay in port because of stormy weather conditions, they are not generating marketable output and GDP is lower. If they put out to sea, however, some fish would be caught (GDP would increase) and some boats would sink (average life expectancy would decline).

10. Wolfson (1996) found for 1990–1992 that the HALE for 15-year-olds in Canada was 7.8 years less than life expectancy (55.6 versus 63.4 years). However, since there is no time series on health-adjusted life expectancy for Canada, we do not know if the rate of increase in the HALE has been greater or lower than life expectancy over time. Neither are data on the HALE available over time for other countries.

11. Implicitly, this procedure ignores both the differential values that individuals might place on changes in mortality probability at different ages and the distribution, by age, of actual changes in mortality probability.

12. This product is released annually by the OECD and can be purchased at http://www.oecd.org. The CD-ROM contains data on the health system and indicators of the health of the population for all OECD countries, as well as macroeconomic and demographic data.

13. The average size of households was calculated from the Luxembourg Income Study micro-data files.

14. Annual average hours worked per working-age person (ages fifteen to sixty-four) depend on the fraction of the population that has employment, the number of weeks per year that employed people typically work, and their average hours of work per week. There are major differences between countries in the proportion of people who participate in full-time paid employment (particularly large differences are observed for married women and men fifty to sixty-four). However, in this chapter, we ignore *how* differences in average working hours are generated.

15. Total annual hours of unemployment are calculated as the product of the number of unemployed and average annual hours per employed person, on the assumption that an unemployed person wants to work average hours. Total unemployed hours are then divided by the working-age population to determine average annual hours of unemployment per working-age person.

16. See Coulombe (2000), who notes that the average depreciation rate for Canada's business sector capital stock over the 1961–1997 period was 10%, compared with 4.4% in the United States.

17. See OECD (2001) for trends in educational attainment and the individual and social outcomes associated with education.

18. The R&D investment series starts in 1960; therefore, the stock of R&D in 1960 is equal to the R&D investment that year, and the series has a base of zero in 1959.

19. The conceptual issues to be dealt with in estimating the costs of CO_2 emissions include whether the costs should be viewed from a global, national, or subnational perspective; whether the costs increase linearly with the levels of pollution; whether the costs should be borne by the producer or the receiver of transborder emissions; and whether costs should vary from country to country or be assumed equally by all countries.

20. A purchasing power parity exchange rate is the rate at which a national currency is exchanged for U.S. dollars so as to leave the price of an identical basket of goods the same in both countries. Purchasing power parity exchange rates are preferred to market exchange rates for living standards comparisons because they account for differences in prices between countries.

21. Recognizing that an additional dollar means less to a millionaire than to a pauper, economists tend to agree that "diminishing marginal utility" is a reasonable assumption.

22. The Gini index is an indicator of inequality that increases as inequality increases. A value of zero indicates perfect equality (every individual in a given society has the same income), and a value of unity indicates perfect inequality (one individual has all the income in a given society).

23. Today, the sex specificity of the 1948 language will strike many people as odd, but Article 2 makes it clear that all rights are to be guaranteed to males and females equally.

24. The term "unemployment insurance" is used here because it is common in most countries, although Canada changed to the term employment insurance (EI) in 1996.

25. However, *rate = incidence × average duration*. Since the poverty rate among single parents is equal to the conditional probability that a single parent will enter poverty and the average duration of a poverty spell, we implicitly account jointly for the duration of poverty spells and for their likelihood.

26. This procedure effectively ignores single male parents, an approach justifiable on the grounds that males make up only about 10% of the single-parent population, and their income loss on divorce is generally considerably less than that of women.

27. To uniformly establish the base year for the indices of all risks of economic security at 1.000 in table 11.4, we have added the constant 2 to the indices of risk of illness, single parenthood, and old age, whose original base was -1.

28. A Microsoft Excel spreadsheet with the required data and programs is available on request from the authors.

29. In addition, we would caution that because we were not able to get, for this chapter, estimates of the income replacement provided under UI in these countries, we may have overestimated the importance for economic insecurity of the rise in unemployment in these countries.

30. But this chapter does not capture the rise in economic insecurity produced by declining UI coverage.

31. In practice, the timing and predictability of work hours (e.g., shift work or mandatory overtime) may be just as important to the possibility of participation in voluntary activities, such as youth sports or choral groups, as the absolute amount of work hours.

References

Angus, R. 1998. CTV/Globe poll of July 1998. Available at http://www.angusreid.com.

Arrow, K. J. 1951. *Social Choice and Individual Values.* New York: Wiley.

Burkhauser, R. V., T. M. Smeeding, and J. Merz. 1996. Relative inequality and poverty in Germany and the United States using alternative equivalence scales. *Review of Income and Wealth* 42:381–400.

Clark, A., and A. Oswald. 1994. Unhappiness and unemployment. *Economic Journal* 104 (424):648–659.

Coulombe, S. 2000. The Canada–US productivity growth paradox. Working paper no. 12, March. Ottawa: Industry Canada.

Daly, M. C., and G. Duncan. 1998. Income inequality and mortality risk in the United States: Is there a link? *Federal Reserve Board of San Francisco Economic Letter* no. 98-29, October 2.

Dawson, J. C., ed. 1996. *Flow-of-Funds Analysis.* Armonk, NY: M. E. Sharpe.

Fankhauser, S. 1995. Evaluating the social costs of greenhouse gas emissions. *Energy Journal* 15:157–184.

Gervais, G. 1994. The size of the underground economy in Canada. Studies in National Accounting, catalogue no. 13-603-MPE, no. 2, Ottawa: Statistics Canada.

Intergovernmental Panel on Climate Change (IPCC). 2001. *Climate Change 2001: The Scientific Basis.* Contribution of Working Group I to the Third Assessment Report of the Intergovernmental Panel on Climate Change, ed. J. T. Houghton, Y. Ding, D. J. Griggs, M. Noguer, P. J. van der Linden, X. Dai, K. Maskell, and C. A. Johnson. Cambridge: Cambridge University Press.

International Energy Association. 2003. *Key World Energy Statistics (2003).* Paris: International Energy Association.

International Monetary Fund. 2002. *International Financial Statistics Yearbook 2002.* Washington DC: International Monetary Fund.

Kendrick, J. W., ed. 1996. *The New System of National Accounts.* Boston: Kluwer Academic Publishers.

Keunig, S. 1998. A powerful link between economic theory and practice: National accounting. *Review of Income and Wealth* 44:437–46.

Lavis, J., and G. L. Stoddart. 2000. Social cohesion and health. In *Teams Work Better: The Economic Implications of Social Cohesion,* ed. L. Osberg. Toronto: University of Toronto Press.

Organization for Economic Cooperation and Development (OECD). 1998. *Flows and Stocks of Fixed Capital 1971–1996.* Paris: OECD.

———. 2001. *Education at a Glance: OECD Indicators 2001.* Paris: OECD.

———. 2003. *Society at a Glance: OECD Social Indicators 2002.* Paris: OECD.

Osberg, L. 1985. The measurement of economic welfare. In *Approaches to Economic Well-being,* ed. David Laidler. Royal Commission on the Economic Union and Development Prospects for Canada (MacDonald Commission), vol. 26. Toronto: University of Toronto Press.

———. 1998. Economic insecurity. Discussion paper no. 88, Social Policy Research Centre, University of New South Wales, Sydney, Australia.

———. 1999. Long run trends in economic inequality in five countries: A birth cohort view. Paper presented at Jerome Levy Institute Conference on Macro Dynamics of Inequality, October 28–29, Annandale-on-Hudson, New York. Available at http://is.dal .ca/~osberg/home.html.

Osberg, L., and A. Sharpe. 1998. An index of economic well-being for Canada. Paper presented at the Centre for the Study of Living Standards Conference on the State of Living Standards and Quality of Life in Canada, October 30–31, Ottawa, Ontario. Available at http://www.csls.ca (under "past events") and as research paper no. R-99-3E, December, Applied Research Branch, Human Resources Development Canada.

———. 1999. An index of economic well-being for Canada and the United States. Paper presented at the annual meeting of the American Economics Association, January 3–5, New York.

———. 2005. How should we measure the "economic" aspects of well-being? *The Review of Income and Wealth,* forthcoming series 51, number 2.

Osberg, L., and K. Xu. 2000. International comparisons of poverty intensity: Index decomposition and bootstrap inference. *Journal of Human Resources* 35 (1):51–81.

Phipps, S., and T. I. Garner. 1994. Are equivalence scales the same for the United States and Canada? *Review of Income and Wealth* 40 (1):1–18.

Sen, A. K. 1970. *Collective Choice and Social Welfare.* San Francisco: Holden-Day.

United Nations. 1948. *Universal Declaration of Human Rights.* New York: United Nations.

———. 1997. *Demographic Yearbook 1997.* New York: United Nations.

United Nations, in collaboration with Eurostat, International Monetary Fund, Organization for Economic Cooperation and Development, and World Bank. 1993. *System of National Accounts 1993.* Series F, no. 2, rev. 4 New York: Eurostat, IMF, OECD, UN, and World Bank.

Usher, D. 1980. *The Measurement of Economic Growth.* Oxford: Basil Blackwell.

Wilkinson, R. G. 1996. *Unhealthy Societies: The Afflictions of Inequality.* London: Routledge.

Wolfson, M. 1996. Health-adjusted life expectancy. *Health Reports* 8:41–45.

World Bank. 1997. *Expanding the Measure of Wealth: Indicators of Environmentally Sustainable Development.* Environmentally Sustainable Development Studies and Monographs Series, no. 17. Washington, DC: World Bank.

Chapter 12

Reallocating Resources across Public Sectors to Improve Population Health

Greg L. Stoddart, John D. Eyles, John N.
Lavis, and Paul C. Chaulk

Recent research on the determinants of health has rapidly expanded and refined our knowledge about the wide range of factors that influence the health of individuals and populations (Evans et al. 1994; Amick et al. 1995; Marmot and Wilkinson 1999; Adler et al. 1999; Berkman and Kawachi 2000; Wilkinson and Marmot 2003; Canadian Population Health Initiative 2004). Even a partial listing of such factors would include influences as disparate as genetic endowment, gender, personal health practices, early childhood development, coping skills, health care, housing, employment and working conditions, education, social status, income, social support, cultural environment, and physical and natural environments. Moreover, the factors are related and do not operate in isolation. Health is the result of complex interactions between the characteristics of individuals and the characteristics of their environments. Context matters.

The gradually unfolding understanding of this complexity presents a formidable challenge to policy makers who attempt to improve both the level and the distribution of population health. They are increasingly recognizing that, to be most effective, initiatives may need to involve several policy sectors simultaneously and that initiatives in one sector can have consequences in seemingly unrelated areas. But recognition is one thing; successful intersectoral policy development is another, and it thus far has proven difficult in all countries (World Health Organization 1997; Lavis and Sullivan 1999; van Herten et al. 2001; Exworthy et al. 2003; Kindig et al. 2003). The reasons for this difficulty are themselves complex, but one significant barrier is often the need to reallocate resources from one sector to another to address better the relative importance of different health determinants in a particular jurisdiction. Policy sectors are often resource "silos," and policy managers in the sectors typically have neither the incentive nor the mechanisms to make cross-sectoral reallocations.

In fact, because of the difficulty in applying a determinants-of-health approach to resource allocation across sectors, there are very few cases internationally for which it has been attempted. To our knowledge, no industrialized country has truly engaged in a formal, national cross-sectoral reallocation exercise aimed at maximizing population health. Attempts at cross-sectoral reallocation have been confined to subnational (state, provincial, or most often local) levels. The government of the Canadian province of Prince Edward Island (PEI) was one of the first governments to design an explicit mechanism to facilitate cross-sectoral reallocation. Here we provide a detailed examination of that experience.

In 1993 the PEI government moved to address the cross-sectoral reallocation problem. As part of a broader attempt at health reform, it passed legislation to regionalize the delivery of health and social services across the province and to provide the regional authorities with "block budgets" that combined the funding for a wide range of programs and services. The expressed intent was to allow the regional authorities the latitude to make management decisions and resource reallocations that they deemed necessary to address the determinants of health and meet local health needs. In this chapter we report on the PEI experience with block budgets and cross-sectoral reallocation of resources for health. We begin with a description of policy development and implementation, and the attempt to establish a process for evaluating health reform. Next, the results of four related studies of cross-sectoral reallocation in PEI are briefly presented and discussed. The results suggest that although some reallocation has occurred, it has been limited at best. In the last two sections we discuss the reasons for such modest effects and the messages from the PEI experience.

Chronology of Health Reform and Regionalization

A maritime province on Canada's east coast, PEI is the smallest Canadian province (with a population of 140,000). In 1991 the cabinet of the provincial Liberal government recommended the creation of a task force to consider the future of health and community services for islanders. At that time the health care system and many community services were managed by many province-wide departments, agencies, and boards, amidst concerns about rising costs and utilization, effectiveness of services in meeting health needs, and lack of community involvement in decision making. The Health Task Force (PEI 1992) recommended a new vision for health policy that emphasized "wellness promotion," need-based planning, community-based services, and local involvement in the planning and delivery of integrated health services. The government response was positive, and the minister of health and social services established a Health Transition Team to recommend an implementation plan for the vision.

In its report (PEI 1993a, i) the Health Transition Team clearly recognized the broad range of influences on health, emphasizing that "health is determined by many factors, such as the environment, social and economic conditions that are outside the immediate control of the health system." Among its ten Principles of Health Reform were ones that affirmed a philosophy recognizing the breadth of determinants of health, highlighted the need for health promotion, and recognized that primary health care should be based partly on the integration of health development with social and economic development (PEI 1993a; Lomas and Rachlis 1996). While recognizing that financial pressures on government meant that reform had to involve the health-care delivery system, the team emphasized strongly, however, a vision for health beyond health care that stressed health promotion, community involvement, and the importance of social and economic determinants of health. The team recommended the regionalization of health and social services, the development of a resource center for health promotion, the development and implementation of community needs assessment by the new regions, and the establishment of a pilot community health centre project (PEI 1993a). The report also contained other recommendations dealing with utilization management, physician payment, and information systems; and the team offered an implementation plan for its recommendations.

The government responded quickly. Within months the provincial legislature passed the Health and Community Services Act (PEI 1993b), largely accepting the principal recommendations of the Health Transition Team report and significantly altering the underlying principles and organizational structure for delivery of human services in PEI. The act created five regional authorities, with population bases ranging from 7,000 to 60,000, each managed by a chief executive officer and an appointed board (with a plan to move to elected boards). Regions were given responsibility for assessing their health needs, setting priorities, allocating budgets, employing service providers, and managing and delivering a wide range of human services. The services included hospitals, home care, mental health, public health, addiction services, child welfare, income security, public housing, job creation and employment enhancement, seniors' social services, community development, probation and correctional services, and various other health and social services (though, interestingly, not pharmaceuticals, physician services, or education). Although regionalization of health services has occurred in other Canadian provinces, no other province has devolved authority for such a broad array of combined health and social services (Lomas et al. 1997).

Most of the provincial Ministry of Health and Social Services staff members were reassigned to the regional authorities, with a small number going to two other, new central agencies created by the act. The Health Policy Council (HPC) was established to set broad health goals and provide advice to the minister, and the Health and Community Services Agency (HCSA) was created to define core services that the regions would be required to provide, set regional budgets and human resource policies, and provide the regions with program development support. The ministry retained responsibility for broad policy guidelines, the agency's overall budget, intergovernmental affairs, and evaluation. Each regional authority was to integrate its service-planning and-delivery responsibilities under a single management structure, which received pooled funding for all services combined in the form of a block budget. The expressed intent of this part of the reform was to empower regional decision makers to address the broad determinants of health through program management and resource reallocations that responded to local needs. In principle, the block budgets afforded wide scope for reallocation; in practice, however, the construction and presentation of them based on existing service and program categories embedded rigidities from the outset.

Although a determinants-of-health approach figured prominently in the health reform philosophy, the reform documents and policy makers also identified several other equally (or even more) important objectives, including more primary and community-based care, improved effectiveness and efficiency through service co-ordination and integration, needs-based planning, increased personal responsibility for health, and increased community involvement in decision making.[1] Policy makers in different parts of the government saw the importance of the objectives differently. Whereas the HPC emphasized addressing the social determinants of health, the HCSA focused on the need for community development and the need to improve integration and coordination while reducing duplication of services. The Ministry of Health and Social Services, influenced by the government's fiscal concerns, emphasized the need for improvements in both effectiveness and efficiency of health service delivery (table 1 in Lomas and Rachlis 1996).

Significantly, at the same time health reform was being implemented and the regions were assuming their responsibilities early in 1994, PEI, like the rest of the Canadian provinces, was entering a period of fiscal retrenchment. Reform gave way to fiscal restraint as an imperative (Lomas and Rachlis 1996). Thus, the regional authorities spent their early years coping with public expenditure reductions of between 5% and 10%, which they felt weakened their effectiveness. On the other hand, during the early years of reform the HCSA invested significant effort and resources to disseminate information on the reform package and especially the determinants-of-health approach, bringing in prominent researchers to speak, conducting workshops, and creating educational materials to support the regions (PEI 1996a, 1996b). Health reform and regionalization became the topics of the day, generating frequent discussion—both pro and con—in the province's newspapers.

In November 1996, the governing Liberals were defeated by the Progressive Conservatives in an election in which the issue of health reform featured prominently. Concerns about the preservation of health care, and especially of small hospitals, surfaced almost daily during the election campaign, with the Conservatives emphasizing their intent to protect the health care system in the reform process. The new government made minor changes to the block-funding envelopes, removing correctional services. It also eliminated the HPC and the HCSA, the latter as part of a move to make regional CEOs directly accountable to the minister. But it left in place the regional governance model (though the minister of the day publicly questioned its usefulness), the commitment to a client-focused, integrated service-delivery system, and—at least in rhetoric—the endorsement of a determinants-of-health approach.

Since then, the Conservative government has been reelected for a second term and has increased funding for acute health care services, child and family services, and home care. At the time of this writing, the regional authorities remain and are moving to a system of partially elected boards. In May 2001 the provincial government released a draft Strategic Plan for the Health and Social Services System and conducted public consultations on it (PEI 2001). Although the recognition of the broad set of determinants influencing health remains, the plan focuses heavily on issues of the demand for and supply of health care, individual responsibility for health, and public confidence in the health care system. The 1992–2001 chronology of policy developments (and also of evaluation activities, discussed next) is summarized in table 12.1.

Evaluation Activities

Although an evaluation component was not built into the reform process itself, both policy makers and stakeholders recognized the importance of monitoring the reforms and assessing their impact. A federal–provincial joint funding agreement between Health Canada and the PEI Department of Health and Social Services (DHSS) provided support for the development and implementation of an evaluation protocol. This led to the establishment of a small group in the department known as the System Evaluation Project (SEP) and collaborative agreements with several Canadian academic researchers interested in health services and policy research. The envisioned evaluation was ambitious. It was to address the reform package's multiple policy goals and involve stakeholders, as well as researchers (both government and academic), in its design. Moreover, it was to include both a formative and a summative component, feeding back information about the process of reform to policy makers, stakeholders, and the public "in real time," as well as producing a series of ongoing reports about the impact of reform.

The methodological and political challenges and the resulting compromises in constructing an evaluation protocol are themselves an interesting subject, though they are not developed here. Through an extensive and intensive set of workshops and consultations, SEP produced a protocol that highlighted fourteen primary and many secondary evaluation questions (PEI 1997, 1998b). The evaluation plan called

Table 12.1. Timing of policy developments and evaluation activities

Date	Policy developments	Evaluation activities
1992	Health Task Force report	
1993	Health Transition Team report (June) *Health and Community Services Act* passed (Oct.)	
1994	Regional Authorities begin operation Provincial fiscal retrenchment begins	
1995		Preliminary work with external collaborators, provincial stakeholders, and steering committee on framework for evaluating health reform Lomas and Rachlis (1996) interview provincial policy makers, regional managers, local stakeholders (July–August)
1996	Governing Liberals defeated by Progressive Conservatives (Nov.)	Federal-provincial funding agreement to design and implement evaluation protocol
1997	Health and Community Services Act amended to abolish Agency and Council	SEP surveys, presentation of preliminary results to government (Jan.–June) Decision-support tools exercise (Dec.)
1998	Correctional services removed from block budgets	
1999		Eyles et al. (2000) interview key informants (Jan.–May) SEP Summary of Results document (PEI 1999) released (July) SEP ends (Oct.)
2000	Conservatives reelected	
2001	Draft Strategic Plan for the Health and Social Services System released for public consultation	

332

for assessments of these questions at one, three, and five years from an agreed-on baseline, using a combination of mail and telephone surveys, focus groups, secondary data sources, and document review. One of the questions was whether or not the regions had taken advantage of block budgets to use cross-sectoral reallocation of resources as a management strategy.

SEP began the first wave of data collection late in 1996 and presented some initial results to the new Conservative government early in 1997, just before the government signaled its policy directions. Over the next two years SEP continued with dissemination activities for government, regional managers, other stakeholders, and the public, culminating with a summary document in 1999 (PEI 1999). But the new government did not view the continued execution of the evaluation protocol as a priority once the deliverables (primarily the evaluation protocol) under the Health Canada agreement were completed and federal joint funding had stopped. The government's message was that it was time for action rather than further study and that all available resources should be going into service delivery. Provincial funding for the second wave of data collection was not made available. SEP was reorganized and renamed, and its staff members were assigned other evaluation responsibilities.

In addition to the limited SEP results, three other sources provide material for reflection on the PEI experience with cross-sectoral reallocation. The first is an examination of block funding in PEI by Lomas and Rachlis (1996), done as part of a larger research project on the role of financial incentives in the Canadian health care system (Giacomini et al. 1996). The second is an exercise conducted by SEP with senior managers of the regions in late 1997 that attempted to identify and develop decision-support tools that would help them make cross-sectoral reallocations (PEI 1998c). The third is a recent follow-up study of progress on cross-sectoral reallocation in PEI by some of the researchers who had participated in the original SEP evaluation (Eyles et al. 2000).

The PEI Experience with Cross-sectoral Reallocation: The Early Days

Lomas and Rachlis (1996) analyzed the first eighteen months of regionalization (all prior to the change in government) through a combination of interviews with key informants in two regions and a review of provincial and regional policy documents and budgets, as well as newspaper clippings. Recognizing that too little time had elapsed to expect major effects, they presented their work primarily as a study of policy implementation. Nevertheless, their observations are interesting, both as insights into the early days of a major policy change and as predictors of what was to come. They found that the regions had used their latitude for cross-sectoral reallocation very cautiously, despite senior managers' and board members' genuine enthusiasm for and commitment to the concept. Reallocations occurred infrequently, and there were few, if any, examples of reallocations in the principal anticipated directions: from acute health-care services to other determinants of health and from institutional to community-based care.

Two specific instances attracted the researchers' attention. In the first, a rural region unsuccessfully attempted to rationalize hospital services by converting one of two tiny, neighboring acute-care hospitals into a long-term-care facility. The proposal antagonized both of the affected communities, drew fierce criticism from physicians and opposition politicians, and resulted in the resignation of the regional board. After a lawsuit and mediation, both sites remained open with acute-care services, even though funds had to be redirected from other regional services to do so. In the second instance, two regions found themselves with a surplus in their income security (welfare) budgets because a major construction project had temporarily raised prosperity above its historical level for the island. One of the regions allocated a large share of the surplus to further job creation, anticipating the end of the construction project. The other region allocated its surplus to acute-care services.

Lomas and Rachlis observed that the regional administrators had generally focused on the easier and more familiar ground of capturing administrative efficiencies in the delivery of existing services, rather than attempting significant innovation or reconfiguration of programs that would have required reallocation. The researchers noted several reinforcing reasons for this cautious approach. Although block budgets and a single management structure facilitated cross-sectoral reallocation, they were also powerful tools for integrating and coordinating teams of providers *within* sectors. Indeed, many front-line managers saw this as their major potential contribution. Coordination and integration were long-standing problems in several service areas—they had been identified as one of the policy objectives of the reform, and they were central to the new regional authorities' client-focused delivery philosophy. Since coordination and integration were also easier to tackle, it was not surprising that they were addressed first.

Public understanding and acceptance of the rationales for reallocation were also a factor. Regional authorities perceived that the general public would need more time and education to understand fully why resources might be shifted away from acute-health-care services in particular. The public mood was in part the result of vocal opposition by physicians and unionized employees (notably, hospital workers) of the regions to large parts of the health reform. Concerns about incomes and jobs were fused with anxieties about the adequacy of health care services in the future. Even in the absence of active opposition, adjusting or renegotiating labor agreements, plus allowing for transition of employment from government departments and central or provincial agencies to the regions, required considerable time.

Actions taken—or not taken—by central bodies in the province also contributed to the regions' caution. The existence of multiple major policy objectives may have diluted the importance of the policy signal about reallocation. Also, the HCSA offered little encouragement of reallocation, perhaps because it was waiting to see how the regions handled other policy objectives requiring less dramatic changes. Nor did either the HCSA or the HPC give the regions specific targets for improvements in health outcomes, a fact that Lomas and Rachlis thought might have motivated the regions to realign their programs. Finally, government fiscal restraint and overall expenditure reductions significantly decreased the scope for discretionary reallocations by the regions after they met the provisions for delivery of core services. The timing of this restraint, coming on the heels of health reform, also fostered some cynicism and mistrust among service providers especially, but also among the public and some regional managers. Regionalization was seen as a convenient way for the provincial government to shift the blame for the effects of its deficit-reduction actions.

Despite the early difficulties, however, the policy makers and regional administrators interviewed by the researchers remained cautiously optimistic that reallocations could be made in the longer term once human resource transitions were completed; the public was more comfortable with reform; and better working relationships and consultative mechanisms between the regions, the central bodies, and providers were established. They emphasized that the magnitude of the reform required a much longer horizon for both implementation and evaluation.

SEP Results

In the first (and what turned out to be the only) wave of its data collection, SEP conducted surveys of several groups early in 1997.[2] The surveys addressed a wide range of topics and were tailored for each group. Regional CEOs and senior managers were asked about several topics, including their experience with cross-sectoral reallocation (PEI 1998b). SEP first constructed a conceptual framework for cross-sectoral reallocation (PEI 1998a). Figure 12.1 displays the health care and social service sectors under the regions' budgetary control. The arrows indicate that cross-sectoral reallocations could occur in four ways: among health-care sectors (A), among social services sectors (B), between health care and social services sectors (C), or between sectors in the health system and sectors in other provincial systems (D). Figure 12.2 adds to the framework the types of resources that might be reallocated and the levels at which reallocation decisions might be made.

The five CEOs and thirty-two senior managers of the regions were asked in a self-administered, mailed survey whether any of the four types of reallocations had been made in their region. If so, they were asked to provide examples. They were also asked about difficulties they had encountered in attempting to make reallocations, and they were given an opportunity for open-ended comments. Seventy-six percent of the surveyed people responded, frequently including detailed comments on their experiences and views, and they indicated that reallocations were

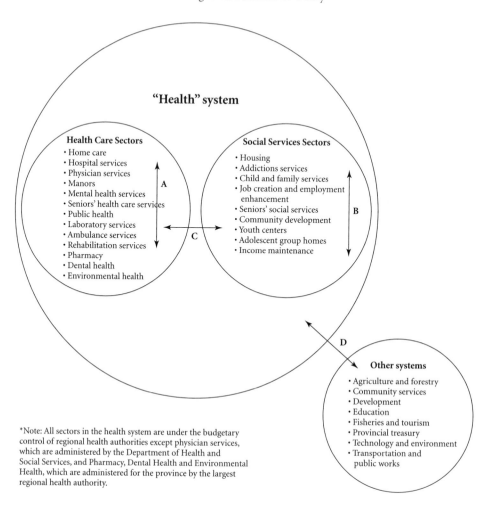

Figure 12.1. Types of cross-sectoral reallocations

Source: Reprinted from PEI 1998a.

occurring. Ninety percent said that their region had reallocated among health care sectors, while 79 percent indicated that their region had reallocated among social services sectors. Seventy-seven percent reported that reallocations between health care and social services sectors had occurred, and 45% indicated that reallocations had occurred between the health system and other systems (PEI 1998c).

On the surface, these findings seemed to indicate a significant increase in cross-sectoral activity over that found by Lomas and Rachlis almost two years earlier. But the actual extent of reallocation was very difficult to determine, due to space and other limitations in the questionnaire design. Respondents were asked only if reallocation had occurred; a single instance would produce an affirmative response.

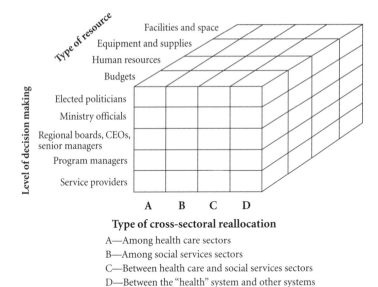

Figure 12.2. A three-dimensional conceptual framework for cross-sectoral reallocation of resources for health

Source: Reprinted from PEI 1998a.

There were no data on the frequency, size, or significance of reallocations. Furthermore, the thirty-seven respondents represented only five unique jurisdictions (the five regions), so respondents were often reporting the same experience, as the list of specific examples made clear. The examples suggested that many reallocations were minor ones and indicated that resources were still flowing toward acute-health-care services, as well as away from that sector. They also supported the earlier observation by Lomas and Rachlis that managers had focused initially on reallocations to integrate provider teams within sectors, rather than on those to reconfigure service delivery across sectors.

Not surprisingly, respondents noted that reallocation was much easier to accomplish on lower-profile programs and that they attempted to give reallocations a low profile generally. One interesting method for doing so was to reallocate people and tasks without adjusting internal budget lines. Managers agreed that "real" resources (i.e., people, equipment, supplies, and facilities) were much easier to reallocate than financial ones because internal budget changes drew attention, whereas the corresponding service-delivery changes often did not.

The respondents' open-ended comments demonstrated continuing concern about the provincial fiscal restraints' effect on the scope for reallocation. Added to this, however, was a new concern about the political climate. Some regional CEOs and senior managers questioned whether they still had a real mandate for cross-sectoral reallocation after the change in government.

By the time the first-wave SEP results were published (PEI 1999), the government's policy directions were firmly established, and it saw little need for investing additional funds to continue to execute the SEP evaluation protocol. Planned follow-up surveys were not undertaken. Nevertheless, the information collected by SEP extends the picture painted by Lomas and Rachlis. Despite their limitations as just noted, the SEP results reinforce the initial assessment that the objective of reallocation had regional support, and they suggest very modest, quite timid progress toward achieving it.

The Decision-support Tools Exercise

This hesitancy and the causes of it became even more apparent in an exercise that SEP conducted for the regions in late 1997. As part of the federal–provincial agreement to fund evaluation of the PEI health reforms, SEP was to assist the regions by developing "decision-support tools" for evidence-based decision making. SEP envisioned the primary focus of such tools to be improvement of the information base for cross-sectoral decision making. It included in this the refinement of a conceptual framework for cross-sectoral reallocation, the specification of basic types of data to be collected for program comparisons (a cross-sectoral cost-effectiveness template), and some initial illustrative display of this information. SEP also saw a need to prepare communities for reallocations through the design of community workshops on the determinants of health, plus a need to reinforce decisions with prepared messages that provided the evidence base for the decision and dealt with anticipated reactions (PEI 1998c).

In December 1997, in one of a series of consultations with the regions, SEP proposed the development of a package of tools dealing with the specified issues, and it was surprised by the regional senior managers' response. Better information was quite low on the managers' list of priorities for support tools, despite the fact that they were not satisfied with the type or quality of information available for cross-sectoral decision making and felt that efforts to improve it might help and would be appreciated.[3] In their view, however, the main barrier to cross-sectoral reallocation was the unsupportive public climate within which they had to make decisions. The managers saw tools to improve this climate, rather than tools to improve the information base, as their primary need (PEI 1998c). They identified a vicious circle involving providers, the public, and politicians, whereby service providers' expressed concerns generated public anxiety, which in turn fed into political processes that inhibited change. They also highlighted the role of the media in sustaining this tense situation.[4] The managers were careful to point out that they understood and accepted some of the principal concerns of providers and the public. For example, aside from fears about loss of jobs and incomes, many hospital workers reported their increasing fatigue as care became more community based, leaving only higher-needs patients in their institutions. In the case of the public, even if people accepted the need for investment in many different activities to improve health, above all they wanted assurances that hospital beds would be available if they needed them.

For these and other reasons, the regions emphasized setting reasonable expectations about the pace of change. Meanwhile, they requested that SEP develop materials that would help them to manage in such a difficult climate. Because part of SEP's mandate was to be responsive to participants in the evaluation, SEP altered its approach to decision-support tool development. Although it did refine and disseminate its conceptual framework for reallocation (PEI 1998a), SEP did not pursue other ways to improve the information base. Instead, it produced three documents for regional managers, covering the following:

- a workshop-based approach to helping service providers and other staff better understand the rationale for reallocation and to involving them in decision making (PEI 1998d)
- a process and a tool for conducting a political/environmental scan of the potential challenges to reallocation (PEI 1998f)
- advice on building a culture of support for reallocation among the media and the public (PEI 1998e)

Updating the Picture, 1998–2000

Eyles and colleagues (2000) have provided the most recent observations on the PEI experience with cross-sectoral reallocation. In late 1998 and early 1999 the investigators conducted in-depth, face-to-face interviews with fifty-eight key informants in PEI, and they held focus groups with subsets of them later in 1999 and in early 2000. The interviewees came from all regions of the province and the DHSS, from all sectors of human service provision, and from all levels of decision making. Respondents were asked about examples of reallocation, the barriers to and facilitators of reallocation, and ways in which the ease of making reallocations was changing over time.

The results were broadly similar to the earlier findings. Although respondents thought that it had become a little easier to make reallocations than at the beginning of reform (five years earlier), they still found it difficult to do so. They were able to give seventy-four examples (many repeating ones in the SEP results) of reallocations, most of which occurred among health care sectors or among social services sectors, rather than between the two, or between the health system and other provincial systems. Most of the examples involved nonfinancial reallocations of staff time, facilities (often, administrative space), or equipment, without explicit

340   Moving from Research to Policy

changes to internal budgets. They reflected often pragmatic management decisions at the margins of program operation. Financial transfers occurred in twenty-five of the seventy-four examples; in eight of those twenty-five cases, funds were shifted from community services to acute hospital care—a direction opposite what had been expected (Eyles et al. 2000).

Many of the study participants felt that their work environment had improved significantly due to regionalization. They reported that the existence of a single regional management structure had made it much easier to share resources and bring teams of service providers together to focus on their patients' and clients' needs. The focus was still on specific individuals or families, however, rather than on groups or the entire population. And the schism between the acute-health-care sector and other health care and social service sectors remained. The perception of those outside the acute-health-care sector was that this sector had benefited the most by reform; those inside this sector felt that they had been the hardest hit by reform.

Although regional governance was unambiguously viewed as a facilitator of real-location, block budgets were not. Some respondents still associated them with fiscal retrenchment, whereas others pointed out that the budgets hindered interregional cooperation. Still others expressed the view that the flexibility of block budgets was illusory, for two reasons. First, in practice, line-by-line budgeting was still used frequently, partly because the change in budgeting philosophy had not been accompanied by a reconceptualization of accounting practices nor investment in new financial-reporting systems. Second, many respondents felt that the regions' decision-making autonomy was less than it appeared. They reported that first the HCSA and later the DHSS (and the minister) had strongly influenced regional resource allocation decisions.

The barriers to reallocation that respondents cited most frequently were familiar ones: lack of overall funding, union agreements, lack of public and media support, and physician opposition. They did not rank poor quality or incomplete information highly among the barriers (Eyles et al. 2000), although they did realize that to enlist support for future reallocations they would need evidence of the effectiveness of those they had already made. Yet again, those interviewed found at least some reasons for optimism. They were proud of the culture and partnerships between organizations that had been created outside acute care and that seemed to be improving integration and coordination of service delivery in their sectors. They saw success on these fronts as a possible precursor to significant program reconfiguration and reallocation. And they believed that time was still on their side, stressing that significant change is likely to take years or decades rather than weeks or months.

Interpreting the PEI Experience: Ideas, Interests, and Institutions

Five years after Lomas and Rachlis's initial assessment of the PEI experience, little seems to have changed regarding reallocation, even if other objectives such as integration, coordination, and partnerships are being met. Although some reallocations have been made, regional managers have found it extremely difficult to implement major changes to move resources to "upstream prevention" from "downstream rescue" (Lomas and Rachlis 1996, 598). The potential for policy and program reconfiguration embedded in the vision of a broad set of social and economic determinants of health contained in the reform documents of the early 1990s remains largely untapped. Why have the effects of regionalization and block budgets on reallocation been so modest? One approach to interpreting the PEI experience is to draw on the traditional political science framework that examines the role of ideas, interests, and institutions in explaining policy action and inaction (Heclo 1974; Goldstein and Keohane 1993; Hall 1993, 1996; Weatherford and Mayhew 1995).

The category of "ideas" includes empirical evidence on which to base action, as well as values or beliefs that may encourage or constrain action. In PEI, the architects of reform accepted not only the new syntheses of evidence about the determinants of population health that were emerging in Canada during the early 1990s (Premier's Council on Health Strategy 1991; Evans et al. 1994; Canadian Minister of Supply and Services 1994) but also the need to balance resource commitments to health care with an increased emphasis on other determinants such as employment, income, housing, and social support. They also attempted to transfer these ideas, along with the basis for them, to the public. In the absence of well-designed before-and-after studies, it is difficult to determine whether these attempts made a difference. However, community-needs assessments and an SEP survey indicated that the public clearly recognized the importance to health of factors other than health care (PEI 1995, 1999; Eyles et al. 2001). Nevertheless, the public also stressed the importance of both formal health care and personal health practices.

The public reaction to the possibility of reallocating resources away from health care suggests that a deeply rooted belief in health care's importance still trumps "intellectual" ideas regarding social and economic determinants' impact. Health care is personal, concrete, and immediate. Other determinants are anonymous, abstract, and distant by comparison, at least for the individual. And the effects of those other determinants will often play out over years, if not decades, whereas the effects of health care can be evaluated in real time. Aside from moments of disaster or crisis, therefore, it is difficult to envision a public becoming as concerned about the social and economic fabric of its communities as it is fearful of not having physician or hospital care when needed.

The "interests" of physicians, hospital workers, and other service providers have also played a key role in determining PEI's pace of change. Although some providers, such as those in community-care or social services sectors, saw themselves or their sectors as gaining through reform, most workers in the largest sector—institutional care—were concerned about the risk of job losses or changes to their working conditions. From the outset, their opposition was strong and vocal. They were joined by many physicians who feared that the combined effects of fiscal retrenchment and a focus on determinants other than health care might leave what they viewed as an already stretched health care system unable to meet basic needs (Lomas and Rachlis 1996; Eyles et al. 2000). The constant presence in the media of these organized and vocal groups of opponents successfully overshadowed the island's few supportive voices and the examples of service-delivery improvements, and it reinforced anxieties among the public.

The policy analysis category of "institutions" includes the design and operation of decision-making structures and the effects of past or concurrent policies. Block budgets for regional health authorities seemed to offer a powerful enabling mechanism for implementing a determinants-of-health philosophy through reallocation of resources—and could still prove to be such. In retrospect, however, there are several reasons in this category that help explain why the capacity for block budgets to encourage reallocation has been underutilized. Fiscal retrenchment by the provincial government immediately following regionalization hampered early reallocation efforts in two ways. First, it reduced the discretionary room that the regions had after providing core services with their lower budgets. Second, it created suspicion among providers and the public about the real purpose of regionalization and block budgeting.

The pursuit of so many policy goals simultaneously—upwards of half a dozen can be found in background policy documents—also affected reallocation in two ways. The sheer number of goals meant that decision makers' attention was divided among multiple, often competing, objectives, all apparently important. Moreover, some (such as improving administrative efficiency) were easier to achieve than others (such as reallocation), so it should not have been surprising that managers moved more slowly on the latter. As Lomas and Rachlis pointed out, block budgets and a single management structure for the regions are as powerful a tool for rationalizing service delivery within sectors as they are for reallocating resources across sectors. Given that rationalizing delivery within sectors through integration and coordination was a more familiar and long-standing objective, and one that meshed with the complementary objective of improving the client focus of services, it is understandable that managers started there.

The structure and activities of central bodies in the province also dampened enthusiasm for reallocation. The regions were given very few specific policy guidelines or targets by the DHSS, the HCSA, or the HPC; and prior to their termination, the roles of the last two were neither clear to nor understood by most of the other parties in the PEI health and social services system (PEI 1998c; Lomas and Rachlis 1996). The change in government in November 1996 was also interpreted as a go-slow signal by regional decision makers, especially after the new minister of health and social services later the next year fired the CEO of the largest region—a CEO unpopular with many physicians—without informing the region's board in advance.

Several specific features of the block budgets and their deployment were also problematic (Eyles et al. 2000; Lomas and Rachlis 1996). The regions' budgets were not based on assessments of their respective populations' health needs; each region received an allocation from the province based largely on the historical flow of funds into, and use of services by, communities within its boundaries. Within the regions, line-by-line budgeting was still used extensively, which frustrated many managers. Also, programs could not carry forward surpluses, so within a region some reallocation took the form of flowing financial resources from programs in surplus to those that had created deficits. Furthermore, the province placed no restrictions on the types of reallocations that could be made. Some managers and observers feel that this has worked to the advantage of the acute-health-care sector, frequently in deficit, as it has been able to absorb resources from community care and social services sectors despite an original policy objective that was just the opposite.

Finally, the significance of union agreements and other issues in the transition of human resources both to the regions from the DHSS and among programs within the regions should not be underestimated. Even in the absence of some of the other influences identified thus far, this factor alone would have caused a significant delay in program reconfiguration and accompanying reallocations.

Final Reflections on the PEI Experience

One message from the PEI experience is that innovation in decision-making structures is tricky business. As the list of problems in the previously mentioned "institutions" category demonstrates, innovations must be carefully designed and implemented so as not to undermine their intended effect—a difficult task. Another message is that changing organizational and decision-making structures alone does not guarantee that desired reallocations can or will be made. Significant reallocation hinges on a supportive climate that includes a clear, strong political signal indicating which types of reallocation are acceptable and which are not. Block budgeting could not hide or resolve the conflicts among interests that are inherent in the redistribution of health resources. It neither changed the incentives for important groups like hospital workers and physicians to oppose reallocations nor altered historical coalitions of interests. A third message is that reallocation away from health care to other determinants of health will always be difficult unless the public's perception of health care's role and contribution changes. Despite the rhetoric of advocates of a determinants-of-health approach to health policy and even with the commitment of managers who embrace this philosophy, reallocation to social and environmental determinants will be almost impossible if it is perceived as "stealing from health care" (PEI 1998c, 7) or if the public perceives the health-care system as underfunded.

The PEI experience contributes to an understanding of the limits of what may be possible with regionalization and block budgets. Some may question whether the small size of PEI prevents any generalization; others may feel that reallocation would be even more difficult in a larger jurisdiction. Perhaps the main point about generalizability, however, is that PEI is only one experience. Policy makers need a pool of case studies regarding block budgets' effects on reallocation in different settings, from which common insights could be drawn.

More vexing is the question of a "gold standard" against which to judge reallocation. In PEI the architects of health reform were clear that they wanted reallocation away from health care and toward other social and environmental determinants (also, within health care, away from institutional and toward community-based care). Perhaps this "normative" statement that this was the way PEI should seek to improve population health is all that is required. But on what basis would one accept the "positive" statement that this was the best way to improve population health? There is very little research on the relative contribution of different types of health determinants (Jerrett et al. 1998). There is certainly no "fantasy equation" showing the independent effect of each type of health determinant, much less the effects of their interactions (Stoddart 1995), and one doubts that there ever could be. At best, it would be context specific. This fact highlights the need for evaluation of reallocations' health effects to be included in future case studies.

Shortly after the completion of this chapter, the PEI government in April 2002 decided to remove secondary acute and specialized services from the regional block budgets. The province's three major hospitals and a provincial addictions center were brought together to form a new Provincial Health Services Authority. Although this will help to stop the acute-health-care sector from absorbing resources from the community-care and social services sectors, it significantly restricts the breadth of the regional block budgets and the scope for reallocation away from acute health care.

Acknowledgments

Several colleagues contributed to the research studies on which this synthesis is based. Jonathan Lomas, Michael Rachlis, Olive Moase, Tina Pranger, Michael Brimacombe, Danny

Gallant, Jo-Ann MacDonald, and Veronica Brown contributed to the System Evaluation Project (SEP) studies, which were funded by Health Canada and the PEI Department of Health and Social Services. Laurie Molyneaux-Smith, Tina Pranger, and Colin McMullan contributed to the project Making Resource Shifts Supportive of the Broad Determinants of Health: The PEI Experience, which was funded by the Canadian Health Services Research Foundation and received additional support from the PEI Department of Health and Social Services, and the McMaster Institute of Environment and Health. These colleagues and agencies are not responsible for the views or statements in this chapter; that responsibility rests solely with the authors.

Notes

1. Further discussion of the philosophy and structure of PEI health reform can be found in Lomas and Rachlis (1996).

2. The groups included members of the central bodies (the HCSA, the HPC, and the DHSS), CEOs and senior managers of the regions, regional program managers and unit supervisors, program support staff, board members and former members, physicians and other service providers, and the general public (PEI 1999).

3. They also expressed some skepticism that high-quality, comparable information relevant to their specific program decisions could be assembled in a timely way.

4. A lack of clearly supportive signals from the central bodies and the ongoing fiscal restraint were other aspects of the environment that managers found intimidating or restrictive.

References

Adler, N. E., M. Marmot, B. S. McEwen, and J. Stewart, eds. 1999. *Socioeconomic Status and Health in Industrial Nations.* New York: New York Academy of Sciences.

Amick, B. C., S. Levine, A. R. Tarlov, and D. C. Walsh, eds. 1995. *Society and Health.* New York: Oxford University Press.

Berkman, L. F., and I. Kawachi, eds. 2000. *Social Epidemiology.* New York: Oxford University Press.

Canadian Minister of Supply and Services. 1994. Federal, Provincial and Territorial Advisory Committee on Population Health. *Strategies for Population Health: Investing in the Health of Canadians.* Ottawa: Minister of Supply and Services.

Canadian Population Health Initiative. 2004. *Improving the Health of Canadians.* Ottawa: Canadian Institute for Health Information.

Evans, R. G., M. L. Barer, and T. R. Marmor, eds. 1994. *Why Are Some People Healthy and Others Not?* New York: Aldine de Gruyter.

Exworthy, M., D. Blane, and M. Marmot. 2003. Tackling health inequalities in the United Kingdom: The progress and pitfalls of policy. *Health Services Research* 38:1905–1922.

Eyles, J., M. Brimacombe, P. Chaulk, G. Stoddart, T. Pranger, and O. Moase. 2001. What determines health? To where should we shift resources? Attitudes towards the determinants of health among multiple stakeholder groups in Prince Edward Island, Canada. *Social Science and Medicine* 53:1611–1619.

Eyles, J., G. Stoddart, J. Lavis, T. Pranger, L. Molyneaux-Smith, and C. McMullan. 2000. *Making Resource Shifts Supportive of the Broad Determinants of Health: The PEI Experi-*

ence. Final report, Canadian Health Services Research Foundation project no. 97-141. Hamilton, ON: Institute of Environment and Health, McMaster University.

Giacomini, M., J. Hurley, J. Lomas, V. Bhatia, P. Grootendorst, B. Hutchison, et al. 1996. *Financial Incentives in the Canadian Health Care System.* Final report, National Health Research and Development Program project no. 6606-5665-303. Hamilton, Ontario: Centre for Health Economics and Policy Analysis.

Goldstein, J., and R. O. Keohane. 1993. Ideas and foreign policy: An analytical framework. In *Ideas and Foreign Policy: Beliefs, Institutions and Political Change,* ed. J. Goldstein and R. O. Keohane. Ithaca, NY: Cornell University Press.

Hall, P. A. 1993. Policy paradigms, social learning and the state: The case of economic policymaking in Britain. *Comparative Politics* 25:275–296.

―――. 1996. *Politics and Markets in the Industrialized Nations: Interests, Institutions and Ideas in Comparative Political Economy.* Cambridge, MA: Harvard University Center for European Studies.

Heclo, H. 1974. Social policy and political learning. In *Modern Social Politics in Britain and Sweden: From Relief to Income Maintenance,* ed. H. Heclo. New Haven, CT: Yale University Press.

Jerrett, M., J. Eyles, and D. Cole. 1998. Socioeconomic and environmental covariates of premature mortality in Ontario. *Social Science and Medicine* 47:33–49.

Kindig, D., P. Day, D. M. Fox, M. Gibson, J. Knickman, J. Lomas, and G. Stoddart. 2003. What new knowledge would help policymakers better balance investments for optimal health outcomes? *Health Services Research* 38:1923–1937.

Lavis, J. N., and T. Sullivan. 1999. Governing health. In *Market Limits in Health Reform: Public Success, Private Failure,* ed. D. Drache and T. Sullivan. London: Routledge.

Lomas, J., and M. M. Rachlis. 1996. Moving rocks: Block-funding in PEI as an incentive for cross-sectoral reallocations among human services. *Canadian Public Administration* 39: 581–600.

Lomas, J., J. Woods, and G. Veenstra. 1997. Devolving authority for health care in Canada's provinces: 1. An introduction to the issues. *Canadian Medical Association Journal* 156: 371–377.

Marmot, M., and R. G. Wilkinson, eds. 1999. *Social Determinants of Health.* Oxford: Oxford University Press.

Premier's Council on Health Strategy, Ontario. 1991. *Nurturing Health: A Framework on the Determinants of Health.* Toronto: Premier's Council on Health Strategy.

Prince Edward Island (PEI). 2001. *Summary Report: Public Consultations on the Strategic Plan for the Health and Social Services System.* Charlottetown: Island Information Services.

PEI, Health and Community Services Agency. 1995. *Community Needs Assessment: The Prince Edward Island Experience.* Charlottetown: Queen's Printer.

PEI, Health and Community Services System. 1996a. *Circle of Health Learning Guide.* Charlottetown: PEI Health and Community Services Agency.

―――. 1996b. *Strengthening Families, Individuals and Communities.* Charlottetown: PEI Health and Community Services Agency.

PEI, Health Task Force. 1992. *Health Reform: A Vision for Change.* Charlottetown: Island Information Services.

PEI, Health Transition Team. 1993a. *Partnerships for Better Health.* Charlottetown: Island Information Services.

―――. 1993b. *Health and Community Services Act.* Charlottetown: Island Information Services.

PEI, System Evaluation Project. 1997. *Vol. 1. A Guide to System Evaluation: Assessing the Health and Social Services System in PEI.* Charlottetown: Department of Health and Social Services.

————. 1998a. *A Conceptual Framework for Cross-sectoral Reallocation of Resources for Health.* Charlottetown: Department of Health and Social Services.

————. 1998b. *Data Collection Instruments for Evaluating Health and Social Service Systems.* Vol. 2. Charlottetown: Department of Health and Social Services.

————. 1998c. *Decision Support Tools for Cross-sectoral Investments in Population Health in the Context of Health System Change.* Charlottetown: Department of Health and Social Services.

————. 1998d. *Facilitating Staff Involvement in the Shift to Cross-sectoral Reallocation.* Charlottetown: Department of Health and Social Services.

————. 1998e. *Preparing for Media Communications about Cross-sectoral Reallocation.* Charlottetown: Department of Health and Social Services.

————. 1998f. *Scan and Plan: Meeting and Managing Potential Challenges to Cross-sectoral Reallocation.* Charlottetown: Department of Health and Social Services.

————. 1999. *Summary of Results.* Charlottetown: Department of Health and Social Services.

Stoddart, G. 1995. The challenge of producing health in modern economies. Working paper no. 46, Program in Population Health, Canadian Institute for Advanced Research, Toronto.

van Herten, L. M., S. A. Reijneveld, and L. J. Gunning-Schepers. 2001. Rationalising chances of success in intersectoral health policy making. *Journal of Epidemiology and Community Health* 55:342–347.

Weatherford, M. S., and T. B. Mayhew. 1995. Tax policy and presidential leadership: Ideas, interests and the quality of advice. *Studies in American Political Development* 9:287–330.

Wilkinson, R., and M. Marmot, eds. 2003. *Social Determinants of Health: The Solid Facts, 2nd edition.* Copenhagen: World Health Organization.

World Health Organization, Office of Global and Integrated Environmental Health. 1997. *Intersectoral Action for Health: Addressing Health and Environment Concerns in Sustainable Development.* Geneva: World Health Organization.

Chapter 13

Taking Different Approaches to Child Policy

Anita L. Kozyrskyj, Lori J. Curtis, and Clyde Hertzman

An extensive body of research now exists—and continues to grow—on the association between socioeconomic factors and health (e.g., Evans, Barer, and Marmor 1994) and in particular, child health and well-being (e.g., Curtis et al. 2001; Phipps 2001; Hertzman 2001; Heymann 2000; Keating and Hertzman 1999; Kohen, Hertzman, and Brooks-Gunn 1998; Human Resources Development Canada [HRDC] 1996). According to an *ISUMA* (2001, 7) editorial:

> Evidence is accumulating into an undeniable critical mass, and governments, at the provincial and national levels, as well as internationally, have been trying to glean the policy imperatives.... In theory, the implications of this research are pretty clear: improving the quality of early childhood development should pay large dividends over time in improved health and human capital.

Has this discourse regarding early child development and population health demonstrably influenced policy directed at the health and well-being of children?

The evidence base for child policies is not well documented. Glouberman and Millar (2003) cited examples of recent Canadian initiatives in early childhood education, which appeared to be a direct response to research on early childhood development. In his book on child policy in Canada, Pless (1995) provided several anecdotes of the penetration of research knowledge, including the virtual elimination of rickets in Quebec, although his book had no shortage of stories that showed lack of policy maker interest in research. Formal evaluations of newly disseminated research on child health are also not plentiful. Philip et al. (2003) described their experience in disseminating information on child inequalities in

Scotland, including their own ethnographic study. Their comprehensive dissemination strategy aimed at a wide range of policy makers in the health, education, and social work sectors generated much interest and activity in the development of child-friendly practices. In a Canadian study on the impact of a local-area profile of child health indicators, Wong and colleagues (2000) found high uptake of the report in program planning and policy development.

As Earle and colleagues (see chapter 14 of this volume), Pless (1995), and others have pointed out, the "strength" of research evidence on its own is insufficient to determine whether there is uptake and in what form uptake occurs. This effect is clearly illustrated if we examine the "purchase" of research evidence on the health and welfare of children and youth in different settings. The same evidence is available to policy makers across the industrialized world, yet as we discuss later, the policies vary dramatically across countries. It is within the context of differing political and value systems that we wish to investigate whether research knowledge contributed to the development of policies that affect the health and well-being of children. To explore the role that research evidence played in the development of child policy, we examine in this chapter a recently implemented child policy in three different countries: (1) the National Children's Agenda in Canada, (2) the State Children's Health Insurance Program in the United States, and (3) the Early Childhood Education and Care Policy in Norway. In setting the stage for this comparative analysis, we take a step back to describe family policy and the social attitudes toward families and children in Canada, the United States, and Norway.

Child Policies in Canada, the United States, and Norway

When addressing policies that may have some impact on children, researchers often refer to child (or children's) policies, family policies, child/family policies, and policies that affect children and/or families.[1] The boundaries between what constitutes children's policies and family policies are often not clearly drawn (O'Hara 1998). Children's policies are usually defined as those that address issues concerning children, but there is no agreement as to what those are (Stroick and Jenson 2000). Family policy is usually defined as a group of polices that focus on parents, children, and the balancing of work and family life (O'Hara 1998). Typically it includes maternity/parental leave, cash transfers (e.g., social assistance, single-parent benefits), taxation (e.g., tax exemptions for dependent children, deductions for child care), subsidized or publicly provided child care, public education, and health care. Policies regarding marriage, divorce, and child support address family situations and are considered family policy by some researchers (Jenson and Thompson 1999; Kamerman and Kahn 1997). Phipps (1999) has focused on policies that affect children but has also included policies that address the family and the labor market, income security, health, and education.

Canada, the United States, and Norway are affluent and industrialized countries but are geographically and culturally different. In comparison with Norway, the two North American countries' populations are relatively young and ethnically diverse (Phipps 2001). All three countries support at least a limited range of programs that assist children and their families, but the range of policies implemented differs dramatically across the countries. In the following discussion we offer a brief overview of the major policies that affect children in these countries (for complete discussions, see Phipps 1999, 2001).

Public Programs to Assist Children

Historically, all three countries have supported public education, and only the United States has failed to provide universal health care for children. None of the countries offers national child-care programs. Norwegian children younger than six years can attend publicly approved child-care centers, with the cost shared between government and parents. U.S. children tend to be cared for in private centers paid for by the parents. Public child care is offered for some vulnerable children in Canada under the federally administered Head Start programs. As of 2001, some Canadian provinces offered universal access to child care. Quebec had a five-dollar-per-day program for children attending centers registered with the government (Phipps 2001). All three countries have tax deductions for child-care expenditures for families who work.

Child Benefits, Child Support Payments, and Benefits for Single Mothers

Both Canada and Norway provide child benefits in cash, whereas the United States does not. In Norway the benefits are universal. Single mothers receive twice the normal benefit, and the benefits increase substantially with family size and the presence of very young children. In Canada benefits are income tested,[2] and there is no substantial extra benefit for single parents or for larger families. There are supplemental benefits for low-income families receiving employment insurance in Canada, and until recently, low-income working families received a supplement.

Child support payments are important sources of income for single-parent families. In the 1990s, in Norway, approximately three-quarters of children in single-parent families received child support payments due to state-provided "advance maintenance payments" if a noncustodial parent did not make payments. In the United States, approximately one-third of single-parent families received child support payments, mainly due to state enforcement of payment from noncustodial parents. In Canada, only one-sixth of single parents reported receiving child support payments.

Norway was the only country in our study that offered a comprehensive set of benefits for single parents. A substantial transition benefit (approximately $12,000

[Canadian] per year) was available to single parents who could not support themselves as a result of child-care responsibilities. It was available until the youngest
child reached the age of ten years. A single mother who gave birth to a child was
entitled to a grant that was in addition to other regular maternity benefits. These
benefits could be collected while the single mother was working or attending
school, in which case she may also have received child-care benefits. In Canada,
single parents received a tax credit, equivalent to the deduction for a dependent
spouse for one child. There were no single-parent benefits in the United States
(Phipps 1999).

Social Transfers, Social Assistance, and Back-to-work Programs

As of the late 1990s, 90% of Norwegian families paid 14% of their disposable
income in taxes, 86% of Canadian families paid 18% of their disposable income
in taxes and 81% of American families paid 11% (Stroick and Jenson 2000). Although fewer American families paid taxes, only 52% of U.S. households with
children received any social transfers, compared with 90% in Canada and 97% in
Norway.

Social assistance is an essential form of income support for poor families with
children, especially poor single-mother families. Just over half of the children in
single-mother families in Canada and the United States received social assistance
in 1994 and 1995. In Norway, only 31% of children in single-mother families
received social assistance, both because rates of labor-force participation were
higher for single mothers in Norway and because single mothers received many
other forms of support. Since 1996, many Canadian provinces have drastically cut
social assistance payments and have implemented back-to-work programs. In 1997,
the United States replaced its Aid to Families with Dependent Children program
(social assistance primarily for single mothers with children) with the Temporary
Assistance for Needy Families, a program that focuses on getting the parent back
to work and puts lifetime limits on the availability of social assistance.[3]

Differences in Core Values between Canada, the United States, and Norway

In his book on the health and the wealth of nations, Keating (1999, 237) has
remarked that "the ability to function as a civic society . . . to generate the human
capital necessary for economic prosperity in the Information Age, and to adapt to
the rapid social and technological changes we now confront depends heavily on
how society organizes itself to support human development." However, the notion
that "it takes a village to raise a child" is not universally understood or accepted.
International comparisons of family policies conducted by Phipps (1998) and
O'Hara (1998) indicate that since the early to mid-1990s, Canada and the United
States have favored the state's minimal interference with the family. Most European

countries offer universal benefits to assist families with children, whereas Canada and the United States do not (Baker 1995; Phipps 1999).[4] Canadian and American children have been treated as private goods—as the responsibility of the family. Norway, on the other hand, has exhibited high levels of government involvement in the support of families, and children have been viewed as public goods and society's responsibility. Canada and the United States have also attempted to minimize labor-force participation disincentives when providing support for families with children, whereas Norway has aimed to support gender equality in the home and the labor force, with a focus on the child (Stroick and Jenson 2000).

A comparison of existing child policies in Canada, Norway, and the United States gives us an indication of the value systems operating in these countries. Although this evidence is relevant and informative for the current discussion, the 1990 World Values Survey has more specific information on the attitudes and preferences of individuals within the three countries. O'Hara (1998) and Phipps (1998, 2001) have summarized some of these data. When asked why people were poor, the most popular answer in Norway was "due to injustices in society." The highest proportion of Americans believed that people were poor because of "laziness." Canadians cited these two reasons equally often. Generally, Norwegians put responsibility for poverty on society, the Americans on the individual, and Canadians, as usual, compromised between the two. Given this evidence, it is not surprising that many of the Canadian and U.S. programs to assist families have been tied to removing negative work incentives and "making work pay," whereas Norway's programs have not.

In summary, there appear to be deep-seated differences in core values across our comparator nations, and those differences may contribute to a continuum of values on the place and importance of families and children in each society. The United States appears to be positioned on the far right, with more "conservative" views: The child is a family responsibility, families are responsible for themselves, and people are the architects of their own difficulties. On the other hand, Norway seems to occupy a position on the left of the continuum with more liberal views. Norwegians view the child—and in some cases, families—as a social responsibility. They believe that individual failures often have as much or more to do with societal injustices as do individual circumstances and that society should be committed to all individuals. The available data have indicated that Canada lies somewhere between these two extremes. Canadians are divided when it comes to determining whether individuals or the society in which they live should bear the major responsibility for their circumstances. There is evidence that, on average, Canadians feel they should take more individual responsibility than is currently the case (Phipps, 1999). Given these differences in ideology or values, it should come as no great surprise that the policies of these societies to support the development of children vary as much as they do.

Specific Examples of Child Policies

We have identified three recently developed child policies in Canada, the United States, and Norway to illustrate whether and how research evidence was a factor in their genesis. Recognizing that policy making is a complex process, we use Kingdon's (1995) three process streams: problem identification, policy formation, and politics. Kingdon was interested in the question of why some issues get on government agendas while others do not.[5] He proposed that when the problems, policy, and politics streams merge, there is an enhanced likelihood of an issue reaching the decision-making agenda. Before that occurs, Kingdon argued, policy ideas "float around," searching for problems or political events that increase the likelihood of adoption, which he called "policy windows."

It is in Kingdon's second category of policy formation (also known as formation and dissemination of ideas) where we have linked research evidence to the formation of each policy under study. Our use of his framework was not intended to provide evidence that a policy window had opened, leading to the implementation of the policy. Rather, the process streams were useful categories to describe the environment at the time of policy implementation, in terms of the availability of research evidence and policy makers' potential access to this evidence, the importance of the problem underpinning the research evidence, and the political environment. This analysis addresses the question of whether research was involved. We were also interested in elucidating the role of research evidence. To this end, we refer to the taxonomy proposed by Earle, Heymann, and Lavis in chapter 14 of this volume, which describes three roles of research: enlightenment, problem solving, and rhetoric.

National Children's Agenda in Canada

On September 23, 1997, the National Children's Agenda (NCA) was announced by the Canadian federal government after concurrence from all provinces and territories except Quebec.[6] The NCA document itself amounted to a statement of strategy that put the cognitive, social, and physical development of children onto the public agenda. Direct funding for these purposes was to wait three more years.

Accompanying the NCA in 1998, under the framework of the National Child Benefit, was the Canada Child Tax Benefit (CCTB), which combined the child tax benefit and the earned-income supplement (HRDC 1997). Provinces were able to reduce family social assistance payments by the amount of the CCTB low-income supplement or tax it. Provinces pursuing the former option were required to re-direct their savings toward improving children's services and support for low–income working families (Jenson and Thompson 1999).

Although the concept of a NCA had yet to be fully developed at the time of its announcement, the essence of the NCA proposition was the development of policies that would ensure that Canadian children develop to their full potential as healthy, successful, and contributing members of society. Children living in low-income families were not the only focus of the NCA.[7] All developmentally vulnerable children, including those with health problems and poor family environments, were to benefit from the NCA strategy. Provincial health and social service ministries were given the task of coordinating future NCA policies and programs.

Contained in the announcement of the NCA was the following statement: "There is strong evidence, including scientific research, that what happens to children when they are very young shapes their health and well-being throughout their lifetime."[8] To fulfill the NCA mandate, the federal government planned to measure and regularly report on readiness to learn in the preschool years. We were interested in identifying the impetus for the federal government's attention to programs that modify early childhood experiences and social environments, rather than simply providing income. As well, we wanted to know how these perspectives had come to be incorporated in the NCA. To help us understand the influence of research evidence in the formation of the NCA, we applied the Kingdon and Earle frameworks to the series of events that had occurred immediately prior to its announcement. Herein we report the outcome of this analysis of events.

IDENTIFICATION OF THE PROBLEM

On November 20, 1996, Human Resources Development Canada and Statistics Canada released the report *Growing Up in Canada,* the first publication of findings from the National Longitudinal Survey of Children and Youth (NLSCY).[9] From this report, Canadians learned that 25% of Canadian children were living in low-income families and that children from these families were at greater risk for emotional and behavioral problems, as were children living in single-parent households (HRDC 1996). Further, the NLSCY indicated that preschool children whose parents had low educational attainment were less school-ready than children whose parents had higher levels of education. Most important, this report illustrated the extent to which early development followed a "gradient pattern." In other words, the probability that a child would be developmentally vulnerable by kindergarten age declined in a stepwise fashion with increasing family socioeconomic status. Although the highest probability of vulnerability was found among the lowest-socioeconomic families, the greatest number of vulnerable children was spread more thinly across the much larger middle class.

One week following the release of the report, there was a first meeting of the Federal-Provincial-Territorial Council on Social Policy Renewal to renew Canada's social safety net.[10] The council proposed to tackle child poverty and defined, as a priority, an integrated child benefit. Two months later the Provincial-Territorial

Ministers of Social Services met to set the objectives of the National Child Benefit (we interpreted this list of objectives as problems that could be solved).[11] The ministers agreed that the objectives of the National Child Benefit, a culmination of family policy that had existed in Canada over the past hundred years, were to reduce child poverty and to promote parent attachment to the workforce. All of the ministers also agreed that the National Child Benefit would require complementary provincial, as well as significant federal investment.

The Federal-Provincial-Territorial Council on Social Policy Renewal met again on January 29, 1997, to continue discussions on the National Child Benefit.[12] The council was presented with a report from the Provincial-Territorial Ministers of Social Services, indicating their agreement to a National Reinvestment Framework that committed provinces to developing programs that would complement the National Children's Benefit.[13] This commitment was to involve provincial investments in programs for low-income children, specifically for programs to help parents on social assistance find work. Once employed, former social assistance recipients would receive the National Child Benefit as a replacement for welfare payments. Provincial dollars saved from reduced welfare payments were to be diverted to antipoverty programs, such as child-care tax credits for low-income families.

According to the published minutes of the January 29, 1997, meeting, the Council on Social Policy Renewal also discussed preliminary plans for a national children's agenda (NCA). Not only would a national children's agenda promote children's well-being, but it would serve as a mechanism for coordinating the activities of provincial social services and health ministries.[14] A Canadian Press newswire, published later that year, identified another problem that could be solved by the NCA. According to the press release, the federal government was waiting for provinces to develop complementary plans to fight child poverty, including the introduction of work incentives for parents on social assistance (Tibbetts 1997a). Despite having agreed to the National Reinvestment Framework, the provinces and territories were slow in developing plans to reform their welfare systems. As of October 1997, only two provinces, Ontario and Saskatchewan, had developed programs to dovetail with the National Children's Benefit (Tibbetts 1997a). Apparently, the federal government was faced with the delicate challenge of trying to encourage provinces to get on with their plans, and the NCA was one tool the federal government could use to help provinces organize their child poverty and welfare reform programs.

At the same time that the Council on Social Policy Renewal was carrying out its deliberations, other federal-provincial-territorial councils were converging on the same policy areas. For instance, the Council of Ministers of Education began to take on a developmental focus in thinking about educational success indicators. More important, however, were the activities of the Federal-Provincial-Territorial Advisory Committee on Population Health, which replaced the Advisory Committee on Community Health in 1992. This change was the result of the already widespread penetration within individual provincial and territorial bureaucracies of population health ideas, ideas which had originated with the members of the Canadian Institute for Advanced Research's Population Health Program (and ultimately published in their book, *Why Are Some People Healthy and Others Not?*) (Legowski and McKay 2000). Because of its commitment to a "determinants-of-health perspective," the Advisory Committee on Population Health took on the issue of early child development as a lifelong determinant of health. More than the Council on Social Policy Renewal, with its focus on compensatory programs, the Advisory Committee on Population Health focused on the issue of "universal access to the conditions for healthy child development." The strategy paper produced by the Advisory Committee on Population Health (Legowski and McKay 2000), more than anything done by the Council on Social Policy Renewal, set the ultimate tone and direction of the NCA.

FORMATION AND DISSEMINATION OF IDEAS

Growing Up in Canada confirmed what federal and provincial reports had previously identified—that child poverty affected health. By the time the planning for the NLSCY was substantially completed in 1993, Human Resources Development Canada,[15] knowing many of the results the NLSCY was likely to find, was already keen to focus on "vulnerable children." Behind the scenes, there was a debate between Statistics Canada and Human Resources Development Canada on this focus. Statistics Canada argued that the NLSCY was too important an opportunity to focus primarily on the vulnerable—that there was a much broader set of issues needing to be addressed. Thus, traditional debates between universal and targeted policies were being conducted with respect to children before any data were produced.

Nevertheless, using data from the NLSCY, *Growing Up in Canada* was the first publication to report on a comprehensive set of developmental indicators for a nationally representative sample of Canadian children in relation to their socio-economic environment (HRDC 1996). The NLSCY was also identified as a key source of information on child readiness to learn.[16] Two earlier publications by the Canadian Institute for Child Health in 1989 and 1994[17] presented data on income variations in low birth weight, childhood mortality, activity limitation, and emotional health. Data on these last three variables were obtained from the Ontario Child Health Study, which at that time was the only population-based longitudinal study of child health (with children surveyed in 1983 and again in 1987) (Cadman et al. 1986; Offord et al. 1992). Other Ontario Child Health Study–based studies found significant associations between low income or single-parent status and childhood psychiatric disorders (Lipman, Offord, and Boyle 1994; Dooley et al.

1998), poor social and educational functioning (Lipman and Offord 1994, 1996), and chronic health problems (Cadman et al. 1986).

Although there is no doubt that the Ontario Child Health Study and the NLSCY were invaluable sources of evidence for informing government decisions to proceed with the NCA, key individuals involved in the NCA's development were also familiar with the social determinants of health literature. During the first meeting of the Federal-Provincial-Territorial Council on Social Policy Renewal, reference was made to the National Forum on Health, which was created in 1994 to advise the federal government on innovative ways to improve the Canadian health care system (National Forum on Health 1997a). To achieve this goal, the Forum conducted nationwide consultations on issues related to health and health care in Canada. Members of the Forum included Canadian academicians Robert Evans and Noralou Roos, both of whom were influential researchers on the broader determinants of health (Evans and Stoddart 1990; Evans et al. 1994; Roos 1995). The National Forum on Health had several working groups, including the determinants-of-health group that had commissioned several research papers on topics, such as children's preschool experiences (National Forum on Health 1997b). These research papers were published alongside the Forum's final report. The presence of the National Forum on Health's determinants-of-health working group gave population health formal recognition as a valuable framework for examining Canadians' health (Legowski and McKay 2000).

POLITICAL ENVIRONMENT

As noted previously, Canadians generally believe that, although society should share some responsibility for children, individuals are responsible for themselves and their families, and children are a private good. The Liberal Party of Canada had lent some credibility to the notion that society was responsible for children and their families in the 1997 election, when issues such as a universal child-care plan had been discussed.[18] But deep cuts in the "social safety net," and particularly in health care, evolved as a major issue in the election.

The Liberal Red Book for the spring 1997 election had pledged to revamp the welfare benefits system to fight child poverty and to stop the next rounds of planned cuts to the Canada Health and Social Transfers to the provinces.[19] Further, Finance Minister Paul Martin had announced the Liberal federal government's intent to double the $850 million in tax benefits for low-income families with children. This money was to be allocated only as resources became available and was conditional on the provinces and territories agreeing to a National Reinvestment Framework.[20] As discussed earlier, under this Framework provinces had committed to moving parents from social assistance to the labor force and reallocating social assistance funds into benefits for children in low-income families, such as earned income and child support supplements. The Framework provided the provinces and territories with the flexibility to design their own programs. Apparently, this flexibility was seen as a key national unity issue for the federal government in its campaign platform.[21] Quebec had decided not to join the Federal-Provincial-Territorial Council on Social Policy Renewal. At the January 13, 1997, meeting of the Ministers of Social Services, the minister from Quebec reminded others that social policies were within Quebec's exclusive jurisdiction and that Quebec would claim an unconditional financial transfer. Providing stewardship, yet giving the provinces more control in the design of their social programs, would have demonstrated to the Quebec populace that the Canadian federation was functioning well.

Similar to the flexible National Child Benefit, some have suggested that the NCA was intended to fulfill the bigger mission of demonstrating national unity. Federal officials were reported as saying that the federal government liked the idea of the NCA because it would show (to Quebec) the federal government's ability to get along with the provinces and territories (Tibbits 1997b). In fact, the Saskatchewan deputy minister had been quoted as saying, "If this county is going to come together under any single issue, can't we come together under the issue of children?"

SUMMARY

Together with the social determinants of health literature, the Ontario Child Health Study and the NLSCY showed unequivocally that cognitive, social, and physical development in Canadian children declined with increasing levels of deprivation and created large differences in children's readiness to learn when entering school. There is strong evidence that creators of the NCA were familiar with the NLSCY findings and well-versed in the social-determinants-of-health literature disseminated by the Federal-Provincial-Territorial Advisory Committee on Population Health and the National Forum on Health. The NCA's goal was to encourage federal–provincial cooperation in the development of programs focused on early childhood environments. By focusing on "universal access to the conditions for healthy child development," the NCA was intended to mitigate the developmental consequences of child poverty and duplication of social services programs.

Applying Earle, Heymann, and Lavis's framework (see chapter 14 of this volume) to the role of research evidence in the NCA's creation, one could argue that that role was one of "enlightenment." New perspectives emerging from the social and early childhood determinants of health literature were considered broadly in the shaping the NCA. However, at the end of the day, the possibility exists that this evidence was also used for rhetorical purposes. The driving factor for the NCA policy could well have been the federal government's desire to demonstrate national unity and to use the state of child welfare as the unifying theme—and the NCA as the instrument. On the other hand, it is counterproductive to overrate a single motivating factor. The evidentiary base as a whole—building from broad population health concepts to the role of early child development as a lifelong determinant of health and well-being—played a prominent, if not definitive, role in motivating new children's policies in Canada.

State Children's Health Insurance Programs in the United States

Three years after the collapse of President Bill Clinton's proposed health security plan, the State Children's Health Insurance Program (SCHIP) was created in 1997 with support from Congress. The Balanced Budget Act of 1997 allocated $24 billion over the following five years to extend health coverage to uninsured children through state-designed programs.[22] This was the largest single commitment to coverage for children since the enactment of Medicaid in 1965. SCHIP enabled states to provide health insurance to children from working families with incomes too high to qualify for Medicaid. SCHIP's goal was to improve child health through access to health care for prevention (e.g., immunization) and treatment purposes. It was created as a block grant to the states, and they were given considerable flexibility in defining benefits. States had three options for expanding health insurance coverage for children—through Medicaid, the creation of a new state program or expansion of an existing one, or a combination of the two (Hill 2000).

In the following sections, we outline the series of events that occurred around the time of SCHIP implementation, such as the publication of research evidence and the introduction of policies aimed at welfare reform. As with the NCA analysis, the problems, ideas, and politics domains of Kingdon's framework (1995) gave us the opportunity to understand how these events could have affected one another.

IDENTIFICATION OF THE PROBLEM

The 1980s in the United States saw the expansion of Medicaid and Aid to Families with Dependent Children (AFDC) benefits to pregnant women and children (Scanlon 1997). In the following decade, amid rising Medicaid costs, proposals were put forward to reform Medicaid through the provision of block grants to individual states, leaving them to define their own benefits (Sardell and Johnson 1998). During the same period, substantial increases in AFDC cases, largely in the number of single-parent families, provided the impetus for discussions on welfare reform that would have limited welfare benefits to two years (Glazer 1995). This impetus was captured in President Clinton's pledge to end "welfare as we know it." The resultant policy changes included the Personal Responsibility and Work Opportunity Reconciliation Act of 1996, which replaced AFDC benefits with the Temporary Assistance for Needy Families (TANF) program. The TANF program emphasized putting welfare recipients to work, setting time limits on the receipt of welfare benefits, and reducing welfare caseloads (Thompson and Gais 2000). The Balanced Budget

Act of 1997 also created the Welfare-to-Work Grants program, which provided the states with funding to meet TANF's work participation requirements (King 1999).

The number of children living in the United States without health insurance had risen steadily throughout the 1990s as private businesses had cut their support for dependent coverage. Since 1989, children had lost private health coverage at twice the rate of adults (Grayson 1998). In 1996, 11 million children younger than nineteen were uninsured; 90% of these children had parents who worked. Almost all uninsured children were from poor, working-poor, and near-poor families (Goggin 1999). Furthermore, the U.S. government's debate around welfare and Medicaid reforms identified for many the potential impact of these policies on children—increases in the number of children without health insurance as previous welfare recipients took on low-paying jobs.[23] That this was identified as a problem by the government was evident in the 1995 and 1996 U.S. General Accounting Office (GAO) reports on health insurance for children, which had been commissioned by the Subcommittee on Children and Families of the U.S. Senate (Nadel 1995; Scanlon 1996). As voiced in President Clinton's statement, proposed welfare reform would have "hurt kids, women and older citizens" (Sardell and Johnson 1998). Moreover, the 1994 defeat of Clinton's health care reform brought to the forefront the plight of all uninsured Americans, including 11 million children—the segment of the population least able to control whether or not it was insured (Karpatkin and Shearer 1995).

Another problem related to the lack of universal health care insurance for American children had come to the forefront by the 1990s: Pockets of children throughout the country remained underimmunized. The Early and Periodic Screening, Diagnosis, and Treatment (EPSDT) program of Medicaid had been implemented in 1967 to ensure that Medicaid-eligible children received comprehensive health coverage, not only for services related to acute and chronic medical conditions but also for a wide range of preventative care such as vision-, hearing-, and dental-screening services and immunizations (Gavin, Adams, and Herz 1998). However, a review of immunization coverage in three urban counties among two-year-olds enrolled in Medicaid found that the proportion of children with up-to-date immunizations peaked at 50% of children born in 1983 and decreased to 44% for those born in 1989. In response to low EPSDT uptake rates, amendments were made to the Omnibus Budget Reconciliation Act in 1989 to mandate coverage of core components of EPSDT and to provide incentives for health care providers' participation (Sardell and Johnson 1998). Despite these efforts, several measles epidemics occurred from 1989 to 1991 among preschoolers in low-income urban areas, predominantly among unvaccinated children (Mason et al. 1993; Atkinson et al. 1992). In response to these outbreaks, Congress approved the creation of the Vaccines for Children program in 1993, the goal of which was to provide free vaccines to uninsured children (Chan 1995). Two years later the success of this program was being questioned.

FORMATION AND DISSEMINATION OF IDEAS

The welfare reform process was heavily informed by academic research on poverty and antipoverty policies (Mead 1992). Intertwined with the welfare reform debate were discussions on the health care of children. Although not focusing on population health, American academic researchers were reporting that children living in poorer families and those without health insurance had worse health outcomes (e.g., Currie 1995; Hanratty 1996). Other research pointed to the positive health impacts of public health insurance (see Currie 1995; Hanratty 1996; Lave et al. 1998). A review of the reports by the GAO[24] published prior to the implementation of SCHIP identified three specially commissioned GAO reports (citing academic research) on the subject of health insurance, access to primary care, and immunization in children. A fourth report, *Health Insurance: Coverage Leads to Increased Health Care Access for Children,* was published three months after SCHIP's implementation. The contents of the GAO reports, which had been commissioned by senators and representatives, appeared in the testimonies of their authors before the House of Representatives.

The first of the two GAO reports on health insurance presented evidence that the number of children without health insurance had grown from 1989 to 1993 but that Medicaid expansion to include low-income children not on welfare had cushioned this increase (Nadel 1995). However, a 1996 update of the GAO report, which included data from 1994, showed that the increase in the number of uninsured children had not, in fact, been stopped by the Medicaid expansion and that 30% of uninsured children were Medicaid eligible but had not been enrolled in the program (Scanlon 1996). Both reports were based on data from the U.S. Bureau of the Census and the Current Population Survey, and they reported extensively from the published literature on the association between lack of health insurance and inadequate health care in children. Both concluded that Medicaid reform would curb eligibility for health insurance and that AFDC reform, encouraging low-income mothers to work (in low-paying jobs), would sever Medicaid eligibility. As the reports noted, health insurance would not be provided as an employer benefit in low-income jobs. The third GAO report on health care insurance in children, published immediately after the implementation of SCHIP legislation, provided further (though after-the-fact) justification for SCHIP (Scanlon 1997). As the title, *Health Insurance: Coverage Leads to Increased Health Care Access for Children,* suggests, the report presented research evidence (e.g., that of Newacheck, Hughes, and Stoddard 1996) showing that health insurance coverage for children resulted in increased use of health care services.

One of the GAO reports specifically addressed the issue of immunization of children. It was published two years after the implementation of the Vaccines for Children program, which was introduced in 1993 by the Centers for Disease Control and Prevention (CDC) to provide free vaccines to uninsured children, on the premise that cost was a barrier to immunization (Chan 1995). This GAO report, *Vaccines for Children: Re-examination of Program Goals and Implementation Needed to Ensure Vaccination,* questioned the CDC's ability to implement the Vaccines for Children program, citing research evidence (including a critique of studies commissioned by the CDC) that cost was not an issue in low immunization rates (Chan 1995). According to the report, many of the preschool children not immunized in the 1990 measles epidemics had had access to free vaccines in public health clinics. The Vaccines for Children program was expected to be costly, yet it could not guarantee immunization of high-risk populations (Chan 1995). The report writers pointed to research evidence on "missed opportunities" for vaccination and suggested that missed opportunities could be addressed through improved Medicaid coverage or health insurance for children.

POLITICAL ENVIRONMENT

President Clinton's Health Security Act of 1993, founded on the imperatives of controlling health care costs and guaranteeing lifetime coverage for all Americans, was rejected by the 103rd Congress in September 1994. Speculation on the reasons · for the failure of Clinton's health security plan ranged from the complexity of the plan and opposition from special-interest groups to beliefs that universal coverage would require additional revenue (Hacker and Skocpol 2001; Barer, Marmor, and Morrison 1995). Those who also speculated on the plan's probable effects had predicted that, in keeping with the American approach to reform, the next strategy would have been incremental reform activity. In this regard, the introduction of SCHIP was evidence of incrementalism in implementing national health insurance in the United States. The newly reelected President Clinton, having invested considerable political capital in the health care reform effort, intended to pursue his health security plan one step at a time. The first step was children. In his words, "Maybe we can do it in another way. That's what we tried to do, a step at a time, until we finish this."[25] Clinton had hoped that states, after having insured children in families with incomes approximately twice the federally measured poverty level, would also enroll parents in SCHIP (Starr 2000).

In the wake of the many roadblocks to the Health Security Plan, what "policy window" had opened to favor passage of SCHIP? The election of a Republican majority to the 104th Congress in 1994 represented a major rightward ideological shift of the House of Representatives (Sardell and Johnson 1998). Throughout the health care reform debate, Republicans had shown far less interest in federally supported health care insurance for all Americans; their agenda was to downsize the role of government (Barer et al. 1995). The outcome of the "Republican takeover" was the radical transformation of President Clinton's proposals for welfare reform (Ellwood 1996). Clinton's welfare reform proposals to support working families through the provision of universal health care coverage were replaced with a proposal to provide welfare block grants to the states, leaving the states to define welfare benefits (Jansson 1997). Under this bill, no federal funds were to be used to provide welfare for children born to teenage mothers or those born to families already receiving assistance. The proposed bill received harsh criticism from the Democrats. Throughout the welfare reform process, the Democrats had paid enormous attention to child health and health care (Mead 1992). With support from Democratic constituents, President Clinton vetoed the Republican pursuit of Medicaid block grants (Sardell and Johnson 1998). In place of President Clinton's proposals, the Republican version of welfare reform was implemented. This included block grants but required states to spend a specified amount of their budget on welfare programs. Welfare recipients were required to obtain work within two years of receiving benefits, but states could exempt 15% of their caseloads (Jansson 1997).

Within two years of the initiation of debate on welfare reform, SCHIP was passed, providing universal health insurance for low-income children and making it easier to implement the work-related requirements. The motivation for SCHIP was not Republican interest in extending health care coverage but welfare reform, spurred on by concerns over rising Medicaid and AFDC program costs, along with a determination by the Republican House to make hard federal budget cuts. However, some have argued that cost was not the only driving force for welfare reform (Glazer 1995; Jansson 1997). Welfare programs had been the target of many previous attempts at reform. Some have suggested that welfare itself had come to symbolize the rise of a permanently dependent population cut off from the mainstream of American society, the decay of inner cities, and the problems of the inner-city black poor. A refrain heard throughout the hearing and debates on welfare reform was the need to invest in the preparation of poor families for employment, so they could eventually become independent (Mead 1992)—a viewpoint illustrating the American value system, noted earlier in this chapter, that individuals are responsible for themselves and their children. Various efforts reflecting this value system were implemented at the state level. For example, Governor George W. Bush fought staunchly to limit the number of children that SCHIP would cover in Texas (e.g., by proposing to set the eligibility level at 150% of the federal poverty level, rather than the 200% that was expected), to prevent more children from getting Medicaid as a "Medicaid spillover" effect.[26] Not only did a Medicaid recipient cost more than a SCHP recipient, but the number of persons receiving Medicaid in Texas had been falling for years—one of Bush's proudest achievements as governor (Green 2000). Bush was not the only politician to view "decline in welfare caseloads" as an indicator of the success of welfare reform. However, Bush's Protestant work ethic apparently could be bought: In the end he agreed to the SCHIP bill in exchange for tax breaks for big oil companies (Thompson and Gais 2000).

SUMMARY

SCHIP was created to provide health insurance to children from working families with incomes too high to qualify for Medicaid. It is not difficult to find documentation that SCHIP was "supported" by evidence that access to health insurance improved health, health care use, and immunization rates in children. However, it is also clear that this search for evidence was strongly motivated by the Republican Congress's desire to make the welfare reform policy work and to halt the decay of America's inner cities. SCHIP would provide health insurance to low-income children when their parents, previous recipients of welfare, became employed.

Our description of events around the time of SCHIP's implementation answers the question of whether reason was used, and it provides some insight into how the use of research evidence was predetermined by a political agenda. However, as Earle, Heymann, and Lavis argue in chapter 14 of this book, it tells us nothing about the role of research in the process. Evidence on the detrimental effects of the lack of health care insurance among subpopulations of American children has been in the public domain for at least three decades (Cauffman, Roemer, and Shultz 1967; Newacheck and Halfon 1986). Certainly, this observation does not support an enlightened role for evidence in SCHIP's creation. The commissioning of the GAO reports around the time of SCHIP's implementation could suggest that research was used for problem-solving purposes. Policy makers were interested in knowing about the current state of health care insurance in the context of previous Medicaid expansions. However, this categorization suggests a linear process—a problem is identified, initiating a search for evidence and culminating in a policy. This was not the case with SCHIP. Lack of health insurance among subpopulations of American children was not a new problem, nor was there lack of evidence to support the introduction of a health insurance policy.

This brings us to the use of research for rhetorical purposes, a category that could easily be applied to SCHIP's implementation. The introduction of a health insurance policy for low-income children, which was obviously grounded in research evidence on the benefits of health insurance in children, would have provided powerful ammunition for the Republican Congress's welfare reform policy. In fact, the SCHIP story shows very nicely Kingdon's notion of evidence "floating about" and searching for policies, and the joining of evidence and policy when the political environment is ripe (Kingdon 1995). Republicans in Congress were cool to Clinton's proposal to fund a health insurance program for uninsured children, but they were aware of the consequences of not reaching a budget deal with the president in 1995 (Goggin 1999). President Clinton was equally anxious to accommodate the Republicans by being willing to support tax and spending cuts. The so-called kiddies' agenda offered a convenient conduit for a bipartisan compromise. Children were a target population for whom sympathy and concern could be easily raised (Hacker and Skocpol 2001). Even more appealing to the fiscally conservative Republicans (and Democrats) was the fact that children were relatively inexpensive to insure. SCHIP was also popular with governors because it was provided as a block grant, rather than as an entitlement. States were to receive a set amount of funds from the federal government, and they could cap enrollment or pare benefits (Starr 2000, 2001).

So although SCHIP was touted as a major victory for the Clinton administration, it was not a universal program like Medicare, but rather a means-tested program. Much of the research evidence, including the GAO reports, identified difficulties (due to, for example, lack of parent knowledge of the tedious application process) that low-income families faced in obtaining Medicaid coverage for their children (Starr 2001; Scanlon 1996). In addition to not conferring benefits on all children, as a universal insurance program would have done, the means-tested SCHIP program was confronted with the challenge of being able to "find" eligible children.[27] Thus, in the end, even the rhetorical use of research evidence to support the SCHIP program was limited. One could in fact, make a case for the complete disregard of research evidence in the development of this child policy.

Early Childhood Education and Care Policy Norway

Early childhood education and care institutions in Norway are called *barnehager* (the English translation is kindergarten).[28] Barnehager have existed in Norway for more than 100 years, and since 1975 they have been regulated under the Barnehage Act. They provide care and education to children, and the costs are shared by the federal government, the municipalities, and parents. Although the Norwegian government provides subsidies for children in barnehage, placement is not guaranteed. A long-standing debate in Norway has been whether young children should be placed in barnehager away from their parents and whether barnehager should be educational or social institutions. In 1998, the Cash Benefits for Small Children Act came into force, providing a benefit to all families with children aged two years or younger if their children did not have a government-subsidized place in a barnehage. Families with children in part-time barnehage were entitled to a partial cash benefit according to the number of hours in the barnehage. Parents could choose whether to stay at home with their children, use some other kind of child care, (e.g., care provided by grandparents), or select a state-subsidized barnehage to take care of their children. The cash benefit was intended to give parents compensation for lack of salary or reduced salary due to a reduction in working hours associated with caring for their children.

Two years prior to this, the National Framework Plan for Barnehager had been implemented as a regulation under the Barnehage Act to establish guidelines for the provision of barnehage services.[29] The guidelines were developed with consultation from preschool teachers, researchers, and representatives from local authorities. All barnehager were required to base their annual plan on this National Framework Plan, which was rooted in the holistic view of the child and stated that cultural and Christian values of Norwegian society had to be represented in the barnehage curriculum. To ensure a common profile of educational programs in barnehager, the National Framework Plan formulated objectives for child development and learning, encompassing areas such as religion, language, and physical activity. The Framework also contained a supplemental section for barnehager caring for Saami children in Saami districts, which recommended increased exposure to the Saami culture and language.[30] The goal of the Cash Benefits for Small Children Act and the National Framework Plan for Barnehager was to improve young children's access to early childhood education, whether this was provided by parents or the barnehage.

From this point forward, we summarize how the goals of the Benefits for Small Children Act and the National Framework Plan for Barnehager were incorporated into policy and how research evidence was consulted in the process. As before, we describe these events under the domains of problem identification, idea formation, and the political environment.

IDENTIFICATION OF THE PROBLEM

Debate on the role of the barnehage in early childhood education and care in Norway has a long history.[31] The concern in the 1990s was over access to barnehage care. Several reports by Statistics Norway indicated that the proportion of children in barnehage had risen considerably since the 1970s, when 3% of children under the age of seven years were in barnehage, to 28% of children in 1985. In 1993, the average barnehage uptake (usage) rates among children aged one to five was 47%, and the rate increased modestly to 60% in 1997. In the 1980s and 1990s, priority was given to barnehage places for older preschool children. The outcome of this policy was lower uptake rates in children younger than three in 1997. In comparison to 50% of five-year-olds, 20% of children one-year-olds and 35% of two-year-olds were in barnehage more than thirty hours a week. There was considerable variation in uptake among local regions, from 30% of children in some regions occupying a barnehage space to up to 90% of children in others. Regions in the south and west of Norway had access rates below 40%. Furthermore, although most children with special needs were in barnehage, only 40% of children from cultural minorities had a place in barnehage.

The insufficient number of barnehage spaces was attributed to a true deficiency in some regions, but in other regions, parent preference was a factor. Regardless, the shortage of barnehager was viewed as an equity problem by a society genuinely concerned about children's rights (e.g., Norway had been the first country to establish an Ombudsman for Children, in 1981).[32] It was anticipated that the demand for barnehage would grow because parents increasingly viewed barnehage as good educational preparation for school. Although no child had a legal right to a place in barnehage, the Norwegian government's goal was to provide, by the year 2000, access to barnehage for all children on a full- or a part-time basis whose parents wanted this service.

Further, the quality of care delivered by barnehager was being scrutinized.[33] Traditionally, barnehager had had great freedom to develop their own programs within the boundaries of the Barnehage Act. In general, Norwegian barnehager were evaluated as providing high-quality care, and most parents expressed satisfaction with this care.[34] However, there were concerns about the physical conditions of some barnehager, such as indoor ventilation, and the qualifications of the staff. A requirement of the Barnehage Act was that individuals responsible for the educational curriculum and day-to-day operation of barnehager (respectively *styrere* and *pedagogisk ledere*) be educated preschool teachers. Following a shortage of preschool teachers, 19% of persons employed as styrere and pedagogisk ledere in 1997 did not have formal training in preschool education. Additional concerns about barnehage care included insufficient emphasis on cultural and Christian values and a lack of standards in the area of child development. The need for barnehager caring for Saami children to provide exposure to the Saami culture and language was also identified as a challenge.

Parallel to issues regarding access and quality of barnehage care was the matter of parents choosing to use barnehage care or to care for their own children. According to a survey conducted by the Ministry of Children and Family Affairs on child care, 49% of parents with two- to three-year-olds reported that they cared for their children themselves and 37% stated that their children had a place in barnehage; far fewer children were cared for by a child minder or another family member.[35] The OECD report on Early Childhood Education and Care Policy noted that Norwegian parents were concerned that they were spending too little time with their children.[36] This parental concern was evident in a survey conducted prior to the implementation of the Cash Benefits for Small Children Act. Most parents with preschool children stated that they preferred to take care of their children themselves. Eighty percent of mothers reported that the cash benefit would lead to reduced working hours for women and to greater freedom of choice for parents with young children.

FORMATION AND DISSEMINATION OF IDEAS

Current early childhood education and care policies in Norway have evolved since the creation of the first kindergartens at the end of the nineteenth century, and they are tightly linked with family policy. Although the evidence for combining education and child care appears to be grounded in Nordic tradition, the rationale for the development of the Cash Benefits Act and the National Framework Plan was supported by evidence from program evaluations and annually collected data from Statistics Norway. Barnehager submit yearly data to Statistics Norway on the number of children accessing barnehage by age group, attendance hours, and special-needs status.[37] Data are also collected on the type of barnehage and the composition of staff. Statistics Norway publishes a compilation of these data in the annual report of child care institutions. It is these statistics that were the source of information[38] for most of the problems identified in the previous section, such as the shortage of barnehage places.

In addition, various parent surveys commissioned by the federal government provided baseline information for the cash benefit policy. For example, a survey of 3,500 mothers with young children, conducted prior to the implementation of the cash benefit policy, addressed the issue of parental choice. The survey indicated that 60% of parents would have used the cash benefit to spend more time with their children.[39] The Ministry of Children and Family Affairs anticipated that the cash benefit would encourage parents to stay at home, reducing the demand for barnehage places and creating places for parents who really wanted to use the service. There was an indication from the 3,500 surveyed mothers that this would occur; 37% of parents with children in barnehage reported that they would use the cash benefit to make other child-care arrangements.

Specially commissioned reports also provided research evidence for the National Framework Plan. The National Institute for Public Health produced two reports on the quality of child care. One report, *Quality in Day Care Institutions,* pointed to the lack of criteria for child development and health. The other, *The Child's Value and the Values of the Barnehage—An Analysis of Knowledge* (Borge 1998), advocated providing choice in the use of cash benefits to support parents staying at home with their children or using barnehage. This report also proposed that parents had a significant impact on child development. Similarly, the OECD report on Early Childhood Education and Care Policy stated that the benefit of parental involvement in child care was supported by "Nordic and international research," which showed that preschool programs had the most positive effect when parents were involved[40] (Andrews 1999). The experience of the Norwegian mother/child service,[41] obtained from interviews with public health nurses, suggests otherwise. Norwegian parents did not consider themselves experts in child rearing (Andrews 1999). Moreover, public health nurses reported that parents with young children in the 1990s asked many more questions about their children's health and development than had their predecessors.

POLITICAL ENVIRONMENT

In Norway the feeling of social responsibility for children and all other individuals is apparent in the political system. Twenty-one different political parties are represented in the parliament, the Storting.[42] The largest party since the 1920s, the Norwegian Labor Party, has been a staunch advocate of the welfare state, promoting rights for all with respect to education and other social services. However, family policies have undergone a big change from the 1960s, at which time they were directed at households that did not function as families (Frones 1997). With the more extensive schooling of women and their increased participation in the workforce, the 1980s gave birth to the educated life career family. This transition in family structure resulted in the growth in the late 1980s of family policies that promoted child care and organized leisure activities for children (Frones 1997). Child care was transformed from welfare for the needy and compensation for working mothers into a requisite part of modern upbringing for the well-educated family. It also became an important benchmark for equality between the sexes. This desire for gender equality is reflected in the fact that 42% of ministers in government are women and that political parties have gender ratios.[43] Strong female representation in government, no doubt, has had a strong influence in the development of the early child care policies discussed in this section.

However, the implementation of the Cash Benefits for Small Children policy and economic support of at-home parents of young children has been credited to the strong commitment made by another party.[44] This is the Christian Democratic Party, which represents 15% of the seats in the Storting since 1997 and is the second largest party. It was founded in 1933 in reaction to public sentiment that the Labor government had betrayed the Christian and moral values of its citizens.

SUMMARY

Norway has a strong tradition of day-care institutions that combine education and child care. It has also introduced many child-friendly policies. The Cash Benefits for Small Children policy and the National Framework were implemented to improve the access to and the quality of day care. The cash benefits policy allows parents to pay for child care or stay at home with their children. Both policies were supported by analyses of Statistics Norway data on barnehager, commissioned reports on the quality of barnehage care, and parent surveys.

In assessing the events surrounding the implementation of these two child-care policies in Norway, it would be easy to argue that research was used for its problem-solving ability to support the Cash Benefits for Small Children policy. The Ministry of Children and Family Affairs' access to statistics on child care from the child care institutions report identified for them the shortage of barnehage places for young children. The policy also addressed the issue of parent choice, although the perception that parents with small children were spending too little time with their children was not grounded on research. As mentioned earlier, to gather evidence that the cash benefit policy would achieve its intended goal, the ministry commissioned a survey of 3,500 mothers. Survey findings indicated that the outcome of the cash benefit would be an increase in the number of parents staying at home to look after their young children. Although the survey represented Norwegian parent preference, unlike the population-based barnehage statistics that are required for funding purposes, we have no information about how representative this survey was.

A stronger case can be made for the use of research evidence in problem identification than for problem solving during the implementation of the Framework Plan. Evaluations of barnehage programs uncovered deficiencies in the quality of care, and those, in turn, were translated into standards of care under the Framework Plan. However, establishment of guidelines to improve quality of care would not have guaranteed implementation or improved outcomes, especially if no mechanisms were in place to monitor adherence to the Framework Plan. In other words, evidence of the solution's effectiveness was lacking. As the Ministry of Children and Family Affairs noted,[45] "It is a challenge to create valid and reliable monitoring, assessment and evaluation to ensure that the intentions of the Framework Plan are implemented in each barnehage."

Based on a single study conducted in Norway, *The Child's Value and the Values of the Barnehage—An Analysis of Knowledge,* the evidence was weak that parents could provide the same quality of educational instruction to their preschool children as had barnehager. No reference was made by the OECD report on Early Childhood Education and Care Policy to the debate in the international literature on the benefits of child care versus parental care in child development (Wilms 1999; Mooney and Munton 1998). Belief in the inherent ability of parents as educators likely reflected the values of the Christian Democratic Party, values which were influential in the implementation of the cash benefits policy. The beliefs of the Christian Democratic Party were strongly conveyed in one of the Framework Plan's objectives to increase emphasis on Christian values in the curriculum of barnehager. Thus, use of the *Child's Value and the Values of the Barnehage—An Analysis of Knowledge* report to support the cash benefit policy is an example of research having been used for rhetorical purposes. Put another way, it is conceivable that the sole purpose of using this research evidence was to persuade those uncertain about the positive outcomes of this policy or those advocating for other strategies, such as policies to increase the number of barnehage places.

Summary and Discussion

In this chapter, we presented an in-depth analysis of recently implemented child policies in three countries—Canada, the United States, and Norway—to address the question of whether research evidence had influenced the formation of these policies. Selected for this purpose were the National Children's Agenda (NCA) in Canada, the State Children's Health Insurance Program (SCHIP) in the United States, and two interrelated early childhood education and care policies in Norway (Cash Benefit for Small Children and the National Framework Plan). We were able to confirm the existence of research evidence that had been used to support the implementation of all three policies. In Canada, findings from the Ontario Child Health Survey and the National Longitudinal Survey of Children and Youth, which reported on the association between child deprivation and development, had been in the public domain during the planning of the NCA. Specially commissioned reports documenting the number of children with no health insurance had been available to U.S. policy makers during the development of SCHIP. In addition, a mountain of evidence on the association between socioeconomic status and (child) health, health care use, and well-being had loomed in the background of many of the Canadian and U.S. discussions. We found that although, historically, Norwegians seemed to have grasped the idea of social responsibility for families and children, research evidence still helped to shape their policy. We accessed statistics on child day-care use and parental surveys to learn about Norway's creation of the Cash Benefit for Small Children policy. We found that research evidence had served a dual role in the development of these policies: It had provided not only information on the extent of the problem but also documentation of the policy's likelihood of being an effective solution to the problem.

We conclude that research evidence played a central role, in all of the jurisdictions under study, in problem identification and policy idea formation. But despite the fact that a common pool of evidence, particularly in the past few decades, had been virtually simultaneously available to all jurisdictions once released, markedly different child policies evolved in the three environments. We contend that this fact is due, at least in part, to the beliefs and values held by individuals within the respective societies. However, as a result of differences in belief systems and values within the countries, governments were also at very different places on the child policy front in the late 1990s, the time frame for our case study. Each of the three countries had developed some collection of social and health policies directed at this vulnerable segment of the population, but the respective collections brought to the forefront different issues regarding children's health and well-being. The United States was still struggling with the very basic needs of providing health insurance and health care for children. In stark contrast, the focus in Canada, which already had universal health insurance, was on moving children out of poverty situations, first through the provision of income assistance to families and later through a more complex set of initiatives that reflected the broader determinants of health, especially those originating in early childhood experiences. Norway, having already attended to both the health care and early developmental needs of its children, was far ahead of both Canada and the United States, and Norwegians wanted to address the issue of choice of child-care arrangements for the very young.

The existing value systems also likely had played a role in the type of research funded and carried out in each country, and thus the nature of evidence available to help policy makers identify problems or respond to problems on the policy agenda. This influence of societal values would certainly be evident in the contrast between, on the one hand, the United States' primary research focus on health care use and the implications of having health insurance and, on the other, Canadian health researchers' recent (during the past decade, in particular) focus on a broader set of health determinants.

Our goal also was to illustrate the interplay between research evidence and other processes important to policy making. Many models for policy making have been advanced (see chapter 10), but we turned to Kingdon's categories of problem identification, policy idea formation, and politics to guide us through the analysis of events when the respective child policies under study were developed. While policy-making and other decision-making processes are similar regarding the importance of value systems and the availability of research evidence, the policy-making process differs substantially because the question of who wins and who loses matters a great deal in public policy making. For this reason, we were particularly interested in describing the respective political environments.

The influence of a political agenda on the application of research evidence was evident in all three case studies. The NCA, which set national guidelines for provincial governments to implement policy aimed at reducing child poverty, was crafted by the federal government at a time when there was concern over national unity. The SCHIP policy of health insurance for U.S. children was advanced in support of a Republican agenda for welfare reform and cost containment. The Cash Benefit for Small Children policy in Norway, providing choice for parents wishing to stay at home to care for their young children, was implemented as a result of the efforts of the Christian Democratic Party, a strong proponent of Christian and moral values.

Taken together, our observations suggest that while research evidence played a central role in getting children's issues on the policy-making radar of these three countries, the political, cultural, and historical environments, along with the core societal values of the populations in question, played a dominant role in shaping the specifics of any policy packages. These observations are informative to researchers who want to influence policies that have health objectives, as well as to policy makers who aim to create policies on the best available evidence.

Also important (and encouraging to researchers) is the recognition that research can take on several roles. In chapter 14, Earle, Heymann, and Lavis strongly advocate that researchers invest the time to learn about the issues important to the electorate and to those making policy decisions. Under the assumption that these problems are important to society, such efforts would engage researchers in finding solutions to problems, an activity that would enhance the likelihood of adoption of their research findings. As illustrated in the case study of Norway's cash benefit policy, the problem-solving role of research can be very effective in producing evidence-based policies. Earle and colleagues also recommend that researchers seek opportunities for the enlightenment role of research, an example of which was provided in our NCA case study. One factor considered influential in the NCA's development was the combination of, first, national survey findings and research on early childhood development and, second, key researchers' concerted efforts to ensure that the results of relevant research were made known to and understood by key policy makers.

Kingdon (1995) has distinguished between visible and hidden participants in the policy-making process. Visible participants include prominent members of government, political parties and campaigners, and the media. Academics and researchers are frequently thrown into the hidden participant group. Kingdon also has referred to the role of "policy entrepreneurs," or individuals inside or outside government who are willing to invest resources to achieve a particular outcome. Although they might advocate on behalf of a problem, they also attempt to link problems, policy ideas, and political events so that a policy window will open. Researchers have the potential to fulfill a policy entrepreneur role by capturing the attention of government officials to ensure that policy windows will open. Advancing research to enlighten the formation of policy places the researcher in a policy entrepreneur role. If researchers actively embraced this role, evidence-based policy making and an increased visibility of researchers as participants in the process would result. The alternative would be to accept either a minimal role or only a rhetorical role for research in the policy-making process.

Notes

The authorship of this chapter was randomly assigned due to the collaborative nature of the work.

1. See, for example, the recent collection of publications by CPRN (at http://www.cprn .ca) addressing this issue.

2. For example, the child tax credit and the child tax benefit.

3. Available at http://www.acf.dhhs.gov/programs/opa/facts/tanf.htm.

4. Beginning in 1945, Canada offered a universal family allowance but moved to a targeted program in 1993.

5. According to Kingdon, for a problem to be recognized, people must be convinced that something must be done to change it. The recognition of a pressing problem may be sufficient for it to gain prominence on the policy agenda, but policy makers pay attention to only a fraction of the problems in their communities. Many ideas are considered in response to perceived problems. The sources of these ideas are many: academics, researchers, government employees, political parties, lobbyists and the media. Only a few ideas survive the policy selection process, which Kingdon likens to biological natural selection. Those that can be easily implemented have a good chance, but the survival of ideas has much to do with the political environment, namely the national mood, election results, changes in government administration, pressures from lobby groups, and the values and turf battles of the governing party. Kingdon uses the recent U.S. health care reform debate to illustrate these phenomena. Proposals for universal health insurance date back to Teddy Roosevelt, but concerns over access to health care heated up the debate during President Clinton's early days. However, the policy stream was in disarray—policy ideas ranged from

a single-payer system to managed competition to incremental implementation. In the end Clinton's proposals failed—some say due to the complexity of his plan and/or strong opposition from special-interest groups that were concerned over the costs of universal coverage.

6. Nonetheless, Quebec permitted a footnote to the agreement saying, in effect, that it was meeting the objectives of the NCA in its own way.

7. Background information on the National Children's Agenda announced in the Speech from the Throne, September 23, 1997. Information is available at http://unionsociale.gc.ca/nca/nca1_e.html.

8. Background information on the National Children's Agenda announced in the Speech from the Throne, September 23, 1997. Information is available at http://unionsociale.gc.ca/nca/nca1_e.html.

9. The NLSCY is a comprehensive, longitudinal survey of a representative sample of Canadian children, which was designed to measure and monitor the development and well-being of Canada's children and youth. The survey is conducted by the Department of Human Resources Development Canada and Statistics Canada, and data are made available for public use. An initial cohort, aged 0–11 years in 1994, is being followed to age 25. To date, there have been four further survey administrations: 1996, 1998, 2000, and 2002.

10. The first meeting of the Federal-Provincial-Territorial Council on Social Policy Renewal was on November 27, 1996. This Council, which has representation from the provinces, territories, and federal government, was created to direct the social union initiative to update Canada's system of social services, including child and family benefits. Information is available at http://socialunion.gc.ca/news/96nov27e.html.

11. This meeting of Ministers Responsible for Social Services was in Toronto on January 13, 1997. Information is available at http://socialunion.gc.ca/news/97jan13e.html.

12. This meeting of the Federal-Provincial-Territorial Council on Social Policy Renewal was held in Toronto on January 29, 1997. Information is available at http://socialunion.gc.ca/news/97jan29e.html.

13. Information on the National Child Benefit is available at http://socialunion.gc.ca/ncb/ncbpamp_e.html.

14. This meeting of the Federal-Provincial-Territorial Council on Social Policy Renewal was held in Toronto on January 29, 1997. Information is available at http://socialunion.gc.ca/news/97jan29e.html.

15. Human Resources Development Canada is the department of the federal government of Canada, which is responsible for employment insurance, pension, child and family benefits, and other social services. In 2003, it was split into two departments: Social Development Canada and Human Resources and Skills Development Canada.

16. National Children's Agenda, "Background Information on Readiness to Learn." Available at http://socialunion.gc.ca/nca/nca5_e.html; Fraser Mustard, who had coauthored, with M. N. McCain, the seminal report *Reversing the Real Brain Drain: Understanding the Early Years Study Final Report* (Toronto: Children's Secretariat, 1999).

17. *The Health of Canada's Children: A CICH Profile* (Ottawa: Canadian Institute for Child Health, 1989); *The Health of Canada's Children: A CICH Profile,* 2nd ed. (Ottawa: Canadian Institute for Child Health, 1994).

18. "Campaign Overview: Liberals Played It Safe, Lost Campaign Momentum." Available at http://www.canoe.ca/FedElection/liberal_overview.html; "Liberal Red Book Gets Second Read," available at http://www.canoe.ca/PastHeadings/apr30_chretien.html.

19. "Campaign Overview: Liberals Played It Safe, Lost Campaign Momentum." Available

at http://www.canoe.ca/FedElection/liberal_overview.html; "Liberal Red Book Gets Second Read." Available at http://www.canoe.ca/PastHeadings/apr30_chretien.html. The Liberal Red Book is a publication of the campaign promises of the Liberal Party.

20. The National Child Benefit. Available at http://socialunion.gc.ca/ncb/ncbpamp_e .html.

21. Canada's federalizing constitution, the British North America Act of 1867, outlines the division of powers between the federal government and the provinces. Under this act, provinces are given jurisdiction for health and social services. In instituting universal health care insurance in Canada in the 1950s and 1960s, the federal government entered into a provincial domain, which meant bargaining with the provinces to achieve the current system of federal transfer payments (tax points and cash) to provinces for health care, but provincially administered health programs. However, each province had to abide by federal criteria (Canada Health Act) to receive payment. Eventually, this payment was lumped together with payments for education and social services (Canada Health and Social Transfer). Tensions between the federal and provincial governments around issues of jurisdiction have occurred historically, especially when substantial cuts were made to the federal transfer payments in the 1990s. Quebec has consistently insisted on making autonomous decisions on matters within its jurisdiction (Facal 1998). Quebec's system of local community service centers (CLSC), which combine primary health and social services, evolved under Quebec's strong provincial leadership (Palley 1987). Quebec has prided itself on its ability to maintain tight fiscal control.

In 1992, the Charlottetown Accord proposed an addition to the constitution that committed the federal government to the social and economic union of Canadians. Until this time, there had been no common principles for the delivery of social services and benefits to Canadians. The accord also proposed to amend the constitution to grant Quebec status as a "distinct society." But the accord failed, and this failure was viewed by Quebecers as a personal rejection by the rest of Canada. Three years later Quebec held a referendum vote on whether to secede from the Canadian federation. The slim majority for the "no" vote (50.6%) for secession indicated to the federal government that it had some work to do in promoting national unity, yet also reconciling Quebec's need for cultural security.

22. "The State Children's Health Insurance Program: Preliminary Highlights of Implementation and Expansion." Available at http://www.hcfa.gov/init/children.htm.

23. In 1997, 675,000 former welfare recipients lost Medicaid coverage—62% of these recipients were children (Starr 2000).

24. A search of GAO's report database, using the keyword *children,* yielded twenty-six publications on issues related to children published from 1994 to 1998, including ten reports and testimonies on vaccination and health care insurance for children. Interestingly, there were twelve reports on poverty and early childhood environments.

25. Quoted in B. Dutcher, "Combating Creeping ClintonCare." Available at http://www .ocpathink.org/economics/CreepingClintonCare.html.

26. SCHIP and Medicaid were inextricably linked because eligibility for one program began when the other ended.

27. In 1999, the states had spent less than 20% of SCHIP funds and had not enrolled about 10 million children. In Texas, only 28,000 children were covered out of 500,000 believed to be eligible (Starr 2000; Schram and Weissert 1999).

28. This information is from the Norwegian Ministry of Children and Family Affairs, "OECD—Thematic Review of Early Childhood Education and Care Policy." Available at http://odin.dep.no.bfd/engelsk/publ/rapporter/004001-990023/index-dok000-b-n-a.html.

29. This information is from the Norwegian Ministry of Children and Family Affairs, "OECD—Thematic Review of Early Childhood Education and Care Policy." Available at http://odin.dep.no.bfd/engelsk/publ/rapporter/004001-990023/index-dok000-b-n-a.html.

30. Saami are indigenous peoples of Norway. Until World War II, Norwegian governing policies towards the Saami population resulted in the suppression of Saami cultural and linguistic rights. Recent initiatives such as the establishment of the Saami Rights Commission and the Saami parliament, have been implemented to redress the Norwegian government's earlier negative policies (Eira 2001).

31. This information is from the Norwegian Ministry of Children and Family Affairs, "OECD—Thematic Review of Early Childhood Education and Care Policy." Available at http://odin.dep.no.bfd/engelsk/publ/rapporter/004001-990023/index-dok000-b-n-a.html.

32. See information from the European Network of Ombudsmen for Children. Available at http://www.ombudsnet.org.

33. Available at http://www.ombudsnet.org.

34. This information is from the Norwegian Ministry of Children and Family Affairs, "OECD—Thematic Review of Early Childhood Education and Care Policy." Available at http://odin.dep.no.bfd/engelsk/publ/rapporter/004001-990023/index-dok000-b-n-a.html.

35. This information is from the Norwegian Ministry of Children and Family Affairs, "OECD—Thematic Review of Early Childhood Education and Care Policy." Available at http://odin.dep.no.bfd/engelsk/publ/rapporter/004001-990023/index-dok000-b-n-a.html.

36. This information is from the Norwegian Ministry of Children and Family Affairs, "OECD—Thematic Review of Early Childhood Education and Care Policy." Available at http://odin.dep.no.bfd/engelsk/publ/rapporter/004001-990023/index-dok000-b-n-a.html.

37. This information is from the Norwegian Ministry of Children and Family Affairs, "OECD—Thematic Review of Early Childhood Education and Care Policy." Available at http://odin.dep.no.bfd/engelsk/publ/rapporter/004001-990023/index-dok000-b-n-a.html.

38. This information is from the Norwegian Ministry of Children and Family Affairs, "OECD—Thematic Review of Early Childhood Education and Care Policy." Available at http://odin.dep.no.bfd/engelsk/publ/rapporter/004001-990023/index-dok000-b-n-a.html.

39. This information is from the Norwegian Ministry of Children and Family Affairs, "OECD—Thematic Review of Early Childhood Education and Care Policy." Available at http://odin.dep.no.bfd/engelsk/publ/rapporter/004001-990023/index-dok000-b-n-a.html.

40. This information is from the Norwegian Ministry of Children and Family Affairs, "OECD—Thematic Review of Early Childhood Education and Care Policy." Available at http://odin.dep.no/bfd/engelsk/publ/rapporter/004001-990023/ndex-dok000-b-n-a.html.

41. The Norwegian mother/child service is a publicly funded program that offers all parents with children and pregnant women mother/child services free of charge. Included are visits by public health nurses and routine examinations by general practitioners. Nearly 100% of Norwegian children receive these services.

42. For further information, see "Norway's Political Parties of the Norwegian Electoral." Available at http://odin.dep.no/engelsk/om_odin/sprn/032005-990426/index-dok000-b-n-a.html.

43. For further information, see "Norway's Political Parties of the Norwegian Electoral." Available at http://odin.dep.no/engelsk/om_odin/sprn/032005-990426/index-dok000-b-n-a.html.

44. For further information, see "Norway's Political Parties of the Norwegian Electoral." Available at http://odin.dep.no/engelsk/om_odin/sprn/032005-990426/index-dok000-b-n-a.html.

45. This information is from the Norwegian Ministry of Children and Family Affairs,

"OECD—Thematic Review of Early Childhood Education and Care Policy." Available at http://odin.dep.no/bfd/engelsk/publ/rapporter/004001-990023/index-dok000-b-n-a.html.

References

Andrews, T. 1999. Pulled between contradictory expectations: Norwegian mother/child service and the "new" public health discourse. *Critical Public Health* 9:269–285.

Atkinson, W. L., S. C. Hadler, S. B. Redd, and W. A. Orenstein. 1992. Measles surveillance—United States, 1991. *MMWR Morbidity Mortality Weekly Reports CDC Surveillance Summary* 41:1–12.

Baker, M. 1995. *Canadian Family Policies: Cross-national Comparisons.* Toronto: University of Toronto Press.

Barer, M. L., T. R. Marmor, and E. M. Morrison. 1995. Health care reform in the United States: On the road to nowhere (again)? *Social Science Medicine* 41:453–460.

Borge, A. I. H. 1998. Barnehagens innhold. In *Barnets verd og barnehagens verdier. En kunnskapsanalyse.* Oslo: Statens institutt for folkehelse, Avd. for samfunnsmedisin.

Cadman, D., M. H. Boyle, D. R. Offord, P. Szatmari, N. I. Rae-Grant, and J. Crawford. 1986. Chronic illness and functional limitation in Ontario children: Findings of the Ontario Child Health Study. *Canadian Medical Association Journal* 135:761–767.

Cauffman, J. G., M. I. Roemer, and C. S. Shultz. 1967. The impact of health insurance coverage on health care of school children. *Public Health Reports* 82:323–328.

Chan, K. W. 1995. *Vaccines for Children: Re-examination of Program Goals and Implementation Needed to Ensure Vaccination.* Washington, DC: U.S. General Accounting Office.

Currie, J. 1995. Socio-economic status and child health: Does public health insurance narrow the gap? *Scandinavian Journal of Economics* 97:603–620.

Curtis, L. J., M. D. Dooley, E. L. Lipman, and D. H. Feeny. 2001. The role of permanent income and family structure in the determination of child health in Canada. *Journal of Health Economics* 10:287–302.

Dooley, M. D., L. Curtis, E. Lipman, and D. Feeny. 1998. Child behaviour problems, poor school performance and social problems: The roles of family structure and low income in cycle one of the National Longitudinal Survey of Children and Youth. In *Labour Markets, Social Institutions, and the Future of Canada's Children,* ed. M. Corak. Catalogue Number 89-553-XPB Statistics Canada (Chapter 7).

Eira, A. J. H, State-secretary, Norwegian Ministry of Local Government and Regional Development. Citizenship–self-government–self-determination. 2001. A comparison of Aboriginal peoples in Canada and Saami in Norway. May 11, 2001. Accessed May 11, 2001 at http://odin.dep.no/krd/engelsk/aktuelt/taler/taler_politisk_ledelse/016091-090006/index-dok000-b-n-a.html.

Ellwood, D. T. 1996. When bad things happen to good policies: Welfare reform as I knew it. *American Prospect* 26:22–29.

Evans, R. G., M. L. Barer, and T. R. Marmor, eds. 1994. *Why Are Some People Healthy and Others Not? The Determinants of Health of Populations.* New York: Aldine de Gruyter.

Evans, R. G., and G. L. Stoddart. 1990. Producing health, consuming health care. *Social Science Medicine* 31:1347–1363.

Facal, J. 1998. Pourquoi le Quebec a adhere au consensus des provinces sur l'union sociale. *Policy Options* (November):11–12.

Frones, I. 1997. The transformation of childhood: Children and families in postwar Norway. *Acta Sociologica* 40:17–30.

Gavin, N. I., E. K. Adams, and E. J. Herz. 1998. The use of EPSDT and other health care services by children enrolled in Medicaid: The impact of OBRA '89. *Milbank Quarterly* 76:207–251.

Glazer, N. 1995. Making work work: Welfare reform in the 1990s. In *The Work Alternative: Welfare Reform and the Realities of the Job Market,* ed. D. S. Nightingale and R. H. Haveman. Washington, DC: Urban Institute Press.

Glouberman, S., and J. Millar. 2003. Evolution of the determinants of health, health policy, and health information systems in Canada. *American Journal of Public Health* 93:388–392.

Goggin, M. L. 1999. The use of administrative discretion in implementing the State Children's Health Insurance Program. *Publicus* 29:35–51.

Grayson, M. 1998. Health care for children. *Spectrum* 71:1–3.

Green, J. 2000. Bargaining chip. *American Prospect* 11:15–16.

Hacker, J. S., and T. Skocpol. 2001. The new politics of U.S. health policy. In *The Nation's Health,* 6th ed., ed. P. R. Lee and C. L. Estes. Sudbury, MA: Jones and Bartlett.

Hanratty, M. 1996. Canadian National Health Insurance and infant health. *American Economic Review* 86 (1):276–284.

Hertzman C. 2001. The case for an early child development strategy. *ISUMA* 1 (2):11–18.

Heymann, J. 2000. *The Widening Gap: Why America's Working Families Are in Jeopardy— And What Can Be Done about It.* New York: Basic Books.

Hill, I. 2000. Charting new courses for children's health insurance. *Policy and Practice of Public Human Services,* 58 (4):30–38.

Human Resources Development Canada (HRDC). 1996. *Strategic Policy Communications* 819:994–1453.

———. 1997. *The National Child Benefit.* Catalogue no. MP 43–372/1997E. Available at http://www.intergov.gc.ca/docs/intergov/ncb/ncbpamp_e.html.

Human Resources Development Canada (HRDC) and Statistics Canada. 1996. *Growing Up in Canada—National Longitudinal Survey of Children and Youth.* Ottawa: Statistics Canada.

ISUMA. 2001. Editorial comment. *ISUMA Canadian Journal of Policy Research* 1 (2):7.

Jansson, B. S. 1997. Reluctance illustrated: Policy uncertainty during the Clinton administration. In *The Reluctant Welfare State. American Social Welfare Policies—Past, Present and Future.* San Francisco, CA: Brooks/Cole.

Jenson, J., and S. Thompson. 1999. Comparative family policy: Six provincial stories. CPRN study no. 8, Canadian Policy Research Network.

Kamerman, S. B., and A. J. Kahn. 1997. *Family Change and Family Policies in Great Britain, Canada, New Zealand and the United States.* New York: Oxford University Press.

Karpatkin, R., and G. E. Shearer. 1995. Commentary: A short-term consumer agenda for health care reform. *American Journal of Public Health* 10:1352–1355.

Keating, D. P. 1999. The learning society: A human development agenda. In *Developmental Health and the Wealth of Nations: Social, Biological and Educational Dynamics,* ed. D. P. Keating and C. Hertzman. New York: Guilford Press.

Keating, D. P., and C. Hertzman, eds. 1999. *Developmental Health and the Wealth of Nations: Social, Biological and Educational Dynamics.* New York: Guilford Press.

King, C. T. 1999. Federalism and workforce policy reform. *Publicus* 29:53–71.

Kingdon, J. W. 1995. *Agendas, Alternatives and Public Policies.* 2nd ed. New York: Longman.

Kohen, D., C. Hertzman, and J. Brooks-Gunn. 1998. Neighbourhood influences on children's school readiness. Working paper no. W-98-15E, Strategic Policy, Applied Research Branch, Human Resources Development Canada.

Lave, J. R., C. R. Keane, C. J. Lin, E. M. Ricci, G. Amersbach, and C. P. LaVallee. 1998. Impact of a children's health insurance program on newly enrolled children. *Journal of the American Medical Association* 279:1820–1825.

Legowski, B., and L. McKay. 2000. Health beyond health care: Twenty-five years of federal health policy development. CPRN discussion paper no. HI04, October 2000, Canadian Policy Research Networks, Ottawa.

Lipman, E. L., and D. R. Offord. 1994. Disadvantaged children. In *The Canadian Guide to Clinical Preventive Health Care.* Ottawa, Ontario: Canadian Task Force on the Periodic Health Examination, Minister of Supply and Services Canada. (Catalogue no. H21-117/1994E).

———. 1996. Psychosocial morbidity among poor children in Ontario. In *Growing Up Poor,* ed. G. Duncan and J. Brooks-Gunn. New York: Russell Sage Foundation.

Lipman, E. L., D. R. Offord, and M. H. Boyle. 1994. Economic disadvantage and child psycho-social morbidity. *Canadian Medical Association Journal* 151:431–437.

Mason, W. H., L. A. Ross, J. Lanson, and H. T. Wright Jr. 1993. Epidemic measles in the postvaccine era: Evaluation of epidemiology, clinical presentation and complications during an urban outbreak. *Pediatric Infectious Disease Journal* 12:42–48.

Mead, L. M. 1992. Welfare reform. In *The New Politics of Poverty. The Nonworking Poor in America.* New York: Basic Books.

Mooney, A., and A. G. Munton. 1998. Quality in early childhood services: Parent, provider and policy perspectives. *Children and Society* 12:101–112.

Nadel, M. V. 1995. *Health Insurance for Children: Many Remain Uninsured despite Medicaid Expansion.* Washington, DC: U.S. General Accounting Office.

National Forum on Health. 1997a. *Canada Health Action: Building on the Legacy.* Vol. 2. Ottawa: Health Canada.

———. 1997b. *Canada Health Action: Building on the Legacy.* Papers commissioned by the National Forum on Health, Determinants of Health, Children and Youth. Ottawa: Health Canada.

Newacheck, P. W., and N. Halfon. 1986. The association between mother's and children's use of physician services. *Medical Care* 24:30–38.

Newacheck, P. W., D. C. Hughes, and J. J. Stoddard. 1996. Children's access to primary care: Differences by race, income, and insurance status. *Pediatrics* 97:26–32.

OECD. 2001. *Organization for Economic Cooperation and Development Health Data.* Organization for Economic Cooperation and Development, France.

Offord, D. R., M. H. Boyle, Y. A. Racine, J. E. Fleming, D. T. Cadman, and H. M. Blum. 1992. Outcome, prognosis, and risk in a longitudinal follow-up study. *Journal of the American Academy of Adolescent Psychiatry* 31:916–923.

O'Hara, K. 1998. Comparative family policy: Eight countries' stories. *Canadian Policy Research Network* (CPRN) study no. 4.

Palley, H. A. 1987. Canadian federalism and the Canadian health care program: A comparison of Ontario and Quebec. *International Journal of Health Services* 17:595–617.

Philip, K. L., K. Backett-Milburn, S. Cunningham-Burley, and J. B. Davis. 2003. Practising what we preach? A practical approach to bringing research, policy and practice together in relation to children and health inequalities. *Health Education Research* 18:568–579.

Phipps, S. 1998. An international comparison of policies and outcomes for young children. CPRN study no. 5. Ottawa: Canadian Policy Research Networks.

———. 1999. Economics and the well-being of Canadian children. *Canadian Journal of Economics* 32:1135–1163.

———. 2001. Values, policies and the well-being of young children in Canada, Norway and the United States. In *Child Well-being, Child Poverty and Child Policy in Modern Nations,* ed. K. Vleminckx and T. M. Smeading. Bristol, U.K.: Policy Press.

Pless, I. B. 1995. *Crossing the Bridge: From Research to Child Policy.* Montreal: McGill University Press.

Roos, N. P. 1995. From research to policy: What have we learned from designing the Population Health Information System? *Medical Care* 33 (12 suppl.):DS132–DS145.

Sardell, A., and K. Johnson. 1998. The politics of EPSDT policy in the 1990s. Policy entrepreneurs, political streams, and children health benefits. *Milbank Quarterly* 76:175–205.

Scanlon, W. J. 1996. *Health Insurance for Children: Private Insurance Coverage Continues to Deteriorate.* Washington, DC: U.S. General Accounting Office.

———. 1997. *Health Insurance: Coverage Leads to Increased Health Care Access for Children.* Washington, DC: U.S. General Accounting Office.

Schram, S. F., and C. S. Weissert. 1999. The state of U.S. federalism, 1998–1999. *Publicus* 29:1–33.

Starr, A. 2000. Chipping away at the uninsured. *American Prospect* 11:18–19.

———. 2001. Children first. *American Prospect* (12 suppl.):40–41.

Stroik, S., and J. Jenson. 1998. What is the best policy mix for Canada's young children? CPRN study no. 9. Ottawa: Canadian Policy Research Networks.

Thompson, F. J., and T. L. Gais. 2000. Federalism and the safety net: Delinkage and participation rates. *Publicus* 30:119–142.

Tibbetts, J. 1997a. Ottawa wants provinces to get on with plans to cut child poverty (no. 3951855). Toronto: *Canada Press NewsWire*, October 2, 1997.

———. 1997b. National children's agenda aims for uniform child services across Canada (no. 3920099). Toronto: *Canada Press NewsWire*, August 24, 1997

Wilms, D. J. 1999. Quality and inequality in children's literacy. In *Developmental Health and the Wealth of Nations: Social, Biological and Educational Dynamics,* ed. D. P. Keating and C. Hertzman. New York: Guilford Press.

Wong, K., S. Gardner, D. B. Bainbridge, K. Feightner, D. R. Offord, and L. W. Chambers. 2000. Tracking the use and impact of a community social report: Where does the information go? *Canadian Journal of Public Health* 91:41–45.

Chapter 14

Where Do We Go from Here? Translating Research to Policy

Alison Earle, Jody Heymann, and John N. Lavis

The chapters in this volume have explored the evidence base, which, for ease of presentation, we call "population health research." This research examines both the fundamental causes of good and poor health status (often labeled the determinants of health) and the mediating factors that may influence relationships between these determinants and health status. Authors here have explored the role of income inequality and labor market experiences (including employment, the structure and organization of work, and work arrangements) and health outcomes; the relationship among food, nutrition, and health at a population level; the role of location, place, and geography in the social production of health; the importance of social conditions over the life course beginning in childhood; the interaction among genetics, the physical environment, lifestyle, and social structure as determinants of population health; and finally the biological pathways that link the socioeconomic environment and health.

The common characteristic among these determinants of population health is that they are fundamentally aggregate-level, social factors over which a single individual—whether a patient or doctor—has little control. The implication of the preceding chapters is that reducing health inequalities is not as simple as requiring every doctor to prescribe a magic pill to all her patients, or to require every individual to exercise more (though this might help as well). Changing, increasing, or decreasing any one of the factors explored in the preceding chapters by definition requires policy change or social intervention. Changing the way that food is distributed, reducing ethnic and racial inequalities, or increasing the availability of more stable work arrangements requires broad-scale institutional and legal change. If policy-level social change is necessary to reduce health inequalities, the next question is how we can influence policy makers and other actors who can change policy and implement programs at a societal level.

Moreover, the translation of research to policy formation is a particular challenge for the types of research discussed in the preceding chapters because this research has implications primarily for public policies that do not have as their principal objective improving the health of the public. Policy makers need little or no prompting to examine relationships between health care financing policy and health outcomes or between occupational health and safety policy and health outcomes. However, they may well need prompting to examine relationships between tax policies and health, between labor-market policies and health, or between early childhood development policies and health.

The last section of this volume has begun to explore what we do know about the translation of population health research findings to policy in specific cases. This concluding chapter will present evidence regarding the use of research in general—an area that has a longer history and a wider range of cases for study—which we hope offers insights for the use of population health research.

Research to Policy in General: What Does Theory Tell Us about the Use of Research?

Research can influence the public policy-making process at many stages: when agendas and goals are set, when policy alternatives are identified, when the costs and benefits of these policy alternatives are weighed, when choices between policy alternatives are made, and when policies are implemented. The answer to the question of whether research does influence the public policy-making process can, however, be disheartening for both researchers and those with an interest in the outcome of the process. Research often plays a limited or no role in the public policy-making process (Allison 1971; Beyer and Trice 1982; Weiss 1980; Hanney et al. 2003), and even when it does play a role, it may be used in ways that send chills up the spines of those who produced and attempted to communicate its implications. On a more positive note, we are beginning to learn more about the conditions under which research is used in what (for now) we will call "constructive" ways (Innvaer et al. 2002).

The public policy-making process shares some attributes with other decision-making processes, such as those in which clinicians are involved. Research and other types of information may play a role. Values, beliefs, personal aspirations, and other influences may also play a role. But the process also differs quite substantially from other decision-making processes. Who wins, who loses, and by how much can matter a great deal in the public policy-making process. The voting public may care deeply about whether one group in society benefits at the expense of another. The rules of the game (i.e., institutional arrangements), including, but not limited to, how decisions get made, can also matter a great deal. Separate executive and legislative functions, for example, ensure both multiple entry points and multiple veto points.

Political scientists have tried to create ideal-type models of the public policy-making process. The rational choice model views this process as basically linear and dependent on the rational behavior of participants (Schelling 1960; Simon 1966). Few people find this convincing. Other more nuanced models acknowledge the limitations of this rationality assumption (Lindblom 1959; Etzioni 1967) and that there may be a more random, spontaneous aspect to policy making that makes timing critical (Cohen et al. 1972; Kingdon 1995). Still others acknowledge the importance of interests and institutional arrangements (Allison 1971; Heclo 1974).

Using these ideal-type models to analyze policy case studies, researchers have documented that policy makers often do not use research in a "rational" way. Instead of being used to help set agendas and goals, identify policy alternatives, weigh the costs and benefits of these policy alternatives, make choices between policy alternatives, or implement policies, research is more likely to be used in less than "rational" ways or ignored altogether. Allison's (1971) now classic analysis of the Cuban missile crisis provides convincing evidence that the information available to leaders about a situation will reflect organizational goals and routines, the political motivations of the participants, as well as the "facts."

More recently, John Kingdon's research examining 247 individuals involved in federal policy in the United States provides a compelling example of the uses and misuses of research (Kingdon 1995). Kingdon's interviews suggest that the researcher–analyst community has little impact on agenda setting. Instead, policy goals are more often influenced by other forces and individuals. For example, during the 1970s the high cost of medical care became a prominent concern of American legislators. Despite the research that health economists and health policy analysts were conducting on this topic, academics did not in this case play a major role in bringing the issue to the agenda. They were, however, among a range of people to whom politicians turned for ideas on how to address it.

Kingdon concluded that among nongovernmental actors, interest groups were reported to have the most important influence on the public policy-making process, with academic researchers following next. Although some politicians, staffers, and bureaucrats look to academic research, there is a full range of opinions on its value in the decision-making process. Some individuals in Washington view academic studies with a great deal of skepticism, whereas others value the work but realize that the recommendations based on it often have practical limitations.

But neither Allison (1971) nor Kingdon (1995) articulate the different possible roles for research in the various phases of the policy-making process. The taxonomy developed by Pelz (1978), a variant of which was later developed by Weiss (1979), offers some helpful framing (see table 14.1). The first way in which research can be used in the public policy-making process can be called a *conceptual* use.

Table 14.1. Possible ways in which research is used

Use of research*	Description	Potential result
Conceptual	Research provides new perspectives emerging from a body of work	Research shapes the political agenda by altering the way policy makers and the public think about and make sense of social issues
Instrumental	Research is used or commissioned to address a particular problem that is already on the policy agenda, identifies policy alternatives, or costs and benefits of policy alternatives	Research influences which policy alternatives are considered and chosen by policy makers
Symbolic or rhetorical	Research findings used to neutralize opponents, convince undecided parties, and provide ammunition for supporters of a policy alternative	Research influences support for policy alternatives
Tactical	Research or an assertion of the lack of research is used tactically to avoid or delay action	Research influences whether issues are addressed by policy

*The terminology for the uses of research is modified from Weiss 1979.

When research includes new perspectives emerging from a body of work, as opposed to the findings of a single study, it can shape the political agenda by altering the way policy makers and the public think about and make sense of social issues. As an example, the growing body of research demonstrating the profound effect of early childhood experiences on health status in adult life has contributed to getting early childhood development onto the Canadian policy-making agenda (e.g., Mustard et al. 2000; see also Curtis and Kozyrskyj, this volume).

Research can also be used in an *instrumental* way in the public policy-making process. Policy makers might use or commission research in specific and direct ways to help address a particular problem that is already on the policy agenda. Research could be used to identify policy alternatives or to identify the costs and benefits of policy alternatives. As an example, policy makers might look to published studies of the health consequences of job turnover in particular demographic groups to determine which groups should be targeted for a new job retention program.

Research can also be used in a *symbolic* or *rhetorical* way, to neutralize opponents, convince undecided parties, and provide ammunition for supporters of a policy alternative. Research on the health consequences of poverty may be used, for example, to gain the support of health activists who might not otherwise pay much attention to a policy debate about whether to reduce income disparities within a population. Weiss (1979) calls this a political use of research. But research, or more commonly an assertion of the lack of research, can also be used tactically, to avoid or delay action. When the findings from existing research do not serve the interests of a particular party or politician, additional research may be commissioned.

What Do Recent Experiences Demonstrate about Whether and How Research Is Used?

Although many individuals and groups have raised questions regarding the influence of population health research, few provide assessments of whether and how this research has been used. When they suggest ways of enhancing the use of such research in public policy-making processes, their suggestions are seldom based on empirical public policy research (e.g., Whitehead 1998). Recently this has begun to change, with some individuals or groups tracing whether and how these ideas have taken root (e.g., Lavis 2004), how groups with vested interests in particular outcomes (e.g., Marmor et al. 1994) or the public more generally (e.g., Blaxter 1997) have responded to these ideas, and how institutional arrangements have helped or hindered the acceptance and use of these ideas (e.g., Lavis and Sullivan 1999). Others have explored the interplay between ideas, interests, and institutions (e.g., Heymann 2000a; Lavis et al. 2001).

In this chapter, we explore the question of why population health research has played a limited role in the policy-making process and what lessons this recent empirical research has to offer about how to enhance the use of population health research in this process. We draw on case studies from the United States, the United Kingdom, Canada, the Netherlands, and Sweden. We begin by describing the ways in which research theoretically can be used in policy making. We then discuss the empirical evidence about whether and how research is currently used in the policy-making process, both generally and in the specific case of population health research. This is followed by a review of what we have learned about the conditions under which research is more likely to be used, from which we derive concrete lessons for both researchers and policy makers interested in enhancing the use of population health research. We conclude with our assessment of the prospects for change.

So has the use of research changed in the decades since these decision-making and research-utilization frameworks were first developed? Evidence would suggest that the answer is "not substantially." But the growing body of empirical evidence about whether and how research is used in the policy-making process offers many helpful insights on how it could change. In this section we review what has been learned over the past decade about the use of research. We draw on examples in which population health research was the primary focus, as well as some from the same policy domain (i.e., health and social policy) but where other types of research were the primary focus.

One approach to studying whether and how research is used takes researchers or policy makers as the unit of analysis. In Canada, Landry et al. (2001) recently surveyed 1,229 Canadian social science researchers to ascertain the extent to which they felt their research was being used. About 56% of respondents reported that their research never or rarely leads to applications, whereas about 16% of respondents reported that their research usually or always leads to applications. But likely only a small fraction of their total output could be considered to be population health research (given that survey respondents were drawn from all areas in social science, not just those studying health) and only some of the applications would be in the public policy-making process (given that applications of research included those by all types of decision-makers, not just those working involved in public policy-making processes).

However, self-reports may overstate knowledge and use of research. Furthermore, an additional difficulty that arises with survey-based assessments of whether research is used in the public policy-making process is that the survey questions typically require respondents to generalize across all of their experiences. These experiences may cross policy sectors (e.g., finance and labor) and policy-making contexts (e.g., strong and weak economies, neoliberal and social democratic governing parties), making it difficult to know whether the summary measure reflects a uniform experience, a true average, or the impact of atypical experiences. As well, it is extremely difficult to get at how research is used without prompts about other competing factors like interests and institutional arrangements.

Detailed case studies provide one means of digging below the surface of survey-based responses. Here we describe eight policy case studies that provide a more fine-grained assessment of whether and how research is used in policy making. These case studies are drawn from the United States (three policy case studies), the United Kingdom (one), Canada (two), the Netherlands (one), and Sweden (one). These policy case studies are described in more detail in source documents. We provide only their most salient characteristics and conclusions here. The case studies are grouped according to whether and how research was used: research was available but ignored, research was used rhetorically, and research was used but not to its full potential. We have yet to find a case study in which population health research has been used to its full potential in the policy-making process.

Ignoring Available Research

Two policy case studies from the United States and one from the United Kingdom provide examples of policy makers ignoring available evidence on program effectiveness. The first two case studies explore a set of policies first developed in the 1960s and 1970s in the United States: the policies were designed to increase human capital through education and training (Heymann 2000a). The programs, summarized below, range from the Head Start program, targeted at preschool children, to the Job Training Partnership Act, aimed at adults ready for employment. With both of these case studies, the research supported expansion of existing programs but policy makers failed to provide adequate access in one case and reduced, then eliminated, programs in the second case.

Numerous studies have shown that well-designed preschool programs have long-term benefits. Early childhood development programs for children living in poverty have been shown to decrease the likelihood of school dropout, unemployment, juvenile delinquency, and teen pregnancy. This research has been well summarized elsewhere (Murnane 1994; Heymann 2000b). Despite the availability and quality of the research showing that early childhood programs are highly cost-effective, the research did not influence policy makers when they were making decisions about the scale at which to continue these programs. There has never been sufficient or sustained support to ensure that there are spaces for all children who are eligible for the programs in the United States.

Research has also shown that training and work-experience programs aimed at increasing human capital in adults such as the Comprehensive Employment and Training Act (CETA) of 1973 can increase wages. For example, Burtless (1994) found that average wages of CETA program participants increased by 25% to 75% of average earnings before enrollment. Estimates by the Congressional Budget Office also showed that the CETA program led to significant increases in annual real wages of women who participated. Despite the demonstrated effectiveness of programs like CETA, in the 1980s overall spending on education and training programs for the poor fell (Burtless 1994). CETA was discontinued in 1982, and was eventually replaced by other programs that have been shown to be less effective. For example, the Job Training Partnership Act (JTPA) which places participants in private sector jobs and is run by "private industry councils," showed gains in wages, but the gains were smaller than those experienced by CETA participants (Blank 1994; Bloom et al. 1993).

The third case study involves the period between the late 1970s and mid-1990s during which research about health inequalities and their likely causes was emerging in the United Kingdom but was being almost completely ignored by policy makers (Lavis 2004). The relevant evidence as it then existed was first brought together in 1979 in the so-called *Black Report* (reprinted in Townsend et al. 1988), a report commissioned by a Labor Government and suppressed, then reluctantly released, by an unsympathetic (and newly elected) Conservative government. More recently, the Variations Sub Group of the Chief Medical Officer's Health of the Nation Working Group, which included members from outside the government in the health policy community and the Office of Population Census and Surveys, produced a report entitled *Variations in Health: What Can the Department of Health and the [National Health Service] Do?* (Department of Health 1995). After almost two decades, perhaps a more appropriate question would have been: What had been done? The answer would have been: Little had been done. Neither the *Black Report* nor the *Variations in Health* report appeared during this period to have meaningfully influenced the public policy-making process.

Using Research Rhetorically

One policy case study from the United States and two from Canada provide examples of policy makers using research rhetorically. The first two policy case studies nicely illustrate the use of research to bolster a policy maker's predetermined position (i.e., a political use of research). The third case study provides an example of policy makers hiding behind calls for more research to justify their inactivity on an issue (i.e., a tactical use of research).

In 1993, U.S. President Clinton made use not of a body of research but of a catch phrase coined by a researcher, David Ellwood, when proposing reform of the income-support program, Aid to Families with Dependent Children (Ellwood 1988). Ellwood had used the phrase, "end welfare as we know it" as a summary of key policy recommendations that emerged from years of research including: raising the minimum wage to provide adequate income without welfare benefits; increasing the need for child support enforcement and when that failed, child support assurance system payments; increases in the availability of child care; and expansion of the Earned Income Tax Credit. President Clinton "borrowed" Ellwood's phrase, thereby making use of research in at least a superficial way but then attached to it a significantly different set of policies than those recommended by Ellwood, in doing so ignoring other research that evaluated state demonstration projects on variations of existing AFDC programs and the plethora of research on the importance of income support to children's outcomes (Ellwood 1996).

In the second policy case study the government of Prince Edward Island drew on population health research to enlist support for their dramatic decision to combine the province's health and social service budgets into a single budget and to devolve authority over these budgets to newly created regional boards (see Stoddart, this volume, for a more detailed description of this case). Researchers had watched the activities of the Ontario Premier's Council on Health Strategy and its counterparts in other provinces and concluded that for a cross-sectoral initiative to bring about improvements in population health, the body had to have decision-making functions (including the ability to reallocate budgetary resources), not just advisory functions (Lomas and Rachlis 1996). But this research was used in Prince Edward Island not at the stage of goal setting or to ascertain the most efficient means to achieve that goal. Instead, it was used to justify and provide convincing ammunition for a decision that had already been reached for other reasons, most notably to facilitate a reduction in the size of government, which could be accomplished in a less visible way with a single pooled budget than with many separate budgets (Lavis 2004).

The third policy case study is also drawn from Canada but involves the federal government instead of provincial governments (Lavis 2004). The constitutional division of powers between levels of government gives Canadian provinces authority over health care issues, but federal legislation (aggregated into a single piece of legislation in 1984, the *Canada Health Act*) provides a funding and related oversight role for the federal government. In order to appear active and attentive to health policy—at a time when opinion polls showed that the public felt the federal government should be playing a more forceful role in this important policy area but the size of fiscal transfers from the federal government to the provinces was shrinking—the federal government and advisory bodies reporting to it invoked the rhetoric of population health (see, for example, the National Forum on Health 1997). Although the federal government had the authority to make institutional and policy changes in line with population health research, the federal government could not point to a single policy or program outside of the health department that could be argued to have been informed by population health research; it instead called for and established priority theme areas in population health research. Funding research was used as a substitute for more meaningful action, even though (compared with the health policy sector) the federal government had both constitutional authority and a fuller range of policy instruments in non–health policy sectors that influenced the health of populations.

Using Research but Not to Its Full Potential

Policy case studies from the Netherlands and Sweden illustrate the use of research but not to its full potential (Whitehead 1998). Both case studies involve a national government's "official commitment to action" on the issue of health inequalities. This commitment includes the establishment of national research programs or commissions of inquiry (which on their own and depending on the circumstances, may be more appropriately categorized as using research symbolically or tactically), official modification of national information systems to facilitate measurement and monitoring of the issue, the publication of government reports, and parliamentary statements that establish the topic as a priority and signal a commitment to policy development. Although statements of agreement to broad policy principles can translate into legislation stipulating specific steps, policy directives, and concrete, real action, in the Netherlands and Sweden, this had not yet happened during the period under study.

In the Netherlands, an "official commitment to action" can be traced back to the late 1980s. In 1987, the Christian Democrat and Conservative coalition government sponsored a national conference of all the major political parties, trade unions, employers, and health sector associations to discuss health inequalities. The outcome of the conference was a five-year national plan of action including a research program directed by a senior official from the Conservative Party and undertaken by all universities in the country. A follow-up conference, held in 1991, was attended by four ministries, as well as employers. On the basis of a consensus agreement that the evidence showed that health disparities in the country had been increasing since 1960, the participants agreed to develop an action program that included a coordinated, integrated approach to action and to institute another five-year research program to investigate causal mechanisms and potential interventions (Mackenbach 1994). The WHO European Health for All targets and the *Black Report* on health inequalities in Britain were cited as having helped to generate awareness of health inequalities and to instigate the development of these conferences (Gunning-Schepers 1989; Mackenbach 1994). Valuable as the conferences might have been, their outcome in real terms for real people's lives has been substantially different from the potential impact of concrete action steps and policy changes that did not occur despite knowledge and acknowledgement of research.

Sweden has a long tradition of supporting the reduction of health inequalities as a broad policy goal. In 1930, research was used in a meaningful way. The government attempted to reduce differentials in infant mortality through changes in housing and social security policies and improved provisions for maternal and child health (Dahlgren and Diderichsen 1986). More often, however, research has not been used to its full potential. In the early 1990s, for example, when Sweden was experiencing an economic recession, a policy bill that promoted equity in health as a "priority" was presented to Parliament. However, the new Conservative–Liberal government did not give the issue high priority. This policy bill, the second of its kind, was in part encouraged by a series of studies showing that manual workers were experiencing poorer health than salaried employees. When a new Social Democrat government was elected, a Parliamentary committee and, shortly thereafter, a commission were set up to focus on how to reduce inequalities in health. In 1996, a Parliamentary bill was passed that established a national research program to provide better data gathering on health inequalities. The justification for this additional intelligence gathering was a series of studies showing that health outcomes are poorer for individuals in manual occupations. Like the Netherlands, Sweden has demonstrated an abundance of "commitment to action" but little action that could be attributed to the use of population health research.

These case studies involving the (non)use of population health research demonstrate that although our understanding of the use of research in the public policy-making process has evolved over the last few decades, we do not have convincing evidence that the actual use of research in the policy-making process has increased in any meaningful way. Clearly, policy makers across different countries and political regimes, and in different policy areas, are often aware of the research community that could inform their decision making, make reference to it, fund it, and organize conferences to facilitate its dissemination. However, an analysis focusing on the critical issue of whether research influences policy at any stage in the policy-making process would yield disappointing results. But just as our understanding has progressed, there is hope that the degree to which research is used can change.

Learning More about the Conditions under Which Research Is Likely to Be Used

Policy case studies can not only help us to determine whether and how research is used but can also provide insights about the more significant challenge of identifying the conditions under which research is most likely to be used. The authors in Section III examine case studies in which policy makers have tried to shape policies that make use of (or apply) an understanding of social determinants of health evidence base. Chapters 12 and 13 ask: In what circumstances have policy makers been able to make use of this evidence base?

In chapter 12, Stoddart and his colleagues explore a case study in which policy makers explicitly aim to structure policy based on the concept from the social determinants of health area that health is multiply determined, and thus successful efforts to improve health are likely to involve the interaction between multiple policy bodies simultaneously, as well as a consideration of consequences of policies in other sectors. Specifically, Stoddart and his colleagues explore the experiences of the Canadian province of Prince Edward Island when, in 1993, the government attempted to follow a "determinants of health" approach to health policy making. Stoddart and colleagues found that although the commitment to the determinants of health approach among advocates and managers within health, environmental, and social sectors was key, public perception that health care sectors were not going to be adequately funded likely prevented true reallocation (or the implementation of new mechanisms that would enable reallocation) of funds to reflect the importance of different social and environmental predictors of health. Thus, the *effective* use of the determinants of health model requires even more than recognition of the tenets—and more than changes in organizational structures— but also a clear, upfront political statement of support for which redistributions of funds will be tolerated and which will not.

In chapter 13 of this volume, Curtis and Kozyrskyj explore what factors influence the uptake of population health research using a comparative approach. The authors examine how historical and cultural factors affected the use of social determinants of health evidence in three policy cases from the late 1990s: (1) Canada's initiation of a National Children's Agenda in Canada; (2) state-level passage of children's health insurance programs in the United States; and (3) Norway's implementation of the Cash Benefits for Small Children Act. Two key findings are highlighted. First, in all three cases, research evidence played a central role in the policy-making process. Second, the nature of the policies that emerged differed in each country, although in each case, policy makers applied findings from the body of evidence that was available at virtually the same time to all. The authors conclude that because these three countries had very different child policies in place in the late 1990's, in part due to differences in core belief systems and values, different aspects of children's health and well-being were the focus of the new child policies.

In addition to these studies, a qualitative investigation of eight provincial health services policies that were developed in two Canadian provinces (Ontario and Saskatchewan) between 1992 and 1999 offers some preliminary insights into the factors that facilitate the use of research (Lavis et al. 2002). This study examined among other policies the establishment of community-based transfer payment agencies for administering and funding midwifery practice groups in Ontario (a governance/jurisdiction issue); the introduction of a needs-based funding formula for the allocation of approximately 60% of health district funding in Saskatchewan (a financial arrangements issue); the establishment of single long-term care access points for admission to long-term care facilities and the introduction of standardized admission criteria for these facilities (a delivery arrangements issue); and the expedited access to human immunodeficiency virus (HIV) prenatal screening (a program content issue).

Some patterns can be discerned in the conditions under which citable research appears more likely to be used. For the three policies in which citable research was a major influence in the policy-making process, policy makers had direct contact with researchers. In two of these three policies, the contact took place through what could be called a "receptor" (Lomas 1997) for research created by the health department. By this we mean that there were specific functions established with explicit responsibility for establishing and maintaining linkages with researchers. In the case of expedited HIV prenatal testing in Ontario, the head of the department's AIDS Bureau, which had been established to improve the department's knowledge of (and responsiveness to) HIV/AIDS–related health issues and community concerns, had developed personal linkages with many HIV/AIDS researchers. In the case of the development of a needs-based funding formula in Saskatchewan, an "expert" working group charged with informing policy development established more formal linkages with researchers by inviting them to join the working group as full members.

For the three policies in which citable research was a major influence in the policy-making process, two could be categorized as professional decisions about program content (HIV prenatal testing and pneumococcal immunization) and one, at least in the policy development stage in which research was used, could be categorized as a technical decision about financial arrangements for which stakeholders' perceptions of the credibility of the decision was perceived to be important to the implementation of the policy (needs-based funding formula). These types of professional or technical "content-driven" decisions may be more amenable to being significantly influenced by research in instrumental ways (i.e., these types of decisions may lend themselves more easily to being informed by research in specific and direct ways, such as to solve a particular problem at hand) than decisions more concerned with, for example, jurisdictional considerations, which are much less often "content driven."

Examinations of single or a small selective group of cases provide valuable insights. No doubt the growing field of study that addresses research utilization will continue to yield new insights as researchers explore alternative methodologies ranging from multivariate regression analyses of survey data derived from large samples of researchers or policy makers (see Landry et al. 2003) to the application of case study methodology across a range of policy domains and policy-making contexts (e.g., Lavis et al. 2002).

At the same time, the ideal way to ascertain the conditions under which research is used in policy making would be to conduct research that samples policies in an unbiased way (e.g., the sample includes both cases in which research is used and cases in which research is not used), that identifies whether and how research is used in the public policy-making process (e.g., research is used in one or more of the policy prioritization, policy development, and policy implementation stages), and that explicitly identifies the conditions that distinguish situations where research is used from those where it is not (e.g., some types of research, some types of interest group support or some types of institutional arrangements facilitate the use of research). Such studies are only now beginning to emerge, though none to date have attempted to deal directly with the use of population health research.

The ability to ascertain the key conditions under which research is more likely to be used will depend on researchers' ability to assess both discrete policy decisions and broader decision trajectories (Mintzberg et al. 1976; Mintzberg and Waters 1990; Langley et al. 1995), to examine the influence of research at each of the many stages of policy making (Kingdon 1995), and to ascertain the influence of research in the context of other competing interests (Goldstein and Keohane 1993; Hall 1996). But only by studying the issue of the role of research in public policy making with as much rigor as we study the determinants of the health of populations will we be able to derive concrete implications for how to better produce, transfer, and facilitate the uptake of population health research.

What Have We Learned?

The field of research on the social determinants of health is gradually maturing, but we are still at an early stage in terms of thinking about how to move the ideas that are emerging from this field into the public policy-making process. In this chapter we have provided empirical evidence that population health research has been used rhetorically (i.e., in a symbolic way). We cannot find well-documented policy case studies in which this research has been used in an instrumental way or in a conceptual way. We turn now to steps that we believe are critical if the utility of research is to increase.

Filling Gaps in Our Research Base

Researchers and research funders need to recognize that there are still areas where our knowledge base is incomplete and therefore not fully able to contribute to the development of policy. It is important that funding agencies identify and target such areas and that researchers respond to the opportunities to work on these often challenging gaps. As has been documented in earlier chapters, the evidence that social conditions affect health status has grown increasingly strong. The necessary next step—addressing the problems that have been brought to light, including poverty, discrimination, and other social inequalities—presents new challenges for researchers and new opportunities for the foundations and granting agencies that fund their research (Heymann 2000a). Successfully changing the social conditions that contribute to poor health status is far from straightforward.

The fight against poverty provides a compelling example. Despite decades of research and proposals on how to reduce poverty, successful strategies have been elusive, and insufficient progress has been made on this complex problem in many countries. A concerted political effort in the United States in the 1960s led to the establishment of a number of programs, ranging from employment and training to housing to income support. The problems varied in their effectiveness. Overall, poverty rates among the elderly declined and stayed down. Political support for programs that provided income for the elderly was maintained. However, political support for programs that provided training, housing, and income to poor families with young children—designed as a targeted instead of a universal benefit—waxed and waned. Some programs undoubtedly failed because they were eliminated before they had a chance to succeed. Other programs, as noted earlier in this chapter, were succeeding and then were eliminated as the politics of programs for the poor changed. Some policies that were enacted were ineffective.

Those policies that failed did so for several substantive reasons. First, programs were often designed as though "the poor" were a monolithic, homogenous population, instead of a diverse and changing group. The determinants of social class are many and complex, and they change over time. Second, programs were often built and then destroyed because of inaccurate assumptions. These assumptions often served important political purposes; they did not help to develop "better" public policy, and they were certainly not grounded in research evidence. They were able to carry the day partly because research on such relevant topics like the actual work experiences of families that received public assistance and the demographic composition of families receiving support from the government was either difficult to produce on a national level, over time, or ran counter to mainstream perceptions. Third, programs were introduced into an environment in which programs interacted with one another in complex and not always foreseeable ways, which made it difficult to determine whether a program was failing because of its innate characteristics or because of the particular context in which it played out. Failure to develop and implement programs in multiple environments often precluded the possibility of determining the role of context.

The case of addressing discrimination reinforces the notion that changing the social conditions that contribute to poor health status is a complex task. A series of public policy initiatives have been introduced in this area in the United States over the last four decades. Most notable were the civil rights legislation passed in 1964 and 1991 that banned discrimination in the workplace (Lehman 1994), as well as affirmative action policies that sought to reduce the long-term effects of past discrimination (Wilson 1996). While antidiscrimination legislation has clearly had an important impact (Holzer and Neumark 2000; Jaynes and Williams 1989), it is also apparent that this legislation has not eliminated employment and other types of discrimination based on race (Alenikoff 1992). And although affirmative action policies provided better opportunities for some minorities, it was largely the more advantaged who benefited, not the most disadvantaged.

Racial and ethnic disparities still exist in the United States today partly as a result of the limitations and failures of past public policy initiatives. But these disparities also still exist because their root causes are resistant to, or difficult to influence through, legislation or affirmative action policies, even if these initiatives are conducted at the local level (Husock 1989, 1990). These root causes include individuals' misperceptions and stereotyping of other groups, which lead to subtle forms of discrimination that are difficult to identify and therefore address.

As these examples demonstrate, the gaps in our knowledge based in terms of both social and health problems has limited researchers' ability to contribute to the development of effective policies. One way that researchers can more effectively shape health policy is by enhancing our understanding of the causes of health problems (see table 14.2). Population health researchers are particularly well positioned for this activity: Their research examines both the causes of good and poor health status in populations (i.e., the determinants of health) and the mediating factors that may influence relationships between these ultimate causes and health status.

Table 14.2. Ingredients for developing successful programs

Understanding the problem	Developing policy responses	Building political support
Understanding the cause of the problem • Including understanding what are the precipitates as opposed to the correlates of the problem Understanding what needs to be changed to address the problem • Mediating factors may be more feasible to address than ultimate causes—it is important to understand when it is necessary to address the ultimate causes	Programs that are effective in a range of political settings and in the context of a range of other initiatives • The other initiatives that will be passed or repealed will be unpredictable Programs that are effective in a range of economic situations • In the long run it is inevitable that any program that is sustained will exist against a backdrop of both strong and weak economic conditions Programs that are effective in a range of demographic settings • Federal programs need to be effective in each state. State programs need to be effective in a wide range of localities Programs that are effective in a range of administrative settings • If the institutional capacity already exists, a program is more likely to be sustained	Sufficient political support to pass • With compromises that will not compromise the effectiveness of the policies • Without changes that will undermine the policy Sufficient political support to sustain the initiative over the time necessary for its effectiveness to become clear

Source: Modified from Heymann 2000a.

Researchers can also more effectively shape policy by suggesting policy responses that are feasible and effective (Lavis 2002). This activity presents a formidable challenge for population health researchers because their research has implications primarily for public policies that do not have health as their principal objective. These include, *inter alia*, tax policies, income support policies, labor market policies, housing policies, some environmental policies, and early childhood development policies. Collaborative research needs to bring together population health researchers with policy researchers from the relevant policy domains. The population health researchers will bring their knowledge of the causes of health problems; the policy researchers will bring their knowledge of the social conditions that give rise to these health problems and of the policy domains that seek to modify these social conditions.

Making Research Relevant and Useful to Policy Makers

For the results of collaborative research to be relevant and useful in the policy sphere, researchers need to use and develop research approaches that are more in line with the perspectives of economic and social policy makers (Heymann 2000a). These policy makers will ask many questions of any suggested policy response, but most questions fall into one of two categories: (1) will the policy work in a range of settings and situations; i.e., is it generalizable? (see table 14.2); and (2) will the policy be politically feasible? If a policy is unlikely to work within particular contexts, for example in particular economic situations like a recession, across most if not all states, provinces or communities, and with existing administrative capacities, then building support will be difficult. And if there are no political rewards, then building support will likely be impossible.

Take the question of whether a policy will work in a range of economic situations. One crucial contribution from researchers would be an examination of the extent to which particular economic conditions influence or could be expected to influence the effectiveness of a program. For example, the welfare-to-work programs developed in the United States in the late 1990s were touted as being highly effective because the welfare rolls fell substantially and the poverty rate did not climb dramatically. These programs were implemented in the context of an unusually strong economy with a record low unemployment rate. These very same programs might have disastrous effects if implemented during an economic recession.

But it is not just the economic context that matters: A policy must also work in a range of demographic settings to be politically feasible. In order to receive ongoing support from a legislative body whose members come from all parts of the country, federal programs need to be effective in a wide range of settings across the country. Similarly, state or provincial programs need to be effective in a range of communities. Researchers often want, but do not always have, access to national, randomly selected, longitudinal data samples. Instead, they often use data gathered in a particular geographic area and time period and from a sample of individuals limited in its diversity.

The political context of change cannot be ignored. Legislators focus on programs with widespread benefits for a good reason: These programs can secure the necessary votes of their colleagues. Moreover, universal programs avoid stigmatizing the populations they are designed to benefit. In contrast, researchers are often wont to propose narrowly focused initiatives that benefit, or address the problems of, a small subpopulation. Researchers need to take the social and political implications of their recommendations in the future as seriously as they have taken the "cost effectiveness" of targeting in the past.

Timing is also critical to any calculation of political feasibility. Ideally a policy will have short-term as well as long-term effects. The political cycle is short: A term in office typically ranges from two to five years in length. Programs that show their effectiveness rapidly are much more likely to be promoted and sustained; those that do not are likely to be cut or modified. Long-term effects, although critically important to the beneficiaries, are unfortunately political gravy. This makes population health related policies, many of which will play out over many years, if not decades, particularly problematic, as their effects may not materialize for many election cycles. It is exceedingly difficult to sell to the politicians of the day, programs whose rewards will accrue to other, as yet unidentified, elected officials.

Enhancing Transfer and Uptake of Research in Policy-making Environments

The policy case studies in this and other chapters in this volume highlight how important it is for researchers to think about how their research will go from book chapter or journal article to policy or program (Heymann 2000a). Since most individuals who are intimately involved in the public policy-making process are not likely to read academic books and journals, researchers must be deliberate in their efforts to see their work reach the public sphere. If researchers do not make a conscious effort to formulate evidence-based policy recommendations and specify the implications for key actors in the policy-making process, only a portion of their work will enter the public debate, and that which does may contribute less than it could have. Publishing one's work and presenting that work to the media are only two of many avenues for influencing the policy process (see fig. 14.1). Transferring research effectively requires more than the passive dissemination of a message through mailings and Web site postings. Researchers and knowledge brokers need to be actively involved with policy makers and influential social actors on an ongoing and sustained basis. Such interactive engagement should be con-

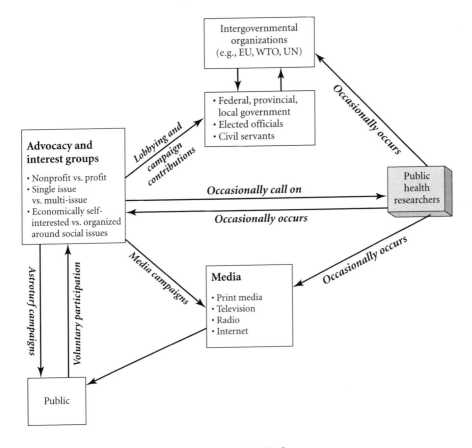

Figure 14.1. Web of influence

Source: Modified from Heymann 2000a.

sidered an integral and necessary part of the research process (Huberman 1994; Lomas 2000).

A number of important factors should be considered when researchers think about transferring their research to policy-making environments. What is the take-home message? To whom should it be targeted and with what investments in targeting them? By whom should it be delivered and with what investments in supporting them? How should it be delivered? (Lavis et al. 2003). The take-home message from a body of research must be compelling and relate to a decision or set of decisions in order to effectively influence policy making. Policy makers listen to academics most when their analyses and proposals are directly related to problems that have already gained their attention. It would therefore behoove researchers to spend time finding out what issues are in the forefront of the minds of the electorate and those making policy decisions (Heymann 2000a). It will be important for researchers to be more aware than most currently are of when a "window of opportunity" has opened and that they are prepared when it happens. Often researchers are generally unaware of the emerging policy issues as they focus on their own specific research. Funding agencies can play an important role in enhancing the chances of dissemination and uptake of research results by ensuring that funds are made available for targeted, more policy-relevant projects in addition to investigator-initiated research.

Measuring the Impact of Translation

Understanding of the challenges inherent in translating population health research into policy is central to our ability to shape the most effective population health policies. But beyond this we must also ask, when research does influence the policy-making process, do we know how to measure success in improving population health?

Vogel and Theorell in this volume describe one approach they have used to examine policy impact. They conduct point-in-time cross-national comparative analyses and longitudinal analyses to assess the link between welfare production strategies and the distribution of health. First, they analyze how the different approaches to social welfare production in the European Union (EU) are associated with different rates of inequality broadly, as well as health outcomes in particular, and second, they describe a longitudinal analysis examining the health and well-being effects of changes in Sweden's social policies over the last two decades. Vogel and Theorell find that clusters of nations that have emphasized a dual approach to improving population health where the state and the labor market both play a role in ensuring the population's health and well-being also tend to have populations that more often report being in good health and with lower rates of illnesses.

In chapter 11 of this volume Osberg and Sharpe follow by asking what measure we could use to evaluate whether economic policies are improving population health. The authors argue that the most frequently used measure of economic status at the national level, gross domestic product, fails to take into account many issues that are important to population health. The authors go on to present an alternative measure of economic well-being that integrates much of the evidence from social determinants of health research, as well as other research regarding the critical factors that affect health and well-being. This index is a broader indicator of economic well-being that includes such things as the degree of income inequality and economic insecurity. Osberg and Sharpe then demonstrate how one can use this alternative measure by examining trends in well-being in several OECD countries as indicated by their more comprehensive measure of economic well-being. The authors document differences in national performance over the last two decades using their healthier index of well-being as compared with using GDP.

Conclusion

Policy makers outside the health sector are beginning to appreciate that the policies they develop can have foreseeable health consequences that need to be taken into consideration. Unless research funders, researchers, knowledge brokers, and policy makers take concrete action, however, the next ten years will see more research being ignored, used rhetorically, or not used to its full potential.

Clearly there are opportunities to improve the contribution that research makes in the policy-making process. In this chapter, we have drawn on empirical research to inform the identification of these opportunities. Researchers need to be purposive about seeking opportunities for enlightenment, not for symbolic uses of research (these will come anyway). The policy case studies used in this chapter, and those more detailed cases that follow, provide guidance to researchers who want to have an impact on policies that have health objectives, as well as on policies that have health consequences. It is no longer enough for researchers to simply make the case that social conditions can have powerful consequences for health and then go back to their research. In many respects that is the easy part of the work. But if it stops there, others might legitimately question why we bother, or why the research receives any public funding to begin with.

References

Alenikoff, A. F. 1992. The constitution in context: The continuing significance of racism. *University of Colorado Law Review* 63:325–372.

Allison, G. T. 1971. *Essence of Decision: Explaining the Cuban Missile Crisis.* Boston, MA: Little, Brown.

Beyer, J., and H. Trice. 1982. The utilization process: A conceptual framework and synthesis of empirical findings. *Administrative Science Quarterly* 27:591–622.

Blank, R. M. 1994. The employment strategy: Public policies to increase work and earnings. In *Confronting Poverty: Prescriptions for Change,* ed. S. H. Danziger, G. D. Sandefur, and D. H. Weinberg, 365–395. New York: Russell Sage Foundation.

Blaxter, M. 1997. Whose fault is it? People's own conceptions of the reasons for health inequalities. *Social Science and Medicine* 44:747–756.

Bloom, H. S., L. O. Orr, G. Cave, S. Bell, and F. Doolittle. 1993. *The National JTPA Study: Report to the U.S. Department of Labor.* Bethesda, MD: Abt Associates.

Burtless, G. 1994. Public spending on the poor: Historical trends and economic limits. In *Confronting Poverty: Prescriptions for Change,* ed. S. H. Danziger, G. D. Sandefur, and D. H. Weinberg, 51–84. New York: Russell Sage Foundation.

Cohen, J., J. March, and J. Olsen. 1972. A garbage can model of organizational choice. *Administrative Science Quarterly* 17 (March 1972):1–25.

Dahlgren, G., and F. Diderichsen. 1986. Strategies for equity in health: Report from Sweden. *International Journal of Health Services* 16:517–537.

Department of Health. 1995. *Variations in Health: What Can the Department of Health and the NHS Do?* London: Her Majesty's Stationery Office.

Ellwood, D. T. 1988. *Poor Support: Poverty in the American Family.* New York: Basic Books.

Ellwood, D. T. 1996. Welfare reform as I knew it. *American Prospect* 26 (May–June):22–29.

Etzioni, A. 1967. Mixed scanning. *Public Administration Review* 27 (December 1967):385–392.

Goldstein, J., and R. O. Keohane. 1993. Ideas and foreign policy: An analytical framework. In *Ideas and Foreign Policy: Beliefs, Institutions, and Political Change,* ed. J. Goldstein and R. O. Keohane, 3–30. Ithaca: Cornell University Press.

Gunning-Schepers, I. 1989. How to put equity and health on the political agenda. *Health Promotion International* 4:149–150.

Hall, P. A. 1996. *Politics and Markets in the Industrialized Nations: Interests, Institutions and Ideas in Comparative Political Economy.* Cambridge: Centre for European Studies, Harvard University.

Hanney, S. R., M. A. Gonzalez-Block, M. J. Buxton, and M. Kogan. 2003. The utilization of health research in policy making: Concepts, examples and methods of assessment. *BMC Health Research Policy and Systems* 1:2.

Heclo, H. 1974. Social policy and political learning. In *Modern Social Politics in Britain and Sweden: From Relief to Income Maintenance,* ed. H. Heclo. New Haven, CT: Yale University Press.

Heymann, S. J. 2000a. Health and social policy. In *Social Epidemiology,* ed. L. Berkman, and I. Kawachi. New York: Oxford University Press.

Heymann, S. J. 2000b. *The Widening Gap: Why American Working Families Are in Jeopardy and What Can Be Done about It.* New York: Basic Books.

Holzer, H. J., and D. Neumark, 2000. What does affirmative action do? *Industrial and Labor Relations Review* 53 (2):240–271.

Huberman, M. 1994. Research utilization: The state of the art. Knowledge and Policy. *International Journal of Knowledge Transfer and Utilization.* 7 (4):13–33.

Husock, H. 1989. Integration incentives in suburban Cleveland. Case Program Series (no. C16-89-877.0). Cambridge, MA: Kennedy School of Government, Harvard University.

Husock, H. 1990. Occupancy controls and racial integration at Starrett City (A, B, C, and Epilogue), Case Program Series (no. C16-90-962.0). Cambridge, MA: Kennedy School of Government, Harvard University.

Innvaer, S., G. E. Vist, M. Trommald, and A. D. Oxman. 2002. Health policy makers' perceptions of their use of evidence: A systematic review. *Journal of Health Services Research and Policy* 7(4):239–244.

Jaynes, G., and R. Williams, eds. 1989. *A Common Destiny: Blacks in American Society.* Washington, DC: National Academy Press.

Kingdon, J. W. 1995. *Agendas, Alternatives, and Public Policies.* 2nd ed. New York: Harper-Collins College Publishers.

Landry, R., N. Amara, and M. Lamari. 2001. Utilization of social science research knowledge in Canada. *Research Policy* 30:333–349.

Landry, R., M. Lamari, and N. Amara. 2003. Extent and determinants of the utilization of university research in government agencies. *Public Administration Review* 63 (2):192–205.

Langley, A., H. Mintzberg, P. Pitcher, E. Posada, and J. Saint-Macary. 1995. Opening up decision making: The view from the black stool. *Organization Science* 6:260–279.

Lavis, J. N. 2002. Ideas at the margin or marginalized ideas? Non-medical determinants of health in Canada. *Health Affairs* 21:107–112.

Lavis, J. N. 2004. A political science perspective on evidence-based decision-making. In *Using Knowledge and Evidence in Health Care: Multidisciplinary Perspectives,* ed. L. Lemieux-Charles and F. Champagne, 70–85. Toronto: University of Toronto Press.

Lavis, J. N., M. S. R. Farrant, and G. L. Stoddart. 2001. Barriers to employment-related healthy public policy. *Health Promotion International* 16 (1):9–20.

Lavis, J. N., D. Robertson, J. M. Woodside, C. B. McLeod, J. Abelson, and the Knowledge Transfer Study Group. 2003. How can research organizations more effectively transfer research knowledge to decision makers? *Milbank Quarterly* 81:221–248.

Lavis, J. N., S. E. Ross, J. E. Hurley, J. M. Hohenadel, G. L. Stoddart, C. A. Woodward, and J. Abelson. 2002. Examining the role of health services research in public policy-making. *Milbank Quarterly*, 80:125–154.

Lavis, J. N., and T. Sullivan. 1999. Governing health. In *Market Limits in Health Reform: Public Success, Private Failure,* ed. D. Drache and T. Sullivan, 312–328. London: Routledge.

Lehman, J. S. 1994. Updating urban policy. In *Confronting Poverty: Prescriptions for Change,* ed. S. H. Danziger, G. D. Sandefur, and D. H. Weinberg, 226–252. New York: Russell Sage Foundation.

Lindblom, C. 1959. The science of muddling through. *Public Administration Review* 14 (Spring 1959):79–88.

Lomas, J. 1997. *Improving Research Dissemination and Update in the Health Sector: Beyond the Sound of One Hand Clapping.* Commentary C97-1. Hamilton: McMaster University Centre for Health Economics and Policy Analysis.

Lomas, J. 2000. Using "linkage and exchange" to move research into policy at a Canadian foundation: Encouraging partnerships between researchers and policy makers is the goal of a promising new Canadian initiative. *Health Affairs* 19:236–240.

Lomas, J., and M. Rachlis. 1996. Moving rocks: Block funding in PEI as an incentive for cross-sectoral reallocations among human services. *Canadian Public Administration* 39: 581–600.

Mackenbach, J. 1994. Socioeconomic inequalities in Health in the Netherlands: Impact of a five year research programme. *British Medical Journal* 309:1487–1491.

Marmor, T. R., M. L. Barer, and R. G. Evans. 1994. The determinants of a population's health: What can be done to improve a democratic nation's health status? In *Why Are Some People Healthy and Others Not? The Determinants of Health in Populations,* ed. R. G. Evans, M. L. Barer, and T. R. Marmor. New York: Aldine de Gruyter.

Mintzberg, H., D. Raisinghani, and A. Theoret. 1976. The structure of "unstructured" decision processes. *Administrative Science Quarterly* 21:246–275.

Mintzberg, H., and J. A. Waters. 1990. Study deciding: An exchange of views between Mintzberg, H., J. Waters, Pettigrew and Butler. *Organization Studies* 1:11–16.

Murnane, R. J. 1994. Education and the wellbeing of the next generation. In *Confronting Poverty: Prescriptions for Change,* ed. S. H. Danziger, G. D. Sandefur, and D. H. Weinberg, 289–307. New York: Russell Sage Foundation.

Mustard, J. F., M. N. McCain, and J. Bertrand. 2000. Changing beliefs to change policy: The early years study. *ISUMA: The Canadian Journal of Policy Research.* Autumn: 76–79.

National Forum on Health. 1997. *Canada Health Action: Building on the Legacy.* Ottawa, ON: National Forum on Health, February 1997.

Pelz, D. C. 1978. Some expanded perspectives on use of social science in public policy. In *Major Social Issues: A Multidisciplinary View,* ed. J. M. Yinger, J. M., and S. J. Cutler, 346–357. New York: The Free Press.

Schelling, T. 1960. *Strategy of Conflict.* Cambridge, MA: Harvard University Press.

Simon, H. 1966. Political research: The decision-making framework. In *Varieties of Political Theory,* ed. D. Easton. 19. Englewood Cliffs: Prentice-Hall.

Townsend, P., N. Davidson, and M. Whitehead. 1988. *Inequalities in Health: The Black Report and the Health Divide*. London: Penguin.

Weiss, C. H. 1979. The many meanings of research utilization. *Public Administration Review* 39:426–431.

Weiss, C. H. 1980. Knowledge creep and decision accretion. *Knowledge: Creation, Diffusion, Utilization* 2:381–404.

Whitehead, M. 1998. Diffusion of ideas on social inequalities in health: A European perspective. *Milbank Quarterly* 76:469–492.

Wilson, W. J. 1996. *When Work Disappears: The World of the New Urban Poor*. New York: Knopf.

Index

health (*continued*)
  prenatal environment and (*See* prenatal period)
  social environment and, 3–4
  stressors and (*See* stress)
  universal cause-and-effect model of, 58–60
  work and, 179–182, 192–194
health care
  costs of, 122
  education and use of, 113–117
  focus on adulthood, 83, 100–101
  health status and, 113–117, 121–125
  life expectancy and use of, 108, 109, 113, 116, 117, 119
  limitations of, 121–125
  preoccupation with, 4, 107–109, 121–125
  privatization of, 282–283, 309–310
  quality of care indicators, 117–119
  regionalization of, 328–331
  socioeconomic status and use of, 110–111, 113–117
  universal, 107–109, 121–125, 224–225, 311
  utilization measures, 111–112
health insurance
  child policy, 359–365
  genetic screening and, 22, 24
  importance of, 124
  income inequality and, 224–225, 228, 230
  State Children's Health Insurance Program (U.S.), 392, 395
  uninsured persons, health consequences for, 124, 223, 360
  universal health care, 107–109, 121–125, 224–225, 311
health policy
  cross-sectoral reallocation of resources and (*See* cross-sectoral reallocation of resources in Prince Edward Island)
  focusing on care *vs.* determinants, 4, 107–109, 121–125
  location-specific, 74–75, 252–254, 259–260
  need for life course approach and, 100–101
  nutrition, 137, 158–161

translation of research into (*See* translation of research into policy)
  welfare systems (*See* welfare production models)
heart disease and cardiovascular disease
  biological embedding and, 39
  genetics and, 17–20
  interactive effects over life course, 93–94
  LDL (low-density lipoprotein) cholesterol and, 19–20
  migrant studies and geographic variation in disease occurrence, 14
  mortality and life expectancy, 241, 243
  neighborhoods, 239, 241–242
  web of causation for myocardial infarction, 18
  work and, 179, 193
hemochromatosis, 21
heritability and genetics, 15–16
hierarchies
  cultural differences in concepts of, 59
  occupational, 1, 91, 176, 179, 180–182
HIV/AIDS, 66–73
  biological, global, and economic factors in West Africa, 71–73
  comparative epidemiology in West Africa, 69–71
  homosexual *vs.* heterosexual spread of, 69, 71
  origins of, 66–68
  social factors and comparative epidemiology in West Africa, 69–71
  translation of research into policy in Canada, 392–393
hormone replacement therapy (HRT), 64–66
housing and health, 125, 228, 259, 270, 272, 286, 327, 329, 341, 397
HPA (hypothalamic-pituitary-adrenal) axis, 44
  case study of life story of, 44–47
  child development, 37
  conceptual model and, 52–53
  interplay with environment and experience over the life course, 47–51
  late life, 39
  latency model of life course relationships, 89

population health (*continued*)
income inequality and, 203, 207–210, 230
intergenerational effects, 46, 47, 86, 101
nutrition and, 135–137
role of health care in, 107–109, 121–125
translation of research to policy on (*See* translation of research into policy)
Population Health Program, ix
post-traumatic stress disorder (PTSD), 77
poverty
elderly persons, 313
food insecurity and, 152–158
income inequality differentiated, 308, 310
policy failures and gaps in research base, 394–395
poverty intensity, poverty gap ratio, and poverty rate, 309
single parents, 312–313
preimplantation diagnosis (PID), 24–25
prenatal period
biological embedding, 36
"fetal origins hypothesis," 90
genetic diagnostic testing, 25–26
latency model, life course relationships, 90
nutrition during, 145–146
prosperity. *See* economic well-being in OECD countries
prostitution and spread of HIV/AIDS, 69
psychological disorders. *See* mental illness
psychoneuroendocrine (PNE) axis, 37, 38, 51
psychoneuroimmune (PNI) axis, 37, 38, 39, 44, 51, 52
public policy. *See also* child policy; health policy; social policy
impact of, 400
influence of research on, 382–385
labor markets, 190–195
nutrition and public health concept, 137
translation of research to (*See* translation of research into policy)

race and ethnicity, 214–215, 395. *See also* genetics

rational choice model of translation of research into policy, 383
reallocation of resources. *See* cross-sectoral reallocation of resources in Prince Edward Island (PEI)
refugee health issues, 74–78
regimes model of welfare distribution, 268–271
regionalization of health care, 328–331
research and policy making. *See* translation of research into policy
rhetorical or symbolic use of population health research, 384–385, 388–389
Rose, Geoffrey, 18–21, 28, 240, 250–254

SAM (sympatho-adrenal-medullary) axis, 38, 39, 44, 51, 52, 178
schizophrenia, 90, 242
Scotland, child policy in, 349
security/insecurity
economic well-being in OECD countries, 309–314
food insecurity, 152–158
job insecurity, 175–177, 186–187, 188, 189
segregation, economic, 227–228, 231
Senegal, HIV/AIDS in, 69, 72–77
sex. *See* gender
sexually transmitted infections (STIs) and spread of HIV/AIDS, 71–72
Sierra Leone, mortality and life expectancy in, 237–238
single-allele or Mendelian conditions, 11, 21
single parents
child benefits for, 350–351
economic well-being and, 312–313
risks to children raised by, 354
social environment
animal studies and, 45–51, 88–89, 205–206
contribution to disease approach, 178–179, 193
cortisol levels and, 39
immune response and, 37, 38, 39, 44
influence on health of variations in, 35–41 (*See also* biological embedding)